MEDICAL RADIOLOGY

Diagnostic Imaging and Radiation Oncology

Innovations in Diagnostic Radiology

Contributors

J. H. Anderson · S. J. Blackband · E. K. Fishman · J. D. Glickson
H. H. Holcomb · W. C. Hunter · J. E. Kuhlman · A. J. Kumar · F. P. Leo, Sr.
H. L. Loats · K. I. Macrae · D. Magid · C. P. Martin · D. R. Ney
D. D. Robertson · A. E. Rosenbaum · S. Uematsu · J. P. Wehrle
D. F. Wong · E. A. Zerhouni

Edited by

James H. Anderson

Foreword by

Martin W. Donner, William R. Brody, and Friedrich Heuck

With 144 Figures, Some in Color

Springer-Verlag Berlin Heidelberg New York
London Paris Tokyo Hong Kong

JAMES H. ANDERSON, Ph. D.
Professor of Radiology
Dept. of Radiology and Radiological Science
The Johns Hopkins University
School of Medicine
600 North Wolfe Street
Baltimore, MD 21205
USA

MEDICAL RADIOLOGY · Diagnostic Imaging and Radiation Oncology

Continuation of
Handbuch der medizinischen Radiologie
Encyclopedia of Medical Radiology

ISBN 3-540-19093-7 Springer-Verlag Berlin Heidelberg New York
ISBN 0-387-19093-7 Springer-Verlag New York Berlin Heidelberg

Library of Congress Cataloging-in-Publication Data. Innovations in diagnostic radiology / contributors, J. H. Anderson ... [et al.]; edited by James H. Anderson ; foreword by Martin W. Donner. p. cm. - (Medical radiology)
Includes bibliographies and index.
ISBN 0-387-19093-7 (U.S.)
1. Diagnostic imaging. I. Anderson, James H. II. Series. [DNLM: 1. Diagnostic Imaging. WN 200 I58]
RC78.7.D53I56 1989 616.07'57- dc19 DNLM/DLC

Typesetting, printing and bookbinding: Appl, Wemding
2122/3130-543210 - Printed on acid-free paper

To Scully, Sparky, Norma, Bob, Bill, and Marian

List of Contributors

James H. Anderson, Ph. D.
Professor of Radiology
Dept. of Radiology & Radiological Science
The Johns Hopkins University
School of Medicine
600 North Wolfe Street
Baltimore, MD 21205
USA

Stephen J. Blackband, Ph. D.
Assistant Professor of Radiology
Dept. of Radiology & Radiological Science
The Johns Hopkins University
School of Medicine
600 North Wolfe Street
Baltimore, MD 21205
USA

Elliot K. Fishman, M. D.
Associate Professor of Radiology
Dept. of Radiology & Radiological Science
The Johns Hopkins University
School of Medicine
600 North Wolfe Street
Baltimore, MD 21205
USA

Jerry D. Glickson, Ph. D.
Prof. of Radiology & Biological Chemistry
Depts. of Radiology, Radiological Science
and Biological Chemistry
The Johns Hopkins University
School of Medicine
600 North Wolfe Street
Baltimore, MD 21205
USA

Henry H. Holcomb, M. D.
Assistant Professor of Radiology
Dept. of Radiology & Radiological Science
The Johns Hopkins University
School of Medicine
600 North Wolfe Street
Baltimore, MD 21205
USA and
University of Maryland Psychiatric
Research Center
Baltimore, MD 21205
USA

William C. Hunter, Ph. D.
Assistant Professor of
Biomedical Engineering
Dept. of Biomedical Engineering
The Johns Hopkins University
School of Medicine
720 Rutland Ave.
Baltimore, MD 21205
USA

Janet E. Kuhlman, M. D.
Assistant Professor of Radiology
Dept. of Radiology & Radiological Science
The Johns Hopkins University
School of Medicine
600 North Wolfe Street
Baltimore, MD 21205
USA

Ashok J. Kumar, M. D.
Associate Professor of Radiology
Dept. of Radiology & Radiological Science
The Johns Hopkins University
School of Medicine
600 North Wolfe Street
Baltimore, MD 21205
USA

Frank P. Leo, Sr. E. E.
Assistant Professor of Radiology
Dept. of Radiology & Radiological Science
The Johns Hopkins University
School of Medicine
600 North Wolfe Street
Baltimore, MD 21205
USA

Harry L. Loats, B.S., M.S., M.S.
Loats Associates, Inc.
1004 Littlestown Pike/Suite G
Westminster, MD 21157
USA and
Research Associate in Oncology
Dept. of Oncology
The Johns Hopkins University
School of Medicine
600 North Wolfe Street
Baltimore, MD 21205
USA

Kenneth I. Macrae, M.D., Ph.D.
Fellow in Nuclear Medicine
Dept. of Nuclear Medicine
The National Institutes of Health
Bethesda, MD 20205
USA

Donna Magid, M.D.
Assistant Professor of Radiology
Dept. of Radiology & Radiological Science
The Johns Hopkins University
School of Medicine
600 North Wolfe Street
Baltimore, MD 21205
USA

Cynthia Paella Martin, M.S.
Medical Editor
Dept. of Radiology & Radiological Science
The Johns Hopkins University
School of Medicine
600 North Wolfe Street
Baltimore, MD 21205
USA

Derek R. Ney, B.S.
Research Assistant
Dept. of Radiology & Radiological Science
The Johns Hopkins University
School of Medicine
600 North Wolfe Street
Baltimore, MD 21205
USA

Douglas D. Robertson, M.D., Ph.D.
Resident in Orthopedic Surgery
Dept. of Orthopedic Surgery
Brigham and Women's Hospital
Harvard Medical School
Boston, MA 02115
USA

Arthur E. Rosenbaum, M.D., F.A.C.R.
Professor of Radiology
Dept. of Radiology & Radiological Science
The Johns Hopkins University
School of Medicine
600 North Wolfe Street
Baltimore, MD 21205
USA

Sumio Uematsu, M.D., F.A.C.S.
Associate Professor of Neurosurgery
Dept. of Neurosurgery
The Johns Hopkins University
School of Medicine
600 North Wolfe Street
Baltimore, MD 21205
USA

Janna P. Wehrle, Ph.D.
Assistant Professor of Radiology
Dept. of Radiology & Radiological Science
The Johns Hopkins University
School of Medicine
600 North Wolfe Street
Baltimore, MD 21205
USA

Dean F. Wong, M.D.
Associate Professor of Radiology
Dept. of Radiology & Radiological Science
The Johns Hopkins University
School of Medicine
600 North Wolfe Street
Baltimore, MD 21205
USA

Elias A. Zerhouni, M.D.
Associate Professor of Radiology
Dept. of Radiology & Radiological Science
The Johns Hopkins University
School of Medicine
600 North Wolfe Street
Baltimore, MD 21205
USA

Foreword

This volume of the new series, "Medical Radiology" addresses the important topic of "Innovations in Diagnostic Radiology". It presents examples of current work of interest not only to the radiological community but to physicians in other medical disciplines and to scientists in general.

The impact of radiology on diagnostic medicine and patient management has been obvious from the beginning of our specialty. However, the evolution of the field is expanding at an astounding rate. During the professional lifetime of one generation of radiologists alone, numerous technologies and procedures have been added to conventional radiography: cross sectional tomography, high resolution nuclear scanning, magnetic resonance imaging, ultrasound, interventional radiology and computer based radiological operations. The optimal interpretation of images obtained by these new technologies requires that we expand our knowledge in physiology, biochemistry and also in our clinical expertise. It also means that radiologists must collaborate closely with other clinicians and basic scientists.

Two introductory chapters set the stage for the current and future challenges in radiology and provide suggestions regarding the successful development of a research program in an academic department. The concept, as presented here, matured over a period of several years and in discussion with junior and senior members of our faculty as well as residents and fellows. When investigation into basic and clinical questions brings together members from different departments of the medical faculty, the Dean's interest in supporting a centralized research resource facility, particularly at its beginning, is heightened. Participation in basic, applied or clinical research should be considered a desirable feature of training programs in diagnostic radiology. The benefits of research experience to young physicians embarking on a career in radiology are numerous, regardless of ultimate career choices. From imaginative investigation of pathophysiological events and of organ involvement in localized or systemic disease, to taking an active role in development, modification, or application of new equipment, time in the research laboratory is well spent as part of trainees' education in radiology.

Whether working alone or as a member of a team, whether results of a project are positive or not, the process of acquiring new knowledge is exciting. The frustration over a failed experiment is a powerful motivator to rethink and perhaps redesign one's experimental approach. The process promotes step by step logical thinking which is carried over in one's clinical work. If followed by success, the investigator's reward are feelings of accomplishment; research induces enthusiasm. Benefits of a good research program collaborating with colleagues from other clinical disciplines or with basic scientists are high motivation, good morale and esprit de corps. These characteristics are almost invariably carried over to the clinical setting. Joint work in research stimulates closer personal ties in patient care.

Martin W. Donner, Baltimore
William R. Brody, Baltimore
Friedrich Heuck, Stuttgart

Preface

Within the past ten–twenty years, technological advances have dramatically changed the image, responsibilities and functions of the diagnostic radiologist. These changes are reflected in a renewed concern for academic department planning relating to patient care, teaching, and research. The antiquated service function image of the radiologist sitting in a room reading stacks of films is being replaced by one of a new breed of radiologist who is more actively involved in the development and application of technology and who participates more actively in the care and management of patients. The computer era and the increasing concern for reducing medical care costs have created both opportunities and concerns for current radiology planners and leaders as well as for the bright young radiologists and trainees who will be the leaders of tomorrow.

Developing individual career objectives or long term departmental plans requires a vision of what the future may hold for diagnostic radiology as a discipline, and for the various imaging and therapeutic modalities currently available as well as for those under development. This volume addresses some of the topics that may contribute significantly to the future of diagnostic radiology. In compiling the chapters, the authors have tried to address the current state of the art and discuss the potential future development of their area of expertise.

The first two chapters of the book discuss current and future challenges for academic radiology and radiology research program development. Both subjects relate directly to the academic growth of diagnostic radiology departments and the continued research and development of the imaging techniques or procedures discussed in the remaining chapters. Chapters three and four are concerned with image analysis techniques and three dimensional image reconstruction. Both areas are receiving increased attention through the use of more powerful computing capabilities and both will receive considerable attention during the next decade. The Nuclear Magnetic Resonance imaging chapter (Chapter 5) provides information regarding the basic principles of magnetic resonance imaging and discusses various Nuclear Magnetic Resonance imaging techniques. Emphasis is placed on developmental trends and potential applications. Nuclear Magnetic Resonance spectroscopy is an area that will receive intense investigation over the next decade and Chapter 6 discusses its current and future role in monitoring tumor growth and response to therapy.

Positron Emission Tomography provides opportunities to image and map functions such as tissue blood flow, blood volume, glucose uptake, protein synthesis and neuroreceptor binding. These topics and others are discussed in Chapter 7. Since its relatively recent introduction, Interventional Radiology has placed the diagnostic radiologist in the unique role of treating patients. This area is now recognized as a true sub-specialty, and Chapter 8 outlines some of the important emerging areas that will be further developed and refined in the near future. The increasingly important diagnostic applications of ultrasound is presented in Chapter 9. The last two chapters of the volume present applications of imaging techniques to study cardiac wall motion and new approaches to CT guided stereotactic brain surgery.

The composition of diagnostic radiology department faculty is becoming more heterogeneous as new technologies emerge and both basic scientists and non radiologists find imaging to be an exciting and important modality in both research and patient care. This diversity in expertise is reflected in the background and training of the chapter authors of this volume. Contributing authors have received formal postgraduate training in such areas as radiology, physiology, mathematics, psychiatry, computer science, biophysics, biochemistry, cell biology, nuclear medicine, electrical engineering, biomedical engineering and neurosurgery. This mix of basic scientists and clinicians working together in collaboration to advance the state of the art in medical imaging should be welcomed and encouraged. It will strengthen the research and development as well as the patient care and teaching components of academic diagnostic radiology departments.

The future for diagnostic radiology is very bright and for this reason, the discipline is attracting some of the most gifted medical school graduates and basic scientists. The contributors of this volume will consider their efforts rewarded if the book helps to stimulate the younger clinicians and scientists seeking direction in a career in imaging and assists in guiding the more senior clinicians and scientists in directing the academic growth and development of their departments.

JAMES H. ANDERSON

Contents

1 Current and Future Challenges for Academic Radiology
JAMES H. ANDERSON 1

2 Diagnostic Radiology Research Program Development
JAMES H. ANDERSON 7

3 Image Analysis
HARRY L. LOATS and HENRY H. HOLCOMB. (With 26 Figures) 23

4 Three-Dimensional Imaging: Advanced Medical Applications
ELLIOT K. FISHMAN, DONNA MAGID, DEREK R. NEY, KENNETH I. MACRAE,
JANET E. KUHLMAN, and DOUGLAS D. ROBERTSON. (With 23 Figures) 47

5 NMR Imaging: An Appraisal of the Present and the Future
STEPHEN J. BLACKBAND. (With 14 Figures) 69

6 NMR Spectroscopy and Its Application to the Study of Cancer
JANNA P. WEHRLE, CYNTHIA PAELLA MARTIN, and JERRY D. GLICKSON
(With 19 Figures) 93

7 Positron Emission Tomography: Current Achievements and Future Projections
DEAN F. WONG. (With 9 Figures) 117

8 Interventional Radiology
JAMES H. ANDERSON. (With 11 Figures) 131

9 Ultrasound
FRANK P. LEO. (With 12 Figures) 155

10 Imaging Distinct Points in Left Ventricular Myocardium to Study
Regional Wall Deformation
WILLIAM C. HUNTER and ELIAS A. ZERHOUNI. (With 11 Figures) 169

11 Toward Computed Image-Controlled Electromechanical Stereotactic
Brain Surgery
SUMIO UEMATSU, ARTHUR E. ROSENBAUM, and ASHOK J. KUMAR
(With 19 Figures) 191

Subject Index 209

1 Current and Future Challenges for Academic Radiology

JAMES H. ANDERSON

CONTENTS

1.1 Introduction 1
1.2 Economic Issues 1
1.3 Image Analysis 2
1.4 Department Divisional Structure 2
1.5 Radiology Training 3
1.6 Loss of Academic Radiologists 3
1.7 Integration of Basic and Clinical Research 4
1.8 Enhancing Academic Image 4
References 5

1.1 Introduction

During the past 10–15 years, clinical medicine and medical research have experienced an unprecedented technological growth. Of all the medical disciplines, diagnostic radiology has likely experienced the greatest impact of this growth. The introduction of computerized axial tomography, for example, demonstrated to the Radiology community the practical application and utility of computer-assisted image acquisition, processing, presentation, and analysis. This major advance, along with the introduction of magnetic resonance imaging (MRI), in vivo nuclear magnetic spectroscopy (NMR), positron emission tomography (PET), digital radiography, and interventional radiology, has dramatically altered the manner in which the radiologist in particular and radiology departments in general function in patient care, teaching, and research. These advances provide diagnostic radiology with unique academic growth and development opportunities that are more available now than ever before.

Indications suggest that medical imaging technology research and development will continue at an even faster rate than previously experienced. As a result, the issues that must be addressed by radiology departments are more complex than those present 20 years ago. At that time, radiology was almost entirely a film/screen-based technology and regulations for health care delivery costs were not focusing attention on high-cost computer-based image technology. In the late 1980s radiology has come to a crossroads; consequently academic departments are now faced with critical decisions that will significantly affect how their discipline will function in the future. Many of the issues that must be addressed now and in the future affect all medical specialties and are not unique to radiology. In fact, because recent advances in medical imaging have made such a positive impression on the medical community and the general public, diagnostic radiology, more than any other specialty, is in a very favorable position to capitalize on the issues in order to further improve academic growth and recognition. Indeed, the future for diagnostic radiology has never been more promising than it is today.

JAMES H. ANDERSON, Ph. D., Dept. of Radiology and Radiological Science, The Johns Hopkins University, School of Medicine, 600 North Wolfe Street, Baltimore, MD 21205, USA

1.2 Economic Issues

Academic radiology departments are responsible for providing high-quality patient care as well as innovative teaching and research programs. Currently, these needs present themselves at a time when economic and social changes in the health care system are placing an increased fiscal burden on academic institutions which are already stressed financially. Academic departments are being asked to economize and restructure clinical services in an attempt to conform with federal regulations on increasing health care costs, the competition of an increasing number of HMOs, the high costs of diagnostic procedures, and cutbacks in medicare reimbursement for teaching and administrative duties. At the same time, university-based radiology departments need to become even more academically oriented and to participate more aggressively in the development and application of new technology. This issue represents a significant opportunity for diagnostic radiologists to exert influence and become more academically involved in defining the true cost-benefit ratio of new imaging techniques. Research funds for such studies are becoming more available.

At the present time, the entire medical community is still somewhat overwhelmed by the relatively recent surge in the development and application of new imaging techniques. Clinical applications of imaging technology are still in their initial growth phase, with the developments occurring rapidly. It is difficult to predict which developments and applications will survive the test of time and which will be able to improve patient care at a cost compatible with the inevitable restructuring of health care costs in the future. This difficulty in forecasting was addressed at a recent international symposium on the impact of new imaging technology on health care, research, and teaching, in which a prevalent theme was the need for comprehensive investigation of the economic implications of new imaging technology (FIGLEY and MARGULIS 1987).

Radiologists must make it their responsibility to scrutinize procedures, techniques, and imaging modalities. They must begin to differentiate between studies that provide meaningful diagnostic information or therapeutic value and studies that provide "pretty" images or information which can be obtained from other less costly methods. Such evaluations will take considerable time, effort, and money, and funding agencies will be prepared to share the costs. For example, the clinical and/or economic value of a new interventional procedure often will require extensive long-term follow-up studies to compare its clinical and economic value with more readily available procedures.

1.3 Image Analysis

As imaging technology becomes more sophisticated and more readily available, the manner in which the radiologist views and interprets images will undergo many changes. In a recent article discussing Future Advance and Directions in Imaging Research, Dr. WALTER ROBB (1988), Senior Vice-President for Research and Development at General Electric, stressed the importance of converting data into information. This paper addressed new opportunities in the fields of digital signal processing, computer-aided imaging and analyses, and artificial intelligence. Dr. ROBB stressed the fact that well funded application research outside of medicine will provide new technology that will have direct application in medical imaging (ROBB 1988). Investments in image analysis technology for both clinical and basic science research can be funneled to enhance or support the routine clinical needs such as transmitting and storing images. Digital radiography may be able to tighten referral networks and help secure hospital patient bases by linking community physician activities and reports to a central digital image system of the hospital (WAGNER 1988). Financial, space, and personnel investments in image analysis cannot help but benefit both research and clinical components in departments of radiology.

As they become more involved in functional imaging, radiologists are introduced to an entirely different data set and approach than previously available through conventional film/screen-based systems. This will provide new areas for academic growth and expose the radiologist to new approaches to become more actively involved in the care and management of the patient. The radiologist will begin to better utilize computer algorithms to analyze images for information about organic disease in addition to information about anatomical detail. Providing functional information such as blood flow, energy metabolism, and oxygen and glucose consumption obligates the radiologist to become increasingly more involved in evaluating the disease process itself. This transition will continue to occur in virtually all areas of radiology.

1.4 Department Divisional Structure

The organization of departments with regard to subspecialization is being reevaluated. The advantages and disadvantages of an organ/system structure versus an imaging modality (technique) structure need to be reconsidered. The increasing emphasis on providing information about the disease process itself and the integration of multidisciplinary components in radiology faculty will also require reevaluation of departmental training programs. Neuroradiology has already addressed this issue by extending fellowship programs to 2 years and pioneering an organ system approach in which neuroradiologists perform angiographic and neurointerventional procedures (POTTS 1988).

1.5 Radiology Training

Radiology departments within academically oriented institutions must take a leadership role in providing both specialized and subspecialization training programs which have emphasis on academic research and teaching. University administrators expect no less and those academic institutions with appropriate resources must set an example for the entire discipline of radiology. A chief mechanism through which they can address this responsibility now and in the future is through aggressive development of academically oriented research training programs. Strong academic institutions should provide academic resident and fellowship programs which are not directed at producing general radiologists. The opportunity for diagnostic radiology departments to provide academically oriented training programs is becoming easier as more emphasis is being placed on extramural funding of medical imaging research.

Although other clinical disciplines such as surgery and cardiology often require research training as part of residency or fellowship programs, radiology has usually not required formal rotations aimed specifically at providing research training or formal exposure to research. For this reason, radiology has fewer physicians actively engaged in careers combining clinical work and basic research as compared to other specialties. Because other disciplines have had such programs in existence for some time, residents and fellows in these specialties accept them as a structured requirement of the training process. Attempts to incorporate formal research training in radiology, on the other hand, are often met with resistance from both faculty and trainees. Continuation of this attitude will not only undermine the academic credibility of radiology in the minds of the university administrators and members of other clinical departments but will also jeopardize the ability of the radiologist to compete with other clinicians for extramural peer-reviewed research funding. Because of increased competition for extramural funding, it is more essential now than ever before that this situation be corrected and research be included in academic radiology training programs. Implementation of a strong research training program requires an environment conducive to academic growth and this requires careful planning with specific short- and long-term goals. Immediate and thoughtful attention must be given to this subject. Important justification for this includes:

1. Radiologists must compete with other medical disciplines in basic research involving the development and application of imaging technology. Although the National Institutes of Health (NIH) provided $ 137 million for medical imaging research in 1987, a substantial amount went to disciplines other than radiology (Hendee 1988). The grant money is available and although awards are very competitive, the opportunities for funding have never been better. More radiologists and basic scientists are receiving training in new imaging technology. Within a relatively short period of time, diagnostic radiology departments will start receiving a greater share of these grants.
2. Because of the recent advancements in imaging technology and interventions, radiology is attracting more of the brightest medical students into residency programs. To maintain this momentum, it is important for academic radiology departments to provide these trainees with superb clinical training, as well as an academic teaching and research environment which will not only advance their own academic careers but will contribute to improvement in the state of the art of medical imaging. Because the national trend shows a decline in the number of students entering science and medicine, radiology may be unique among the specialties in attracting these bright, young scientists and physicians (Weaver 1988). This represents a major positive factor for the future academic growth of radiology.
3. The capability of radiology departments to retain control over imaging studies will depend on their academic and research credibility relative to that of clinicians in other departments. Radiologists are becoming more aware of this and positive steps are being taken to improve training programs to prepare radiologists to become more academically competitive.

1.6 Loss of Academic Radiologists

Radiologists should be concerned that so few residents and fellows who leave academic training programs ultimately pursue academic careers. Although the financial burden of a medical school education and the physical burden of extended residency and fellowship programs may tend to "burn out" many individuals, the lack of academic role models in the radiology faculty also contributes to the loss of academic radiologists. In addition, many clinical and research faculty members who serve as role models are themselves leaving academics for private practice largely because of financial considerations and the lack of adequate research time and/or facilities (HESS 1988). This situation is not unique to radiology. The opportunities for academic career development in diagnostic radiology have been significantly enhanced with the growth of interventional radiology, computer-assisted imaging, and NMR/MRI. If role models are leaving academia for private practice because of a lack of research time and/or facilities, inadequate attention has been given to developing an environment conducive to academic career development. This is an issue that must be addressed by all academic clinical departments.

1.7 Integration of Basic and Clinical Research

Although most research and development of hardware and software will be accomplished through industrial efforts, applications research and probing questions of biological or medical significance will be, as always, the domain of academic institutions. The responsibility inherited in this task requires a major effort to integrate basic and clinical research. It also requires the cooperation and collaboration of physicians, biochemists, engineers, physicists, physiologists, statisticians, mathematicians, computer programmers, and biologists. During the past 12 years, as many Ph. D. basic scientists have been appointed to clinical departments in the United States as have entered basic science departments in medical schools (MCKNEALLY et al., 1986). Radiology departments and many nonimaging specialists are actively and aggressively recruiting basic scientists into faculty positions. As new people are recruited into radiology departments, major decisions will need to be made about program development and investments in salaries, equipment, research projects, and space. Decisions will also need to be made about the specific areas most worthy of pursuit and the intregration of the research with teaching and patient care activities.

An active, productive research program enhances both the teaching and clinical care activities of a radiology department. However, research programs must be fiscally responsible. Funding levels for basic research often cycle with changes in funding priorities. This normal fluctuation should be expected and anticipated. However, departmental support of research for which there is continued lack of peer-reviewed funding creates financial and morale problems for clinical departments and does little to enhance academic credibility in the view of university administrators and other non-radiology-based clinicians and basic scientists.

The importance of research in medical imaging was recently summarized by Dr. ROSS WEAVER of the Office of Technology Management, American Medical Association. Dr. WEAVER strongly feels that research in radiology is an important national resource. He said, "The priorities are clear: actively recruit the brightest and the best, fight to protect funding sources, and demand that the research equipment be updated and modernized. The time to begin is now, for there is a great deal to lose by the research environment in particular, and in the health of the American people in general" (WEAVER 1988).

The role of the basic scientist in radiology departments will expand while the training and diversity of departmental faculty members will change as more basic scientists are needed to support the technological developments that will continue to impact on the growth of radiology. This trend will not only continue but will also become more important than ever before for full integration of the interests and activities of these individuals with clinical faculty. To be able to pursue and develop ideas to bring benefits to patients, basic scientists must be exposed to clinical problems. If these basic scientists fail to be integrated into the academic program, and if their activities are not combined with those of the radiologists, they will align themselves with clinicians from other departments who have financial and scientific interest in medical imaging. Although multidisciplinary interaction is scientifically valuable and should be encouraged, it should not be the result of alienation of the basic scientist by the clinical radiologist. In many instances the basic scientist can act as a bridge linking radiologists with other clinicians who share common research interests.

1.8 Enhancing Academic Image

There is no doubt that the development and application of new technology will progress, with or without radiology. If radiology departments do not recognize this, the credibility of the radiologist will deteriorate while imaging techniques and patient populations will be usurped by other medical disciplines. Further growth mandates that radiology departments structure their academic programs in a manner similar to those of other clinical disciplines. Although this restructuring may require a change in philosophy, it should not compromise quality clinical care or place heavy financial burden on the radiology department.

The tendency for radiology departments to be looked upon as primarily "service departments" has previously diminished university administration support for radiology research. University administrators are beginning to expect more from academic radiology departments because of the recent advances in imaging technology, the infusion of more basic scientists in radiology, and the interest that nonradiology departments are showing for imaging and profitable interventional procedures. Federal funding for imaging research has increased significantly over the past 15 years and more radiology departments are obtaining federally funded research training grants to assist in research training for both the basic scientist and the radiologist. NIH funded $ 137 million for medical imaging research in 1987 (Weaver 1988). This represents a nominal increase in funding dollars of 10% annually for the past 10 years. Grants supporting radiology research have increased in number at a rate of 6.1% annually during the past decade (Weaver 1988). Basic scientists within radiology are beginning to compete more actively for federal-funded research support of work in which radiology clinicians are becoming increasingly involved.

The time for radiology departments to establish stronger academic programs and provide proper role models for the younger trainees has never been more opportune than it is today. Departments must meet this challenge by providing the environment and incentives conducive to academic career development of faculty members. The challenge to improve the academic functions of radiology departments and the need to develop and reward role models cannot be ignored if radiology is to be actively competitive in the years to come.

It is time basic scientists and clinicians in radiology stop complaining and start competing. Many of the most important contributions in medical science and patient care during the past two decades have involved imaging. Innovations in diagnostic and therapeutic radiology will continue to be made, much to the increasing appreciation of the medical and general public. Radiology is attracting the brightest young scientists and physicians. Now is the time to channel their energy in a productive manner into further expansion of imaging and imaging research. The future of these young people should be the future of radiology; this should not be compromised nor their energy and enthusiasm dampened. The time has never been better for academic radiology to flourish. The future of the discipline depends on radiology departments assuming a more active responsible role in training future academic radiologists who will continue to expand the field.

Those factors that may strengthen or weaken the role of academic radiology as a discipline will affect all aspects of departmental programs, including patient care, teaching, and both clinical and basic research. Economic issues, technology development and application evaluation, departmental divisional structure, training programs, integration of basic and clinical research, and academic image all relate to one another and cannot be addressed as separate issues independent of the others.

The remaining chapters in this book address more specific areas of imaging with an emphasis on future development and application. The manner in which these technologies enhance the future role of radiology in patient care is dependent to a large degree on the manner in which they evolve in relation to many of the issues discussed in this chapter. Ultimately, the crossroads at which radiology sees itself can be traversed successfully, but only if radiology departments within academically oriented institutions assume the leadership role intended for them and take advantage of this "window" in time when opportunities for academic growth and achievement are most apparent.

References

Figley MM, Margulis AR (1987) The impact of new imaging technology on health care, research, and teaching: An international symposium. AJR 149: 1111-1126

Hendee WR (1988) Critical review of article "Setting research priorities for the next decade." Invest Radiol 23: 563

Hess TP (1988) Defections and lack of support undermine radiology research. Diagn Imag Clin Med 10: 63-72

McKneally MF, Mulder DS, et al. (1986) Facilitating scholarship: Creating the atmosphere, setting, and teamwork for research. In: Troidl H, Spitzer WD, et al. (eds) Principles and practice of research. Springer, Berlin Heidelberg New York, pp 36-42

Potts DG (1988) Coherent radiology planning. Invest Radiol 23: 552

Robb WL (1988) Future advances and directions in imaging research. AJR 150: 39-42

Wagner JL (1988) Author's reply to critical review of article "Cost containment and computerized medical imaging: Meeting one another's needs?" Invest Radiol 23: 554

Weaver RH (1988) Setting research priorities for the next decade. Invest Radiol 23: 561-563

2 Diagnostic Radiology Research Program Development

JAMES H. ANDERSON

CONTENTS

2.1	Introduction	7
2.2	Departmental Commitment	9
2.3	Role of Department Chairman	10
2.4	Planning the Research Program	10
2.5	Specifically Defining Short- and Long-Term Goals	11
2.5.1	Long-Term Goals	11
2.5.2	Short-Term Goals	11
2.6	The Role of the Basic Scientists	13
2.7	Getting and Keeping Clinicians Involved in Research	14
2.7.1	Migration to Private Practice	14
2.7.2	Research Time	14
2.7.3	Research Training	14
2.7.4	Personnel Assistance	15
2.7.5	Other Incentives	15
2.8	Integrating Basic Research and Clinical Activities	15
2.9	Multidepartmental Collaboration	15
2.10	Funding	17
2.10.1	Basic Sources	17
2.10.2	Extramural Peer-Reviewed Funding	17
2.10.3	Industrial Support	17
2.10.4	Private Funding	17
2.10.5	Departmental Pilot Grants	17
2.10.6	Balance in Funding Programs	18
2.11	Research Training	18
2.11.1	The Importance of Research Training	18
2.11.2	Residents	18
2.11.3	Faculty Members	19
2.11.4	Clinical Fellows	19
2.11.5	Basic Scientists	20
2.11.6	Research Training Grants	20
2.12	Animal Facilities	21
	References	22

2.1 Introduction

Providing recommendations regarding developing and maintaining radiology research and research training facilities is a difficult task because no two departments have the same goals, resources, commitment, faculty composition, or philosophy. There is no ideal model and every department must address issues specific to their own particular goals and needs. However, concern has been generated in the radiology community regarding the role, development, and expansion of research programs and many of the issues that need to be considered are germane to all departments. The primary purpose of this chapter is to provide information which may be of value to the reader charged with the responsibility of addressing research-related issues in a clinical radiology department.

The decision to develop or expand the research program in any clinical department must be made with a firm understanding of the degree of commitment that is necessary. This commitment must permeate throughout the entire department and be part of a larger commitment to total academic excellence stressing superior patient care, teaching, and research. The success of a program will eventually be judged on the quality and not the quantity of work. The research program must be an integral part of department activities, and form a symbiotic relationship with clinical and teaching components. Although high-quality, clinically relevant research does not necessarily require major resources, it does require a strong departmental commitment to ensure its excellence and to maintain its proper perspective in the department and the institution.

During the past 15 years, the manner in which radiology departments view the development or expansion of research facilities has changed. This change has largely been related to the significant rapid advances in medical imaging technology and the manner in which these advances have altered the role of the radiologist in patient care and the training and composition of departmental faculty. When visiting radiology departments 15 years ago, it was not uncommon to be guided through one or two small, cramped rooms that constituted the "dog lab" or "physics lab." These facilities were usually used by one or two faculty members. In most cases, the laboratory did not constitute an integral part of an established, goal-oriented departmental research

JAMES H. ANDERSON, Ph. D., Dept. of Radiology and Radiological Science, The Johns Hopkins University, School of Medicine, 600 North Wolfe Street, Baltimore, MD 21205, USA program. These laboratories were usually equipped with secondhand or discarded clinical equipment and staffed by technicians who had additional responsibilities as X-ray technologists in the clinical department. Funding almost always came from clinical revenue or industry and very few received support from extramural peer-reviewed sources such as governmental agencies, foundations, or large private funding sources. However, the radiology researchers were usually very dedicated and much of their work laid the foundation for modern-day applications such as in interventional radiology. At that time, most radiological imaging involved film-screen technique, research was not a major focus in most departments, and university and hospital administrators did not look upon most radiology departments as research-oriented resources.

Although such facilities still exist today, the trend is changing towards many radiology departments being concerned with developing more active, comprehensive, and formal research and research training programs. This involves major financial investments for renovation, equipment, personnel, and space. However, if some individuals are discouraged from developing or supporting a major research program because of the potentially prohibitive cost, the following factors should be considered:

1. People and not equipment or facilities are responsible for successful research programs.
2. Well designed clinical and basic research projects in medical imaging have a much greater chance of receiving extramural funding than was the case 10–15 years ago.
3. Most successful radiology research programs focus attention in only one or two specific areas of work.
4. Government research funding agencies will usually reimburse equipment use and maintenance fees for expensive imaging equipment used for research.
5. Multidepartmental generated funds can be a major source of income to purchase equipment and finance technical support salary.
6. Industry often provides reduced purchase prices or even free equipment for research laboratories.
7. The university and other departments benefit both academically and financially from image research laboratories and should help provide funding.
8. Highly successful, productive, clinically applicable research can still be done in relatively simple facilities. For example, good basic research in interventional radiology can be performed with X-ray equipment including little more than a fluoroscope, an overhead tube, and a film changer.
9. Strong academic programs with well equipped research facilities will attract academically strong clinicians and basic scientists who can support their own research projects through extramural sources. Strong academic programs attract strong academic people.

Because of the diversity of departmental goals, capital, and research interests, it is impossible to make specific recommendations regarding space, equipment, and personnel needed to develop or expand existing facilities. However, careful consideration must be given to space and equipment requirements not only for the immediate needs but also for those of the future. One of the most important factors to consider in planning radiology research facilities is maintaining flexibility and balance to meet changing needs relative to technology development, faculty research interests, and funding sources. Although some departments have invested heavily in personnel and resources directed towards a single specific area such as digital angiography, magnetic resonance imaging (MRI), and interventional radiology, it is those programs that maintain flexibility and balance that will continue to be productive over an extended period of time. If properly planned, this can be done without diluting areas of research that may experience temporary but clinically important periods of intense investigation. Investing heavily in research and development during this initial technology and application research phase can be highly productive and rewarding. However, if such investment totally jeopardizes other more conventional areas of work, the long-term results may not be in the overall best interests of the department or faculty.

If major investments in manpower, equipment, and facilities are heavily directed towards a very specific area of work, the results should be designed to benefit other clinical and basic research areas in the department. For example, computerized image acquisition, presentation, transfer, and analysis will form an important contribution in radiology departments of the future. This applies not only to larger academic institutions but also to the smaller community hospitals. Radiology departments cannot ignore the importance of this developmental trend. Research and development investments in image analysis will have widespread application in all clinical and research areas of the department. If academic institutions invest in centralized image analysis centers, they will be contributing to the development of the state of the art and protecting their investment for future widespread research applications.

The need to address the research issue seems to be almost universal in today's academic radiology departments. This requires an analysis of the department's previous research activity, the experience and background training of the clinical and basic science faculty, and the overall departmental goals, philosophy, and resources. In addition, very practical issues relating to space, equipment, and money must be addressed. However, even with all these variables, specific areas of concern common to all departments can be identified. Essentially, the following areas of concern seem common:

1. What is needed to provide an academic atmosphere conducive to research?
2. Should efforts be concentrated on one or maybe two areas of research, or should more be considered?
3. How much and what type of space is needed to provide an adequate research facility?
4. How many and what type of people should be hired and what should be the role and responsibility of basic scientists?
5. How does one get and keep physicians involved in research?
6. How should the research program be funded?
7. Should radiology research facilities and/or equipment and personnel be shared with other departments?
8. Should research programs include training components, and if so, at what level?
9. What type of facilities are needed if animal research is part of the program?

The remainder of this chapter will address these basic issues and provide suggestions which may be of value to those concerned with implementing a more active research component in their academic radiology program.

2.2 Departmental Commitment

Although academic radiology departments may encourage research, few have made the commitment to rank this a high-priority objective (Maynard 1986). This is largely related to apprehensions regarding inadequate space, equipment, funding, and the availability of necessary personnel. There is also concern that a commitment to research may be intimidating to faculty members who have no research experience or particular desire to become involved in research. In such situations, it is best to start conservatively and focus on individual strengths. This may represent a particular strength within a section of the department or a major institutional strength where radiology may become more involved. In either case, a commitment must be made to develop and support academic development in that area. For example, if ultrasound represents the strongest or potentially strongest academic section, focus attention on supporting the growth in this area. This may require providing one or two faculty members with more research time, recruiting a specific individual to further enhance the academic development of the section, or providing initial start-up funds to support specific projects or purchase equipment (Maynard 1986). This initial financial support should not require a major drain on departmental resources.

If the institution has a strong program in neurosciences, capitalize on this strength and become more supportive of radiology's role in the development of the program's research projects.

In this early research development phase it is particularly important to require focused attention on an area of development and provide maximum support, require academic accountability, and monitor progress. It is also important during the early stages of program development to provide positive reinforcement for academic excellence. If a department commitment is made to developing academic strength in one area, the future growth of this area will most likely develop through its own procurement of extramural funding. The success of this development will influence academic growth in other sections. In summary, capitalize on departmental or institutional strengths, support productive individuals, and develop a departmental commitment to the academic success of the project.

An important factor in developing a research program is creating the proper academic environment through commitment and personnel recruitment. Providing faculty with academic time for research and creating an academic atmosphere is more important than monetary investments in research equipment. The individual most responsible for creating and maintaining an academic environment is the department chairman.

2.3 Role of Department Chairman

Academic department chairman must strive to develop a departmental environment conducive to academic growth. Important reasons for this include:

1. Academic departments have the responsibility to train and prepare young residents and fellows for academic careers. The strength of a program or an institution is often measured by the future success of its trainees or graduates.
2. An academic atmosphere in a clinical department stimulates an inquisitive approach to solving problems. This enhances the teaching program and promotes young physicians to think logically (Selye 1975).
3. Academic pursuits encourage multidisciplinary approaches that transcend from the research environment to the clinic.

The department chairman plays the most important role in creating an academic environment and in establishing and maintaining an active research program. His or her commitment must be recognized at all levels of the department and the university. The department chairman must set priorities, delegate responsibilities, provide incentives as well as positive reinforcements, and require accountability. The chairman must be a primary role model, place a high priority on academic productivity, and set personal examples of encouragement for scholarly research (McKneally et al. 1986). He or she must take the responsibility of creating the environment conducive to a productive research program. An environment conducive to research must first be conducive to providing superior patient care and a strong teaching program. An inappropriate and excessive emphasis on research with a casual attitude towards acknowledging and rewarding excellence in patient care and teaching will lead to faculty jealousy, competition, and isolation (Chiu and Mulder 1986). Such an environment does little to create faculty role models who are essential in influencing younger staff members and trainees to remain in academics. All decisions regarding departmental growth and development should center around the concept of integrating patient care, teaching, and research activities.

The chairman must maintain a participating management role. As the department leader, the chairman must encourage multidisciplinary collaboration and be effective in influencing others in order to achieve the long-term goal of improving academic quality. This includes influencing not only clinicians, basic scientists, and administrators within the department of radiology, but also other departmental chairman and university administrators.

It is also important for department chairman to ensure interaction between basic scientists and clinicians. Such interaction prevents sequestering clinical and research activities into separate components. It provides the basic scientists with a better understanding of problems faced by clinicians in conducting clinical research or in translating results from basic research into practical clinical applications. The interactions also strengthens the clinicians' support for basic research. McKneally (1986) reflected on these issues when discussing the collaborative relationship between basic scientists and surgeons. He said "The surgeons brought a refreshing vigor; a tendency to rise early, and enthusiasm for the expeditious completion of experiments to the environment of the basic scientists. Conversely, the intellectual vigor of the physiologist had a positive impact on the scientific thinking of the surgeon."

Weekly research/clinical conferences by themselves cannot provide this much needed interaction. It is more important to foster an atmosphere where clinicians and basic scientists meet regularly in small groups to discuss their respective activities or common areas of interest. Basic scientists should be required to participate in the residency and fellowship selection process and to take part in the resident training program. This may involve presenting lectures relating to their research and providing assistance to trainees interested in basic research. The chairman's presence at departmental research conferences, involvement in research conferences of other departments, and active positive reinforcement and support of quality academic achievements by radiology faculty members help to create an environment that emphasizes academic growth and facilitates and expedites research. The chairman must provide an academic environment that is motivating.

2.4 Planning the Research Program

The basic ingredients that must be blended to ensure the development of a successful research and research training facility are essentially no different than those common in the development of a program in industry. Major considerations include (1) formulation of a specific plan or goal, (2) creating the environment for the project, (3) having a commitment to the successful completion of the project, (4) providing the essential people to participate, (5) providing adequate short- and long-term funding.

Industrialists would not consider entering into an area of expansion without adequate planning, but physicians and scientists often overlook this basic principle in developing research programs. Although concepts and goals can be generalized verbally, it is imperative that a plan be drafted in writing. This is necessary in order to be very specific in defining short- and long-term goals. Exactly what is to be accomplished must be carefully defined (long-term goal). A list of specific short-term goals may help to clarify what exactly must be addressed to accomplish the long-term goal.

2.5 Specifically Defining Short- and Long-Term Goals

2.5.1 Long-Term Goals

A written plan should be developed outlining how the long-term goal will be accomplished via a series of specifically defined short-term goals. Clear-cut decision making must follow an organized plan to achieve the desired goal. Long-term goals should have a timetable of 3–5 years. Examples of long-term goals may include:

1. The development of a comprehensive multimodality imaging research resource
2. The implementation of a degree- and/or non-degree-seeking research training program
3. The development of a state of the art image analysis center

2.5.2 Short-Term Goals

Although long-term goals may be less specific, short-term goals should address clearly defined, tangible issues that can be accomplished within a very specific time frame. For example, short-term goals to help create a more academic environment may include:

1. Initiating weekly or bimonthly departmental research conferences
2. Developing a departmental program to provide faculty with funds to support pilot research projects
3. Organizing a departmental research committee to assist faculty in identifying extramural funding sources
4. Initiating journal clubs or critical review sessions to evaluate the scientific merit, methodology, and value of published articles
5. Organizing seminars and conferences where researchers from other departments discuss their work and its possible interactions or applications in radiology
6. Recruiting either basic scientists or academic clinicians to address a specific need or objective

Department faculty members should be assigned to each specific short-term goal and be made accountable for its successful completion. The department chairman should meet regularly with the individuals to monitor progress in accomplishing each short-term goal. All of the above contribute to building an environment more conducive to academic growth and represent specific actions that can be easily monitored for success.

A flow chart can be useful for outlining the relationship between long- and short-term goals. The order in which short-term goals are sequenced can be an important factor in determining the success of the program.

A practical example of this strategy is illustrated in the development of one major component of our own departmental research program. The plan was formulated in 1980. At this time, the departmental cardiovascular research division consisted of a cramped 800 sq ft laboratory supplied with inadequate, outdated X-ray equipment. The long-term goal was to develop a modern cardiovascular and interventional radiology research facility that would be radiology based, but yet serve as a core resource to provide X-ray imaging capabilities for all medical school departments. The main problems were obtaining space and providing funds for renovation and equipment purchase. The following short-term goals were defined with each goal having a completion date set:

1. Evaluate radiology and nonradiology departmental X-ray imaging needs – current and future
2. Formulate basic concept of the function and structure of a research facility based on needs
3. Gain multidepartmental support for the concept of building a multidisciplinary X-ray imaging laboratory
4. Present initial concept to the dean
5. Formulate specific plans for space, equipment, funding, and personnel
6. Present formal proposal to the dean
7. Obtain formal department financial commitments

8. Obtain industrial pledges
9. Present final proposal to dean
10. Begin construction

Evaluating the existing and future X-ray research imaging needs of our own department as well as those of other departments was comparable to a market survey analysis. This step was essential since the facility could not be developed if the department of radiology had to provide total financing. Also, a large comprehensive X-ray research facility that did not receive adequate use would be detrimental to the image of the departmental research program. When it was determined that many departments could benefit from a centralized X-ray imaging laboratory, a preliminary plan outlining the structure and function of the facility was prepared. The next short-term goal was to obtain more specific support from potential users. This short-term goal was the most important since potential users were now required to be more specific in outlining their degree of support and projected use of the facility. At this time, it was important to gain the confidence of the various potential users and convince them that the department of radiology was not soliciting their support merely to subsidize the radiology laboratory or its research program, but to develop a comprehensive facility that would benefit their own research and improve their capabilities to obtain extramural funding.

Gaining confidence required a nonaggressive approach in which an emphasis was placed on (1) maintaining our own active research interests, (2) assisting other radiology and nonradiology department users in their imaging research needs, (3) educating collaborators in the value of more sophisticated imaging for their current and future research requirements. In working with nonradiology departments an emphasis was placed on providing collaborative research support as opposed to providing a service where major concerns centered around immediate financial reimbursements or coauthorship on publications. Our own laboratory research interests often coincided with those of other departments and a policy of open collaboration was established. The approach was successful and nonradiology users and potential users of our small, inadequate X-ray research laboratory realized the value of supporting a larger, more comprehensive facility. The approach of providing scientific collaboration for multidepartmental research imaging projects and maintaining our own active research program was important in gaining the trust and confidence of other departments. This approach also strengthened the concept of multidisciplinary approaches to research.

The University was initially approached with the plan in the form of a preliminary proposal outlining the need for a facility by multiple departments within the institution. A preliminary budget for space renovation and equipment purchase was developed and a request for space (4000 sq ft) was made. During the next 6–12 months, potential users of the facility were contacted for monetary support pledges. Because the proposed budget approached $ 1 000 000, a schedule was developed to spread the payments over 5 years. The large initial outlay of funds for renovation and equipment purchase was accomplished by borrowing money at the current interest rate from the University. At the same time that multidepartmental support was being negotiated, contacts were made with industry to assist with equipment donations or purchase price reductions. The multidepartmental commitment to the project and the scope of the project proved instrumental in convincing industry of the value and importance of their contributions. The final plan, which included a complete description of the facilities, a detailed 5-year payment plan, and industrial support commitments, was presented to the University. The University approved the project and identified the required space. The time from initial concept of the idea to final University approval was 2 years. The facility was developed in the 3rd year and successfully financed over the subsequent 5 years. It is important to emphasize that the long-term goal was accomplished because specific tangible short-term goals were outlined and sequenced in a logical manner.

The practice of requiring specific written short- and long-term goals is central in developing an academic program at all levels in the department. Each division head within the department must develop their own short- and long-term academic development goals. The department head with the assistance of a departmental academic development committee should review these divisional goals to ensure that they complement and contribute to the overall academic direction of the department. This approach will only be successful if each division is required to account for its progress in accomplishing the goals. Division chiefs will also be providing faculty members with a mechanism to gauge their own individual academic career development. A common complaint of faculty in clinical departments is that they are not fully aware of the requirements for academic promotion. The individual faculty members's academic career development and promotion track is linked directly to the divisional and departmental academic and research development progress. Requiring individual faculty members to document in writing their own short- and long-term academic career development goals, and meeting with each member frequently to review progress in achieving these goals, is the most efficient manner to make them accountable and responsible for their own career development and at the same time create an overall departmental atmosphere that stresses academic progress and growth. The role that research plays in this growth will be obvious to each faculty member and this in turn will help provide the divisional chiefs and departmental chairman with an environment conducive to support research efforts.

2.6 The Role of the Basic Scientists

Although it is not well appreciated among nonradiologists, basic scientists play major roles in academic radiology. Medical physicists contribute to X-ray and ultrasound physics and engineering research, take major roles in the radiology residency teaching programs, and have the responsibility of maintaining equipment quality control standardization and radiation health measures. In addition, radiobiologists have major input into radiotherapy programs and chemists have always been actively involved in nuclear medicine programs. However, with the introduction of computer-assisted image formation and analysis, interventional radiology, and MRI and spectroscopy, demand for computer scientists, biologists, physiologists, biophysicists, mathematicians, engineers, and chemists became very apparent and the basic science faculty of academic radiology departments is now much more diverse. The reluctance of many scientists to join clinical departments is changing, as existing new possibilities for research develop and funding becomes more available. In the future, academic radiology faculty will become even more of a blend of basic scientists and clinicians. The clinician/basic scientist barrier, which often interferes with collaboration, is beginning to break down and both groups of professionals are realizing the productive nature of interaction and collaboration.

The basic scientist has multiple responsibilities in a radiology department research program. The primary responsibility is to carry on his or her own active and productive research program. This is very important and must be reinforced. They must obtain peer-reviewed extramural funding in a manner comparable to basic scientists with primary appointments in nonclinical departments. Without their own base of research support, clinical department basic scientists tend to be satisfied with just providing assistance to other researchers in need of help. If this becomes a primary function, basic scientists rapidly develop the reputation of being highly paid technicians and/or managers. This does little to foster their academic growth and eventually will prove detrimental both to the career development of the scientist and to the image of the departmental research program.

It is an important responsibility of the basic scientist to assist in research facilities and program planning and to assist and train clinicians in establishing their own research projects. The philosophy of providing research training goes far beyond that of providing a 3–6-month rotation in the "research lab." Although examples can be cited where residents, fellows, or faculty members inexperienced in research have successfully completed good research projects during a 3–6-month block of time, the examples are an exception rather than the rule. More specific information regarding research training is provided later in this chapter. However, it is important at this point to stress that the basic scientist has the responsibility of guiding the inexperienced resident, fellow, or staff member in basic concepts of the scientific method. This essentially involves helping the individual to define the research hypothesis clearly and to carefully construct methods to test the hypothesis. These two basic steps constitute a major and very important effort in research.

A radiology department's ability to grow academically will never be realized if basic scientists and basic research laboratories function in isolation to clinical programs. Radiology departments cannot meet their responsibility to academic medicine by supporting basic science research facilities that do little more than act as "window dressing" to satisfy the requirement of having a research laboratory. The academic growth of a clinical department is dependent upon a strong collaborative, responsive interaction between the clinician and the basic scientist. Basic scientists should be recruited with a clear understanding of their responsibilities to their own career development and to the long-term academic goals of the department.

2.7 Getting and Keeping Clinicians Involved in Research

2.7.1 Migration to Private Practice

One of the major current problems in radiology is the migration of academic faculty to private practice. This trend is not new and is not limited to radiology departments, but because there are fewer radiologists engaged actively in research as compared to some other clinical specialties, the problem seems to be more acute. Economic factors play the major role in enticing active productive academic radiologists to private practice, but a second important factor is the lack of an academic environment provided by many radiology departments. This is unfortunate since the opportunities for research development in radiology departments have never been greater than they are today. Most radiologists, even those actively engaged in research or academic career development pursuits, cite lack of sufficient research time as a major obstacle in being academically productive. Additional factors that interfere with radiologists doing research include perceptions of insufficient training or experience in laboratory work and inadequate facilities and/or personnel to provide advice or help.

If radiologists consider research to be an issue that must be addressed for the future of the discipline (KEATS 1986; NELSON 1983), specific steps must be taken to remove the obstacles that block academic career development progress. Academic salaries can never compete with those of private practice, so if economic issues are the only reason why an individual leaves academics, there is very little that the department chairman can do. However, the other issues, i.e., adequate research time, insufficient training, personnel assistance, and adequate incentives are issues that can and must be addressed. The issues pertain to both keeping productive radiology researchers in academics as well as getting more clinicians involved.

2.7.2 Research Time

The department chairman must protect research time for those clinicians who show research productivity. Although most academic radiology departments provide faculty members with specific days each week or blocks of time each year for research, the system is often improperly used and the time spent is often not adequately monitored. Faculty should be accountable for time provided as "research days." Those who do not use their research time for the intended purpose should perform clinical studies during the time in order to provide adequate coverage for those who use the research time for its intended purpose. This approach requires that clinicians who do not engage in research will not have their academic career development jeopardized and that they will be recognized and rewarded academically for superior teaching and patient care skills. A two track tenure system for academic promotions should be considered (KEATS 1986). University-based hospitals/ medical school administrators need to be more practical about faculty composition in clinical departments and recognize that academic excellence is based on a strong combination of superior patient care, excellent teaching, and both clinical and basic research.

All clinical departments need a core of physicians whose primary concern is patient care. These individuals often form the blackbone of the clinical work of the department and their future in the academic system must be protected. The academic contributions of the radiologist in clinical research and in teaching are often not appropriately recognized, especially by university promotion committees. Clinical research is essential to better understand the disease process and to evaluate the application and value of imaging techniques. Its value compared to basic research should not be minimized by promotion committees. Also, the future of medicine is in the hands of the teachers as well as the basic research "innovators." Good teachers are essential to inspire and guide young residents and fellows. A two track tenure system would not discriminate against physicians primarily concerned with patient care and teaching and would greatly improve morale when solid, primarily patient care related physicians face promotional consideration (KEATS 1986). If a two track system is implemented, research time could be more appropriately allocated to those individuals oriented towards research track careers. If sufficient research time is provided, there is no reason for any faculty member to be academically nonproductive (KEATS 1986).

2.7.3 Research Training

Very few physicians have had formal research training or extensive on-the-job laboratory research experience. Academic institutions can best provide such training and if radiologists are to be competitive in the research arena, more departments must initiate research training programs. The research experience promotes growth and knowledge and enables the investigator to foster and stimulate training in others. The net result is enhanced scientific credibility for the department, the university, and the discipline (PUTMAN 1986). A more detailed discussion of research training is found later in this chapter.

2.7.4 Personnel Assistance

As previously indicated, radiology departments with active basic science research components must make the basic scientists and their support personnel more sensitive to the needs of physicians desiring to pursue research. Speaking from the viewpoint of a surgeon, CRUESS (1986) stated that a true symbiotic relationship can develop between the clinician and basic scientist. The basic scientist can play a major role in educating the clinician and can come to appreciate the problems faced by the clinician and understand the knowledge bases required (CRUESS 1986).

2.7.5 Other Incentives

Incentives can also be used to reward academically productive individuals. People require incentives to do their best and those who fulfill the entire role of academician should be amply rewarded (KEATS 1986). Such incentives may include:

1. Providing additional "research time"
2. Providing salary support for a technician to assist the physician
3. Providing additional travel funds to productive individuals to attend more meetings relating to their work
4. Assigning productive individuals a greater role in directing and shaping future academic growth in the department
5. Providing departmental and institutional recognition to those academically productive individuals
6. Promoting those individuals who demonstrate academic development

2.8 Integrating Basic Research and Clinical Activities

Clinical departments with the most successful research programs stress integration of basic science and clinical activities. This includes: (1) an emphasis on departmental research conferences which integrate both clinical and basic research projects, (2) structuring courses or symposia around both clinical and research-related topics, (3) providing basic scientists with input into major programs such as residency and fellowship training, faculty recruitment, departmental business decisions, and departmental long- and short-term planning programs. Every major decision within academic departments should be made with a consideration as to how the decision will contribute to academic growth. Basic scientists who are involved in the decision-making process will develop a closer personal relationship with the clinical faculty and will have a much greater investment in the success of departmental development.

2.9 Multidepartmental Collaboration

The concept of interdepartmental collaboration in both conducting and financing research is becoming more prominent in radiology. The rationale for this cooperative approach reflects:

1. The broadening research base in radiology
2. The increased use of imaging by researchers in nonradiology departments
3. The cost of providing high-quality imaging equipment
4. The expanding role of the radiologist in areas of interventional radiology and nonconventional X-ray imaging
5. The increasing trend in subspecialization seen in all medical disciplines

Medical school administrators need to be better informed on the technological advancements that have occurred in radiology in the past 15 years and how these advancements have contributed to improve patient care. In addition, these same administrators need to appreciate the institutional value of a centralized image and image analysis research resource. Academic radiology departments should invite university administrators to medical image development seminars and take advantage of university publications to inform readers of the impact of recent imaging technology on patient care. It is naive to assume that university administrators are aware of the advances in imaging technology or the manner in which imaging research facilities could benefit the entire university community.

The presence of a technologically advanced imaging research facility, whether it be for X-ray imaging, nuclear magnetic resonance (NMR) spectroscopy, or image analysis, provides the university with a core resource that enhances extramural funding and research programs of all departments. In addition, the facility will enhance the ability to recruit academically oriented faculty, help attract industrial collaboration, and contribute to the university's capital research equipment investment which will factor into calculating extramural grant indirect cost recovery. Institutional and departmental strategy that fosters collaboration and joint projects increases the scientific vigor of the whole institution (McKneally et al. 1986). Because of these factors, the university should contribute financially to the facility.

The future of radiology research and the role that the radiologist will play in shaping this future will be enhanced if a spirit of interdepartmental research and research funding collaboration is encouraged. The fear that either scientific interaction or sharing of financial responsibilities for the development and operation of imaging research facilities will result in radiology departments losing control of the research base is unfounded as long as radiology departments and researchers maintain a high profile in their own research and properly manage the resource. In many cases, interdepartmental collaboration may provide a possible solution to the dilemma of providing sufficient expertise to develop a research program and at the same time, provide sufficient funds to renovate space and purchase equipment. A better understanding of the necessity of encouraging interdepartmental interaction comes from a closer examination of the following points.

1. The Clinical and Research Base of Medical Imaging is Expanding. The clinical as well as the research base of radiology is rapidly expanding with the increasing applications of interventional radiology in nonvascular areas, and the recent interest in image analysis and metabolic studies using NMR spectroscopy and positron emission tomography (PET).

Expansion of both the clinical and research applications of radiology necessitates more emphasis on an interdisciplinary approach to research. Radiology departments should profit both scientifically and in terms of grant support by such interdepartmental interaction.

2. There is an Increased Use of Medical Imaging by Researchers in Nonradiology Departments. Researchers with primary appointments in nonradiology departments are realizing the value of medical imaging in their research programs. This trend involves both clinicians and basic scientists. During the period 1987–88, 16 different departments or divisions utilized our diagnostic X-ray research facilities. In some cases, requests were for simple fluoroscopic guidance for catheter placements. In other instances, X-ray imaging formed the most important part of the data collection process.

The use of radiology research equipment by nonradiology researchers should be encouraged. However, it should be emphasized that in all cases, actual operation of the equipment should be performed by radiological technicians or staff trained in the equipment operation and radiation safety protection.

The approach of encouraging the use of medical imaging in nonradiology department initiated research enhances the value of the research facility, provides valuable support for the work of others, and improves interdepartmental relationships. However, the most important result is that it stimulates true scientific collaboration and provides radiology researchers with access to techniques, methods, procedures, and assistance of the other workers. In addition, the financial support base of the research facility is strengthened as scientists from other departments can budget equipment use and maintenance fees into extramural grant application budgets.

3. The Cost of Providing High-Quality Imaging Equipment for Research Cannot Always Be Borne by One Department. Very few radiology departments can afford to equip research facilities with the most modern imaging equipment. In special development and application work, industry may provide this equipment, but this does not apply to all research imaging equipment. An important mechanism to assist in providing such high-cost equipment is to share the expenses with other nonradiology department users. In most cases, user costs can be budgeted into extramural grant budgets. If properly managed, such an arrangement can significantly help to reduce the costs of developing or maintaining a facility (Fischer and Morris 1987).

2.10 Funding

2.10.1 Basic Sources

The long-term stability of a clinical department's research programs requires four major sources of support which include: (1) peer-reviewed National Institutes of Health (NIH) or other large extramural funding sources; (2) industrial support; (3) foundation/private gift support; (4) departmental pilot project grants for faculty members. Each of the above sources fulfills a particular need in the long-term financial operations of a technology-based research laboratory.

2.10.2 Extramural Peer-Reviewed Funding

Peer-reviewed, extramural funding such as that obtained from government-supported research organizations like the NIH or the National Science Foundation should form the major source of research support. Even if other sources of funding are adequate to support the research program, it is important to establish a strong extramural, peer-reviewed funding base. In addition to the monetary aspects, such support provides peer recognition of the research and establishes the credibility of the program within the scientific community. In addition, extramural, peer-reviewed support provides considerable indirect costs to the university for overhead operational expenses. A departmental research program's overall recognition will be significantly enhanced if it has a solid track record of this type of research support. In addition, the ability of individuals to generate this funding base is a major consideration in evaluating the research career development of faculty members. The best mechanism to ensure this type of funding base is to hire basic scientists and clinicians who have extramural peer-reviewed grants or who are strong candidates for obtaining grants. Individuals who desire to do continuing research without assuming the responsibility of competing for outside peer-reviewed funding are not enhancing their own career development and their work will soon become a financial drain on the department. This is particularly true for basic scientists where a proven track record of peer-reviewed extramural support is often a prerequisite for academic promotion.

2.10.3 Industrial Support

In a technology-oriented research area such as medical imaging, industrial support of research programs is essential. Although industry may provide only money for specific research projects, it is much better for long-term developmental purposes to concentrate industrial support in terms of equipment and technology development. It is difficult and/or impractical for industry to develop their own equipment or technology applications research center. Having access to a university environment and the wealth of specialists in both research and clinical areas is a very important objective for equipment manufacturers. It is essential that radiology research programs emphasize the need to form cooperative interactions with industry. This symbiotic relationship is essential in order for the university to have access to costly, advanced equipment and more importantly, to have direct access to industrial engineers who are responsive to the needs of both the basic and clinical researcher. Departments that have made the most significant contributions in NMR/MRI, digital imaging and interventional radiology have had a close working relationship with industry. Future advances in computer-assisted image analysis will require similar relationships.

2.10.4 Private Funding

Private funding forms the third component in the overall research funding program. Private funding can encompass gifts from alumni or local or national groups, and donations from grateful patients who have a desire to support research efforts. Private funding levels are usually less in monetary value than peer-reviewed extramural support. These funds should be used to support pilot projects to provide younger staff members with sufficient research data to test or evaluate a research project or idea or to provide preliminary data to support extramural peer-reviewed grant applications. Although private funding can be substantial, it should not be used to replace the extramural peer-reviewed grant sources.

2.10.5 Departmental Pilot Grants

The department should provide faculty members with small ($ 2000–$ 5000) pilot or seed grants. Like private funding, these grants should be targeted for those faculty members who desire to test an idea or generate preliminary data that can be used to support future extramural grant applications. This type of support is an obligation of the department to encourage investigative activity and enhance faculty members' career developmental potentials. Although the grants should be small to modest in their budgets, faculty members should be required to submit a formal application. The application should not be as extensive as that required by extramural agencies, but it should be complete enough to ensure that the faculty member presents his or her objective, specific aims, rationale, methods, and data analysis in a logical written format. The process of clearly and succinctly formulating a research proposal is one of the most important factors in training individuals in the scientific method and ensuring a rational, logical approach to their research.

2.10.6 Balance in Funding Programs

Long-term financial stability of a radiology research program requires a balance in the above support sources. All four areas of support, i.e., peer-reviewed NIH funding, industrial support, private funding, and departmental support, should complement one another and each should be used specifically for their respective value to the program as a whole. Programs that rely solely on one of the above funding mechanisms will sooner or later be subject to funding shortages and the consequences can be significant with respect to the continued operation of a productive research program.

2.11 Research Training

2.11.1 The Importance of Research Training

Not all academic radiology departments can or should consider research training as an integral component in their research program. However, as a discipline, radiology is in desperate need of clinicians who have research training exposure. In specialties other than radiology, research training as an essential component of residency or fellowship programs has been more readily accepted. TAVERAS (1986) feels that research in academic departments of radiology has not developed as rapidly or as strongly as it should have and that the most important reason for this is the purely clinical traditions and environments under which radiology training programs developed (TAVERAS 1986). CRUESS (1986) indicates that there is no doubt about the absolute necessity of providing research opportunities in the training of academic surgeons. He states that it is the only way in which the inquiring mind needed for academic creativity can be developed. Even if a clinician does not practice research after spending 1 year in the laboratory, the experience should make him or her a better physician. The training may help develop critical analytical skills, encourage the use of the scientific approach, stimulate the thought process, and be of value in critically reviewing the literature.

2.11.2 Residents

It is the responsibility of those departments that have adequate personnel and facilities to begin incorporating research training in their residency programs. This is essential if radiology is to compete with other medical disciplines in the future development and application of medical imaging and interventional procedures. Most radiology residencies offer little research experience in the scientific underpinnings of the discipline (HENDEE 1988). A residency confined principally to clinical procedures with perhaps occasional encouragement to become involved in a clinical case study does little to stretch the minds of young radiologists. A stronger commitment to research is needed in the training experience (HENDEE 1988).

In most instances, the problem is not so much an issue of whether research training should be incorporated, but how it can best be accomplished and at what level. Attempts to incorporate "research rotations" in residency training programs often meet with problems of a practical nature. The most prevalent problem is that there is just not enough time to do adequate research in a program that is already filled with necessary clinical rotations. Requiring that a resident spend a preset amount of time in bench or laboratory research may not be the solution. There will always be individuals who will find time for research either in the evenings or on the weekends. However, these individuals are rare and they possess a motivation that is not characteristic of the typical resident. One approach to the problem is to create an academic development requirement in the program that is flexible enough to meet the needs of most residents and not compete with their clinical training. This will require special attention to scheduling conflicts and a sincere commitment from the faculty to make the program work. Residents would be required to define and complete a project that would complement development of their own career development plans. Areas of concentration could include bench or laboratory research, but could also include active participation in a specific well defined clinical research project, learning specific techniques or procedures such as building or modifying surface coils, concentrating efforts in NMR spectroscopy, enhancing computer use and programming skills, or evaluating economic issues in radiology. The requirement should complement the clinical training. It should stimulate the resident to apply the knowledge to improve patient care. If the radiology faculty members are academically oriented in clinical or basic research, most residents will naturally associate themselves with an ongoing project. It is then the responsibility of the faculty member to act as a preceptor and role model for the resident. The concept of role models is important. Trainees are motivated to pursue academic careers when they perceive a positive effect of the knowledge and skills acquired in the laboratory on the performance and personal satisfaction of their role models (McKNEALLY 1986).

Each trainee should be required to specifically define the area of work, prepare a proposal outlining the work, and prepare a written report describing the results of the work. An oral presentation of the work should also be given at a departmental conference. The performance of the resident in completing this requirement should be weighed as heavily as the performance in acquiring skills in any of the clinical rotations in the residency program.

Incorporating an academic development rotation in the residency program will require special attention to scheduling conflicts and appropriate clinical care coverage. This will most likely involve increasing the number of residents and this may require additional departmental financial support. Flexibility in the program must be maintained since all resident projects may not be ideally suited for a 6-month block of time. In some cases, the rotation may be more appropriate early in the training program whereas in other cases, it may be more appropriate towards the end of the residency. In some cases, the work may carry over the 6-month block of time. There is no reason why the rotation could not involve spending time at another institution where a specific technique or area of work could be developed. All of the above variables must be considered and managed. The success of a resident academic development rotation will require a major departmental commitment and very careful planning.

2.11.3 Faculty Members

Academic radiology departments have the responsibility to provide faculty members with the environment and opportunities to pursue both clinical and basic research. Although one should not force faculty to engage in research, it should be strongly encouraged. The major problem in most academic clinical departments is providing adequate time and financial support for the work. Time away from clinical responsibilities for research often necessitates hiring extra personnel to provide clinical coverage. Departments that have a sincere commitment to improving academic programs must recognize this financial obligation. PUTMAN (1986) feels that in order to remove the apparent stigma attached to scientific research in academic radiology, a certain percentage of annual revenues must be assigned to creating and maintaining research laboratories and recruiting gifted individuals who wish to devote protected time to the pursuit of sound research.

2.11.4 Clinical Fellows

The most appropriate time to incorporate a research component in the clinical training program may be at the fellowship level. At this point in time, young radiologists have been exposed to the subspecialties and should be developing their interest and careers in a particular area. The fellow's attention is more focused and the role research may play in academic career development is more obvious. If research is to be a part of the fellowship program, careful fellow selection criteria must be employed. The fellow must be made aware of what is expected and a clearly defined focus area of work must be outlined prior to beginning the fellowship or very early in the program. Faculty preceptors must be identified, and guaranteed time away from clinical responsibilities must be provided. Initially a two track fellowship program may be of value. One track would be specifically directed towards clinical training. The second track would be 1 year longer and provide dedicated time for research. The two track system may be more appropriate for programs that are in the initial phase of incorporating research training as a component in the fellowship program. A two track system could also be considered for residency training, but this would require an extra year beyond that of the normal residency program.

The most effective manner to incorporate research into the fellowship program is through an extramurally supported training grant mechanism. More information regarding training grants is provided later in this chapter.

2.11.5 Basic Scientists

Pre- and postdoctoral training programs are the best method to introduce basic scientists to career opportunities in medical imaging. Although physics and engineering students may be aware of radiology and medical imaging related careers, those in study areas such as mathematics, biology, physiology, and chemistry have few preceptors, mentors, or role models to guide them. This is unfortunate since basic science graduate Master and PhD programs are ideal sources to train and expose these young people to the tremendous opportunities that are available. Although few clinical departments offer predoctoral degree-seeking programs at the Masters and PhD level, there is no reason why research thesis projects in the conventional basic science departments cannot incorporate medical imaging themes or components.

For example, in our own program, a PhD candidate in biology utilized CT reconstruction techniques to study cochlear morphology in marine mammals. This work led the individual to direct career objectives in image analysis. A biomedical engineer interested in cardiac dynamics helped develop a radiographic technique to monitor 3-D motion in the heart. Similar techniques were adapted by a radiologist to evaluate motion involved in swallowing. Encouraging basic scientists to utilize imaging in research provides a strong, solid resource that will enhance and expand the research program of any radiology department.

It is the responsibility of both the clinical and basic scientists in radiology departments to seek out and nurture the development of these students. This requires a radiology department research program that encourages multidisciplinary interaction and an active program to inform both medical and basic science graduate students of the opportunities that exist. This responsibility has been made much easier since radiology department programs in NMR and PET have heavily incorporated basic scientists in their work. Basic scientists in radiology departments must develop grant funding mechanisms and basic science department cross-appointments in order to ensure a steady flux of both pre- and postdoctoral basic scientists into imaging research projects. The future of medical imaging research depends heavily on the success of this approach.

2.11.6 Research Training Grants

Research training grants provide the most important resources for improving the academic training program in clinical departments. These NIH-sponsored grants provide salaries or stipends for clinicians or basic scientists engaged in research. The programs are administered through the various institutes with the NIH and include such agencies as the National Cancer Institute and the National Heart, Lung, and Blood Institute. This form of support is particularly important since the long-term success and stability of a research program in a clinical department requires implementing some form of research training component. Compared to other specialties, such as surgery and cardiology, radiology is far behind in providing research training in residency and fellowship programs. This situation is becoming more acute as the number of basic scientists in radiology departments is increasing because of the introduction of NMR/MRI, PET, and image analysis. Although it seems natural for these basic scientists to remain in radiology-based programs, it is obvious that they will migrate to non-radiology-based departments that actively support research and pre/postdoctoral programs.

The research training grants are granted to departments and are structured to provide the trainee with an environment conducive to research productivity. Grant application format varies from institute to institute within the NIH, but they usually require a description of the proposed program indicating faculty, administrative structure, facilities, and research opportunities, i.e., specific ongoing projects, resources, and information regarding trainee selection. The ability of many nonradiology clinical departments to provide residents and fellows with 1–2-year laboratory research rotations is because of the availability of these grants.

The research training program can be structured at both the pre- and postdoctoral level. Many departments have both of these. The predoctoral program requires a structured degree-awarding (MS or PhD) component and for this reason, most clinical departments do not comply, since degree-awarding capabilities usually require vigorous structured course work in the basic sciences. However, many clinical departments utilize existing degree-awarding programs from other basic science departments for course work requirements and provide the trainee with a thesis research project directly relating to radiology or medical imaging. This has been the primary mechanism for training medical physicists who in many cases eventually seek employment in diagnostic radiology departments. The importance of radiology departments becoming more involved in predoctoral training grant programs relates directly to the new breed of basic scientists who are applying their background to radiology-based technology. The availability of predoctoral students is essential for the research and academic development programs of basic scientists with primary or secondary academic appointments in radiology departments. The presence of basic scientists and graduate students in radiology departments is also very important in providing support, facilities, and a teaching source to clinicians. Basic scientists with primary academic appointments in clinical departments of radiology can act as preceptors or advisors for predoctoral students if the basic scientist obtains an academic cross-appointment in a degree-granting department.

The postdoctoral component of the research training program provides salary support for PhDs and MDs engaged in a 1–2-year postdoctoral fellowship. The same program could be used to provide radiologists with a 1–2-year block of time for research prior to or immediately after the clinical fellowship. A well structured postdoctoral research training program is the most logical and productive method to provide both the clinician and basic scientist with experience, techniques, and publications that will be essential for their career development and their ability to compete for extramural funding.

At the present time (1988) the National Cancer Institute alone supports 135 research training programs in the United States. Of the 135 programs, radiology departments have 24. These grants provide research training to radiologists and basic scientists in such areas as NMR imaging and spectroscopy, radiation biology, imaging physics, and diagnostic imaging. It is time all academic radiology departments consider these grants. More information regarding application requirements, format, and deadlines can be obtained by writing to the specific institute within the NIH or by contacting your institutional research office.

2.12 Animal Facilities

In planning most medical imaging research facilities, issues regarding the use and care of animals must be addressed. The institutional animal care personnel must be involved in all decisions involving the use of animals or planning of facilities where animals may be used. It is particularly important to consult with the veterinarian staff early in the laboratory or research program development planning process. One should not be overly conservative in estimating future animal needs. Particular attention must be given to the design of sterile surgical facilities, since specific requirements regarding air handling, lighting, wall and floor coverings, surgeons' scrub area, and postsurgery recovery area must be met if federal- or government-supported research is to be done.

Practical suggestions regarding the use of animals in imaging research facilities include:

1. Long-term Storage. Although short-term (1–8 h) animal holding areas are usually necessary near research imaging facilities, long-term animal housing should not be an integral part of the imaging laboratory facilities unless it is absolutely necessary. The ideal situation is to have animals housed in supervised facilities in the immediate vicinity of the laboratory. If long-term housing areas are to be incorporated into the research facility, special attention must be given to federal regulations regarding personnel training and room characteristics. Also in some institutions, investigators who desire to maintain their own long-term animal housing area may be required to hire their own personnel for these services.

2. Animal Preparation Room. The imaging rooms should not be used to initially prepare animals for study, i.e., anesthetizing animals or shaving them for surgical procedures. A 100–200 sq ft room immediately adjacent to the imaging room should be used for these purposes.

3. Survival Surgery. If survival surgery is to be performed, approved facilities must be employed. Such facilities must meet standard codes with respect to size, ventilation, construction, etc. The institutional animal resource division should be consulted regarding surgery suites.

4. Temporary Anesthesia Recovery Area. A small 100–200 sq ft room for animal surgery and anesthesia recovery should be provided adajcent to the imaging rooms.

5. Laundry. A small area (50–75 sq ft) should be designed for laundry purposes. This is particulary important if surgical procedures are anticipated.

The use of animals in research has always been a controversial issue. Within the past 10 years, organized groups have effectively lobbied at the local, state, and federal level to impose greater restrictions on the use of animals for research. In many respects, legislation resulting from pressure of these groups has corrected substandard practices relating to the use of animals in research. On the other hand, these same groups have influenced other legislative decisions that have severely limited animal research activities and jeopardized important medical research. Indications are that further restrictions will be enacted in the near future. Investigators must be more aware of the issues relating to the use of animals in research. More attention must be given to alternatives to animal research and to the proper use of appropriate animal models. Although it is beyond the scope of this chapter to discuss these issues at length, several recent publications are recommended to better understand the important issues relating to animal research and the appropriate choice of animal models. These publications include books entitled *Effective animal care and use committees,* edited by ORLANS et al. (1987), *Animal models in cardiovascular research* by GROSS (1985), and a recent publication entitled *Experimental surgery and physiology: Induced animal models of human disease,* edited by SWINDLE and ADAMS (1988).

References

Chiu RC-J, Mulder DS (1986) Roles for the surgical investigator. In: Troidl H, Spitzer WO, McPeek B, Mulder DS, McKneally MF (eds) Principles and practice of research: Strategies for surgical investigators. Springer, Berlin Heidelberg New York, p 20

Cruess RL (1986) Philosophy of surgical research. In: Troidl H, Spitzer WO, McPeek B, Mulder DS, McKneally MF (eds) Principles and practice of research: Strategies for surgical investigators. Springer, Berlin Heidelberg New York, p 18

Fischer HW, Morris TW (1987) The imaging research laboratory: The rationale for sharing of equipment. Invest Radiol 22: 71–72

Gross DR (1985) Animal models in cardiovascular research. Martinus Nyhoff Publ., Boston Oordrecht Lancaster

Hendee WR (1988) Critical review of article "Setting research priorities for the next decade." Invest Radiol 23: 563

Keats TE (1986) Faculty research productivity: The chairman's dilemma. Invest Radiol 21: 945

Maynard D (1986) A piece of the action. Invest Radiol 21: 944

McKneally MF (1986) Research challenges and solutions in the United States. In: Troidl H, Spitzer WO, McPeek B, Mulder DS, McKneally MF (eds) Principles and practice of research: Strategies for surgical investigators. Springer, Berlin Heidelberg New York, p 336

McKneally MF, Mulder DS, Nachemson A, Mosteller F, McPeek B (1986) Facilitating scholarship: Creating the atmosphere, setting, and teamwork for research. In: Troidl H, Spitzer WO, McPeek B, Mulder DS, McKneally MF (eds) Principles and practice of research: Strategies for surgical investigators. Springer, Berlin Heidelberg New York, p 36

Nelson JA (1983) Training a research radiologist or, where are the Young Turks? In Eric C. Milne (ed) Models and techniques in medical imaging research. Praeger, New York, p 3

Orlans FB, Simmonds RC, Dodds WJ (eds) (1987) Effective animal care and use committees. Scientists Center for Animal Welfare, Bethesda, Maryland

Putman CE (1986) A rare talent – The search for clinical scientists. Invest Radiol 21: 383

Selye H (1975) History, philosophy and sociology of science. In: From dream to discovery. Arno Press, New York

Swindle MM, Adams RJ (eds) (1988) Experimental surgery and physiology: Induced animal models of human disease. Williams & Wilkins, Baltimore

Taveras J (1986) Subspecialization in radiology. What approach should we take? Invest Radiol 21: 91

3 Image Analysis

HARRY L. LOATS and HENRY H. HOLCOMB

CONTENTS

3.1 Introduction 23
3.2 Background 24
3.3 Clinical Relevance 25
3.4 Advanced Quantitation Techniques 25
3.4.1 Morphology/Morphometry Analysis 26
3.4.2 Texture Analysis 28
3.5 Multi-image Registration and Analysis 29
3.5.1 Coordinate Reference Systems and Atlases 30
3.5.2 Image Registration 30
3.5.3 Image Overlay, Rescaling-Resampling 34
3.6 Statistical Pattern Recognition, Feature Recognition, and Signature Analysis 36
3.6.1 Tissue Segmentation 39
3.6.2 Corrections for Feature Contamination (CSF Pixel Deletion) 40
3.6.3 Hybrid Color Display 40
3.7 Three-dimensional Reconstruction, Display, and Measurements 41
3.7.1 Areas and Volumes by Thresholding 42
3.8 The Impact of Future Image Analysis Hardware Developments on Radiology 43
3.9 Prospects for the Future 44
References 44

3.1 Introduction

Image processing and analysis are having a significant impact on many scientific fields, especially biomedical research. Though digital imaging techniques are used in many radiology applications, particularly the acquisition, preprocessing, and display phases, insufficient use of their quantitative potential has been made. The majority of analyses are done by visual inspection and comparison of film images. The quantitative information which can be derived from other imaging modalities is largely ignored.

Radiologists routinely inspect black and white (B/W) images and focus on aberrant or altered anatomic features and/or textural abnormalities. Texture analysis relates to local variations in image properties which can subtly change the appearance of structural features in the image. The more general texture analysis techniques relate to gray level dependence. Subtle alterations in the structure of a lesion related to physiologic effects can manifest as changes in the distribution of contrast in individual lesions leading to perceivable localized textural differences in the image. For example, LEBIHAN et al. (1988) showed that variations in the diffusion/perfusion flow in individual volume elements (voxels) of magnetic resonance images cause differential signal attenuation. In the case of tumor lesions this results in variations in the texture of the image.

Radiologists employ a memory-oriented data base which they compare with each image or with previous images from the same patient. Nonquantitative but powerful visual heuristic pattern recognition rules are employed. However, it has proven to be very difficult to transfer and reproduce these algorithms in the computer. Recent advances in artificial intelligence are steadily improving this deficit.

Even for imaging modalities that are acquired in a digital format, direct inspection of films of the digital image remains the gold standard. The transformation of B/W images to color-scales is not universally recognized as being useful, due in part to the large time "investment" in rebuilding the radiologist's data base required to analyze color images.

The emphasis on display and visual perception is one of the key reasons why digital image archiving systems, termed "picture archiving and communication systems" (PACs), have not reached their potential except in larger installations where the economies related to image storage and transmission are sufficient for justification of the generally large costs. The main test is whether the digital display can equal the quality, contrast, and resolution of the

HARRY L. LOATS, B.S, M.S, M.S, Loats Associates, Inc., 1004 Littlestown Pike Suite G, Westminster, MD 21157, USA, and Research Associate in Oncology, Department of Oncology, The Johns Hopkins University, School of Medicine, 600 North Wolfe Street, Baltimore, MD 21205, USA
HENRY H. HOLCOMB, M.D, Dept. of Radiology and Radiological Science, The Johns Hopkins University, School of Medicine, 600 North Wolfe Street, Baltimore, MD 21205, USA and University of Maryland Psychiatric Research Center, Baltimore, MD 21205, USA

film. This requires display resolutions of 2048^2 pixels (picture elements). Cost comparisons are made against relatively inexpensive automated light-box technology.

Light-box technology permits rapid visual inspection of many B/W images with minimal time delay in a quasipanoramic mode. This technology cannot, however, transform images; the range of meaningful information is markedly reduced as a consequence.

However, the effective use of digital analysis as a radiology protocol need not replace visual inspection of films. Indeed the cost of high resolution digital display of the resolution of the light box is currently limiting the acceptance and utilization of the pure PACs. The role of digital analysis can enhance the visual techniques in isolating and quantifying the features in the images, particularly for features which are not directly visible.

Image processing techniques are employed in different degrees in image preprocessing, restoration, and display, but are not routinely under the interactive control and guidance of the radiologist. Important quantitative morphologic measurements are relegated to manual measurement techniques. Image processing and analysis techniques developed in other fields have not been transferred to radiology applications.

Surprisingly few of the procedures that are required to supplement conventional radiology protocols necessitate new techniques. What is required, however, is the emphasis on technology transfer of existing image analysis techniques from other scientific disciplines like space technology and the use of low-cost hardware currently being developed for the much larger general microcomputer market. For example, the development of feature identification and classification used to identify land resources from multispectral satellite imagery is directly applicable to multiecho magnetic resonance imaging (MRI) analysis of tumors. The computer algorithms developed by the National Aeronautics and Space Administration (NASA) are directly applicable and available from the NASA Technology Transfer program at little or no cost. The interpretation and analysis of sea-surface roughness patterns routinely accomplished by the National Oceanic and Atmospheric Administration have direct application to texture analysis in chest X-rays and for interpretation of ultrasound imagery.

The promise of digital radiology with its large potential improvement in objective image quantitation, lowered radiation dose, and film processing and archiving cost reductions is largely unfulfilled and has not made a significant impact on radiologic operations patient care. Recent developments in low-cost computer image analysis, coupled with its rapidly accelerating performance/cost ratio, will play a significant role in changing the way radiologists analyze images. This chapter discusses future developments in image processing and analysis; we expect them to have significant impact on radiology operations and positive impact on patient care.

3.2 Background

Most radiologists perform limited quantitative measurements on visually identified anatomic structures or anomalies. This analysis is performed on high resolution film images displayed on relatively inexpensive light-box viewers. For digital imaging modalities such as computer tomography (CT) or MRI, the radiologist works with low to medium resolution digital cathode ray tube displays. Various simple computer-assisted techniques are often incorporated to measure changes in identified lesions or other structural features.

Studies have shown that radiologists rapidly scan the total image and then fix on a limited number of critical foci for short time periods. Analysis consists of visual identification and review of suspect regions. The analysis of diagnostic images has proved to be very difficult. LODWICK (1983), reporting on a study involving a large number of image classes, indicated that error rates in the detection of disease were on the order of 20%, resulting in diagnostic errors of between 10% and 15%. Studies with enhanced spatial resolution and contrast did not significantly improve these numbers since they were mostly related to pattern recognition of diseased tissue.

KUNDEL and NODINE (1987), reporting on studies at the Pendergrass Radiology Laboratory of the University of Pennsylvania, indicated that radiologists make errors in detecting lung cancers about 30% of the time. Their study focused on the effect of the mode of observation on error type. The radiologist typically examines an image in two steps. The first step provides a global impression of the image. In the second phase, the radiologist examines certain areas of the film in more detail to confirm the information obtained in the global phase. Neither of these phases lasts for extended periods of time. They indicate that about 10% of the errors are related to lack of adequate coverage. Their work showed that examinations of film relate to clusters of fixation, each of which affects the ultimate decision. They concluded that it took approximately 18 such clusters to cover the entire film. Review of the sites on the film showing the most viewing activity on the first pass often leads to decision changes.

Quantification of individual anatomic structures is accomplished by identifying "regions of interest" (ROIs) and obtaining the average value of raw or calibrated units within the region. These regions are manually generated by tracing the apparent border of the structure directly on the images. The spatial positions and characteristics of these ROIs are generally not saved for future reference, thus limiting the ability for post facto analysis and the development of signature data bases. A signature is an explicit set of morphologic, texture, and single or multiple mode intensities uniquely related to specific anatomic or target features such as tumors. Signature data banks, when developed and verified, can be used to automatically classify various types of radiology images.

The manual approach limits the precision and reproducibility of measurements because of four factors. First, structural images like X-ray, CT, and MRI have significant obscuring artifacts and distortions. Second, features defined in structural images by nonpathologic textural characteristics have low relative contrast. Their boundaries are difficult to define, if they exist at all. Third, in functional images like positron emission tomography (PET) and single photon emission computed tomography (SPECT), with relatively poor spatial resolution (5 mm for the best PET scanner; 10–15 mm for typical SPECT systems), the delineation of a structure's edge is difficult and often misleading due to functional abnormalities and partial volume effects. Fourth, functional images such as ^{18}F-deoxyglucose PET metabolic maps only show structures whose physiologic or biochemical functioning is high enough to be distinguished from nonfunctioning or "background" areas.

Virtually all of today's image processing computer systems offer general image processing quantitation routines, including image arithmetic, moderate edge detection, and various utilities that have applicability to ROI analysis. These techniques are slowly finding their way into radiology. Their rapid integration is slowed by the lack of stand-alone workstations and the lack of radiology-specific software for existing high performance imaging workstations.

3.3 Clinical Relevance

The clinical relevance of image analysis is illustrated with four clinical problems that are best addressed with advanced, microcomputer-based, image analysis strategies: atrophy measurement, localization for stereotaxic surgery, PET/MRI image registration for tumor characterization, and diagnostic group assignment. Each of these techniques requires digital images. Most applications require some degree of cross-image registration and redirected sampling.

In the examples related to atrophy, the primary inputs come from morphology measurements and edge enhancement and detection. Stereotaxic applications require registration with external fiducial controls and then superposition of images on a feature-identified image. External atlases may also serve as templates. For the multimodal image applications, in addition to registration, careful consideration must also be given to image data resampling to accommodate the several levels of resolution between the various imaging modalities. For the functional images the impact of digital image processing is immediately evident in the requirement to transform the raw data into physically or biologically relevant information.

As clinical disease or experimental-related digital annotated group image data sets become available and accessible, it will become possible to generate composite normal and case-related image data sets. These will provide the capability to generate "significance images" for functional imaging modalities.

3.4 Advanced Quantitation Techniques

The capacity to use quantitative image processing is currently conditioned by the preponderance of visual inspection protocols and therefore has been restricted to fixed and limited routines such as simple thresholding, contrast enhancement, and fixed convolution filters. The advanced imaging workstations which are slowly being introduced into radiology environments concentrate mainly on impressive but nonquantitative display features, and offer only limited quantitation capability.

Advanced quantitation techniques can be divided into two broad categories: texture and morphology. Texture analysis and discrimination play a vital role in diagnostic imaging and offer great potential for digital image analysis. Radiologists utilize texture to discriminate subtle disease features. Current visual techniques do not extract quantitative and reproducible texture measures. Morphology theory, which came out of the work done on cellular automata in the late 1960s, analyzes images in terms of shapes and size. These techniques employ elementary morphologic patterns called structuring elements. Morphology theory and currently evolving computer firmware models of these techniques provide automated image segmentation which is important for area and volume measurement of structures and for texture-based pattern recognition (Bartoo et al. 1988).

Cortical atrophy measurements illustrate the utility of advanced quantitation. Cortical atrophy is characteristic of normal aging but is often accelerated in several pathologic conditions, including Alzheimer's disease, parkinsonism, schizophrenia, and multi-infarct dementia. MRI permits highly accurate separation of cerebrospinal fluid from brain tissue. Gray/white tissue partitioning is also enhanced through this technique. Computerized image analysis greatly facilitates quantitative volumetric determinations of sulci, ventricles, the total brain, total cranial capacity, gray tissue, and white tissue.

A new method of characterizing atrophy is through cortical shape. As sulci enlarge the cortical surface becomes more "complex." This means that simple shapes such as ellipses and circles no longer adequately characterize its elaborate invaginations.

Atrophy in one diagnostic group (e.g., young schizophrenic patients) is likely to have significantly different meaning than that for another group (elderly Alzheimer patients). By accurately measuring variations in tissue texture, density, and shape, radiologic consultants are more likely to provide clinically relevant judgments.

3.4.1 Morphology/Morphometry Analysis

Morphology techniques are used to analyze images in terms of shapes and sizes using predefined patterns called structuring elements. The result of morphologic processing is to produce binary type images. These images replace the gray scale values present in the original images with a binary pattern of logical ones and zeros in which the ones represent membership in a designated class and the zeros indicate nonmembership. Morphology assessment utilizes alterations in the gray scale or calibrated values of image pixel elements based on various size local neighborhoods.

Morphology transformation is analogous to discrete convolution kernels used to perform simple global processes like image smoothing, etc. The major difference is that where convolution uses mainly addition and multiplication operators, morphology transformations use the basic logic operators, e.g., union (OR), intersection (AND), difference (XOR), and complement. These operators are supplemented by the transformation operators – rotation, translation, and reflection.

In addition to the simple operators, morphologic operations also include the compound operators of dilation and erosion which are used to conformally expand or contract shapes within the image. Erosion is performed by moving the specifically shaped structuring element over the object in the scene to produce a new object containing all points for which the structuring elements fit within the original object. This is important in eliminating small and sometimes false bridges between separate objects in the scene preparatory to automated classification. Dilation is the reverse of the erosion process.

Morphologic techniques are very useful in anatomic feature identification pattern matching procedures which lead to automated image segmentation. An important aspect of these morphologic operators is that they are relatively easy to incorporate into inexpensive real-time image processing firmware. The use of morphologic processes can directly modify the measurement of areas, volumes, and shapes related to pathologic conditions.

In addition to the direct measurements of area and length, it is often important to introduce objective analysis techniques of anatomic features. Quantitative shape analysis permits the systematic analysis of structural changes in temporal image sequences.

The shape of an anatomic feature can be described by:

$$R(\Theta) = R_o + \sum_{n=1}^{\infty} R_n \mathrm{COS}(n\,\Theta - \Phi_n) \qquad (1)$$

This function decomposes the aggregate shape into contribution of primary shape elements. Figure 1 illustrates the Fourier shape decomposition technique and the primary shapes which are used to generate the total shape.

The first coefficient in the series, R_o, is equivalent to the average radius of the feature about its centroid, i.e., a centered circle having an area equal to total area of the feature area. The remainder of the coefficients, termed harmonic amplitudes, R_n, de-

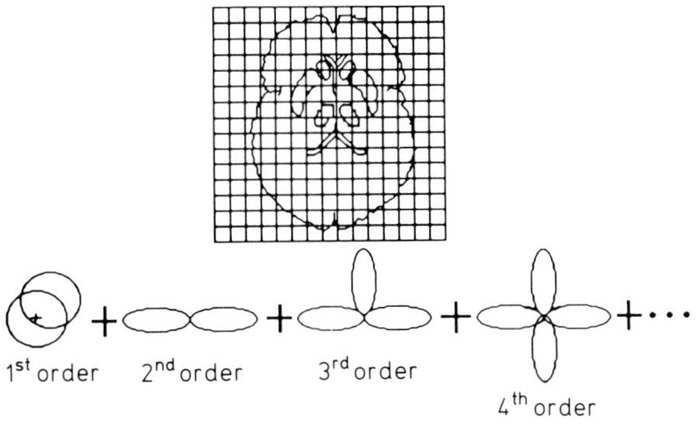

Fig. 1. Fourier shape decomposition determines the contribution of simple shapes to those that are more complex. Shape analysis of the third ventricle will indicate a higher contribution from the third order harmonic component than would an analysis of the caudate nucleus, which is predominantly first and second order. Pathologic processes such as edema, tumor, and cell death are likely to have different effects on feature shape

fine the contribution of successively more complex elementary shape features. For example, the first harmonic amplitude, R_1, describes the contribution of an offset circle, the second, R_2, that of a figure eight, the third, R_3, that of a trefoil or three-lobed figure, etc. The R coefficients are computed based on a polar coordinate decomposition of the boundary of the anatomic feature.

Figure 2 shows the application of the Fourier shape decomposition technique for some simple shapes and plots the magnitude of the harmonic amplitudes. The harmonic amplitudes are plotted versus normalized components which represent the contribution from the characteristic shapes defined in Fig. 1. Note that this type of Fourier shape decomposition is analogous to the more frequently used Fourier technique which decomposes gray scale images into spatial frequency components.

A circular or oval shape yields a series expansion whose form is dominated by the first and second order harmonics while pyramidal shapes yield a series expansion which exhibits a strong contribution from the third order (three-lobed) harmonic term. By extension, the spectra of the harmonic amplitude can be used to describe and quantitate complex biologic shapes such as the ventricles or the sulci for age – or disease – related studies.

The angles, Φ_n, are the phase angles related to each harmonic and are measures of the rotational orientation of the various contributing harmonic shapes. Thus, the angles, Φ_n, can serve as shape-specific measures of orientation. The phase angle of the 2nd harmonic can be used most often to define general orientation.

The Fourier technique provides a capability to analyze the shapes of complex structures such as the entire cortical surface or a single lateral ventricle. The procedure is described as follows.

The cortical surface or ventricular perimeter is identified using an automatic boundary finding routine. The polar coordinates of these boundaries

Fig. 2. Harmonic amplitudes plotted against normalized components reveal the contribution of various simple shapes to those more geometrically complex. The increasing contribution of higher order components suggests that measurements of cortical surface shape may vary with severity of atrophy or developmental arrest

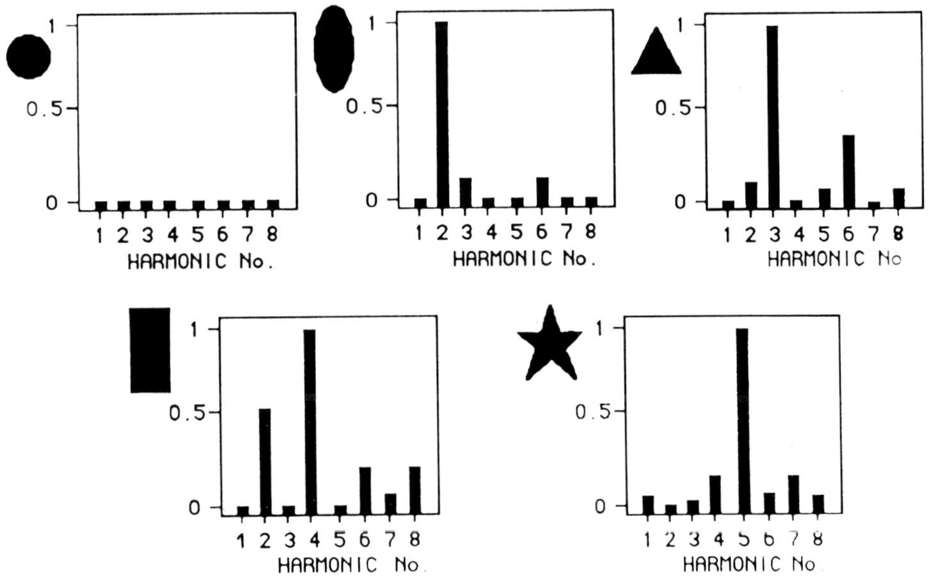

are calculated. The harmonic amplitudes and phase angles that describe that shape are computed.

Complex, multilobed structures are described by higher level harmonic terms than those that are relatively smooth, ovoid, or ellipsoid. The more distant and discontinuous the arms or lobes of the shape, the higher the phase angles will be that describe the relationships of those lobes. This suggests that a deeply invaginated, atrophic cortical surface will be best described (high amplitudes) by high order harmonic terms. This is illustrated by comparing the shape harmonics of two cortical surfaces (Fig. 3).

Shape analysis of ventricles is likely to indicate how these spaces physically respond to tissue loss. This is demonstrated in the comparison of two ventricles below. The enlarged ventricle has lost the sharp turns and acute angles characteristic of the normal ventricle. Figure 4 illustrates ventricular shape comparison.

Detection of abnormalitites in shape, volume, activity, or location similarly require a valid normative data base. It is, however, the "significance" of the change or abnormality that requires integration of clinical information and image comparison measurements. Given that a real change, or abnormal single measurement, in ventricular volume has been verified, the "clinical relevance" of that change can only be assessed through multivariate pattern assessment.

Fig. 3. MR images, 3 mm thick, obtained from a normal 52-year-old male volunteer, on the *left*, and a 50-year-old woman suffering from Alzheimer's disease, on the *right*, indicate marked differences in cortical surface morphology. A comparison of serial planes taken from these two subjects reveals that the eighth harmonic is significantly greater in the patient with Alzheimer's disease

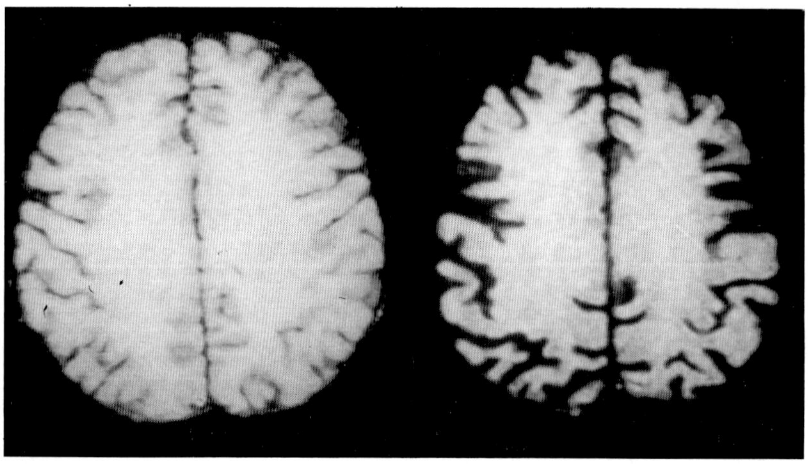

Ventricular changes are likely to have dramatically different implications in different clinical populations. Elderly patients are likely to have different ventricular volume changes than are children. Metabolic changes in the globus pallidus have a different significance in a patient with a history of psychosis than a patient with head trauma.

Quantitative image comparison requires:

1. Stereotaxic transformation and scaling. The image must represent the same proportional position in geometric space.
2. Systematic measurements of relevant structures and identification of abnormal features.
3. Multivariate feature comparisons between the case and its reference set.
4. Assignment of probabilities and weights to the feature comparisons.

3.4.2 Texture Analysis

Texture is the pattern of gray scale values which constitute the image. Local changes in the image texture for a given object or region within the image are indicative of important but oftimes subtle physiologic changes and are often the source of a radiologist's identification of an image anomaly or suspect region. Texture measures define invariant correlates of the global or local smoothness/roughness of the image. Since textures often vary locally and are not uniformly defined over distinct anatomically defined regions, visual analysis of their location, extent, and strength is difficult.

Radiologists often use various texture descriptors such as "spotted," "spongy," "honeycombed," or "fluffy" to describe the appearance of suspect features in the image. These are generally "fuzzy" de-

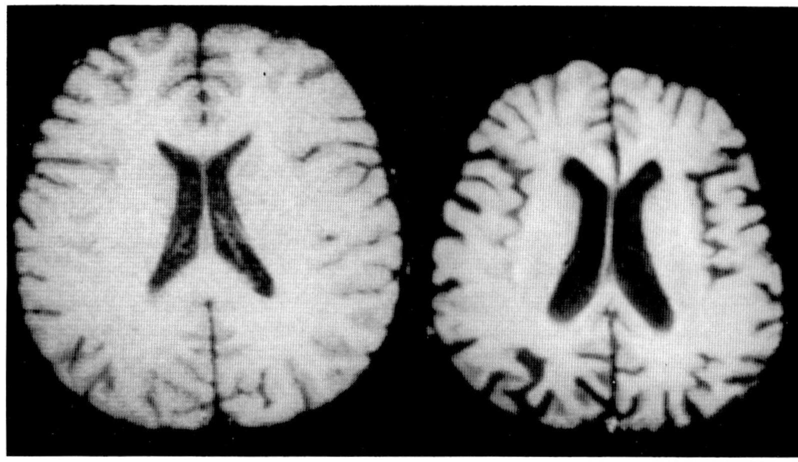

Fig. 4. Shape analysis of ventricles, using MR images, demonstrates the loss of sharp angles in the patient with Alzheimer's disease. By combining area, perimeter, and centroid measurements with shape analysis, a more complete characterization of the pathologic process is provided

scriptors (KANDEL 1986) and are not easily translated into objective measures. Computer digital procedures, however, can easily determine primary and second order texture measures such as energy, entropy, correlation, and local homogeneity from the gray level dependencies.

Exploratory studies over the past several years (NGUYEN and QUINQUETON 1982; PICTIKAINEN and ROSENFELD 1982; PEARCE 1987) have indicated that the computer procedures often define areas of altered texture better than human observers. The major problem with completely automated texture classification is related to which decision is appropriate. However, the use of hybrid techniques where the computer is used to classify an image based on texture, jointly used with atlas - or human - guided anatomic feature identification, would significantly improve disease identification based upon texture measures. The potential for earlier identification of subtle effects could have a beneficial effect on patient care and enhance the utility of radiology diagnostics.

3.5 Multi-image Registration and Analysis

Stereotaxic neurosurgeons rely heavily on atlas images for guidance. These "average brains" do not match an individual patient's brain in size or shape. For example, when a neurosurgeon prepares to lesion the nucleus ventralis lateralis in a young patient with unilateral parkinsonian tremor, he must rely extensively on the atlases of SCHALTENBRAND and WAHREN (1977), SCHNITZLEIN and MURTAGH (1985), MATSUI and HIRANO (1978), or TALAIRACH et al. (1967). This reliance on the atlas versus the individual used as his or her own atlas presents several problems. The difficulty in registering the coordinates of the atlas accurately with the "matching" coordinates of the patient represents a considerable handicap to the neurosurgeon which can be minimized by using matched images.

Image overlay and registration using the patient's own structural images like MRI or CT with their high resolution, permit the surgeon to have much improved accuracy and confidence. These techniques in conjunction with three-axis stereotaxic and/or three-dimensional display further increase the utility of image analysis.

Stereotaxic coordinate transformation from one image set to another has several problems, including size and shape incompatibilities. Conformal mapping permits the surgeon, with radiologic intervention, to find loci in his patient that correspond with specific points in the atlas. This guided map distortion is facilitated by MRI, which readily provides three-dimensional, high contrast images. The radiologist obtains coronal, sagittal, and horizontal MR images. Similar images, proportionally matched (% distance from the midline to cortex edge, intercommissural axis to cortical vertex edge distance, and intercommissure midpoint), from the patient and atlas are rescaled to provide similar sizes (the atlas is rescaled to match the patient's MRI set). Once corresponding points have been chosen to map the atlas onto the patient's image set, algorithms developed from the field of conformal mapping (complex analysis) provide the rules of transformation (Ratib et al. 1988).

Once mapping (rescaling/reshaping) has occurred the neurosurgeon and neuroradiologist can accurately specify the precise coordinates in the patient that correspond to a locus in the atlas. Validation of this method depends on physiologic studies: electrical stimulations, electrophysiologic recording, and quantitative behavioral measurements (tremor, rigidity, bradykinesia).

High resolution structural images can be used to spatially interpret lower resolution functional images. This is particularly important in the interpretation of functional (e.g., metabolic) PET images which have relatively low resolution and are also strongly affected by partial volume effects. Important anatomic structures in the brain can be analyzed from registered CT and MRI images. Computer-assisted techniques for combining images from multiple imaging modalities are currently in development, and have not been adapted for general use in clinical environments.

3.5.1 Coordinate Reference Systems and Atlases

Images can be registered to appropriate coordinate systems and atlases. For example, various researchers have proposed using reference atlases and a reference coordinate system to identify structures in the brain. This approach is particularly important for relating functional images, such as PET, with relatively low spatial and feature resolution to higher resolution structural images, e.g., MRI and CT. For brain imaging, this approach makes the assumption that a given subject's brain anatomy matches either the atlas or the coordinate references. While this is not always achievable, the use of valid coordinate systems for post facto interpretation is an important aspect of precise quantitation and will become more prevalent. This technique gives rise to two important clinically relevant features: (1) the production of composite "normals" to which disease characteristics can be statistically compared and (2) the development of anatomic libraries of normal and disease state.

Using image feature comparison profiles, clinical and research evaluations concerning the "significance" of various comparisons can be produced. "Significance" estimates are dependent on group characteristics. For example, in order to predict the "significance" of a change in structure volume or metabolic activity between measurements at two or more time points, one must estimate the "normal" or "central" group's observed change on a similar time interval. Volumetric changes in head trauma patients and metabolic changes in stroke, tumor, dementia, or psychosis are relevant examples.

Digitized cross-sectional atlases of the head and body are used and displayed (with structure identification) along with the primary images. Standard ROI templates will be available which match with images from reference atlases. A significant benefit of this approach is to provide a capability to use the high anatomic resolution of MRI imaging to provide registered anatomic structure ROI templates for sampling. This will provide a significant increase in the precision and accuracy of quantitation. Careful attention to geometric correction of the structural (MRI) image would be required.

3.5.2 Image Registration

Registration of images from different acquisition modalities is accomplished by digitally matching the position of externally located fiducials in each imaging modality. These fiducials comprise small-bore tubes filled with appropriate markers: Panopaque or Renografin for CT, gadolinium or vegetable oil for MRI, and a suitable radionuclide (e.g., Tc-99m for SPECT; F-18 for PET) for ECT.

Registration of human brain images has been accomplished between PET and MRI using a head mask specifically tailored for each patient, with small fiducial tubes located on the periphery (Fig. 5). Using either sagittal scout images from MRI or lateral skull films, the glabella-inion (GI) line is identified from visible bony landmarks on the skull. The bicommissural line is identified on the MRI or estimated on the lateral skull film. This axis (Fig. 6) provides a normalized coordinate geometry for later statistical correlation.

When acquiring MRI images the fiducial tubes are filled with an appropriate marker such as vegetable oil which is clearly visible in both T_1 and T_2 images (Fig. 7). The registration technique has been applied to PET/CT/MRI and histologic sections to sample and correlate images related to implanted animal tumors (Fig. 8). This technique improves image analysis even if registration is not available, due to repeated sampling and image enhancement procedures. Figures 9 through 11 show the location of fiducials on typical MRI and CT images.

The orientation and geometric relationship of the functional image data to the MRI/CT fiducials can also be defined relative to a line marked on a fixed

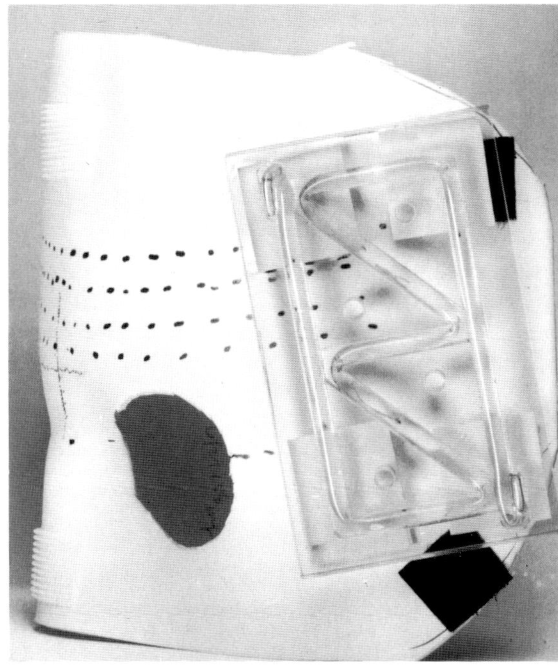

Fig. 5. When multiple imaging modes or multiple image sets are anticipated, a thermoplastic face mask is individually fitted to conform optimally to the person's face. Particular attention is given to the bony orbit to assure a tight apposition of the mask to this part of the head. Using double-sided adhesive squares, we then attach the acrylic registration systems to each side of the mask. The thin tubing embedded in the acrylic block is filled with vegetable oil, a substance easily captured with T_1 and T_2 MR imaging protocols (see Fig. 7). When performing PET, we can fill the tubing with ^{18}FDG and water. The unique geometry of the registration system readily permits identification of the image plane's intersection with the mask. Having identified that plane on the mask, we then inscribe it with an indelible felt tip marker. That line is subsequently used to align the PET detector system with the subject's head

head restraint, which is aligned by existing laser orientation system. Software utilities are used to register the fiducials and to establish a stereotaxic coordinate reference system required for reproducible image data bases. Insertion of three-dimensional coordinates follows the rules generally described by Fox et al. (1985). Holcomb et al. (1988a) have adapted this scheme for MRI using the following procedures:

1. Sagittal and horizontal "scout" images are initially acquired to provide orthogonal reference overlays. In Figure 12 are sagittal views with serial transaxial images; also shown is a horizontal image with serial sagittal placement lines. These scout films and another image (Fig. 13) indicate the relative locations of all planes, their distances from one another, and key bony landmarks.
2. From the sagittal view, obtained in the midline plane, anterior and posterior commissure reference points are located (Figs. 6 and 14).
3. The x, y, z coordinate origin (0) is found by locating it in the midpoint of the AC-PC axis (y and z axes), and in the midline (x axis). The midpoint of the AC-PC line constitutes the z axis 0 reference (Fig. 15).
4. Once the x, y, z origin has been established the only additional information required is the slice thickness and interslice gap for the complete transformation of all pixels to their respective sterotaxic coordinates. Measurement of the image plane angle is made on the sagittal scout image.
5. This method permits measurement standardization with respect to brain location. It is, for example, useful to know where the caudate's center of mass is located three-dimensionally in a patient with Huntington's disease. By knowing a

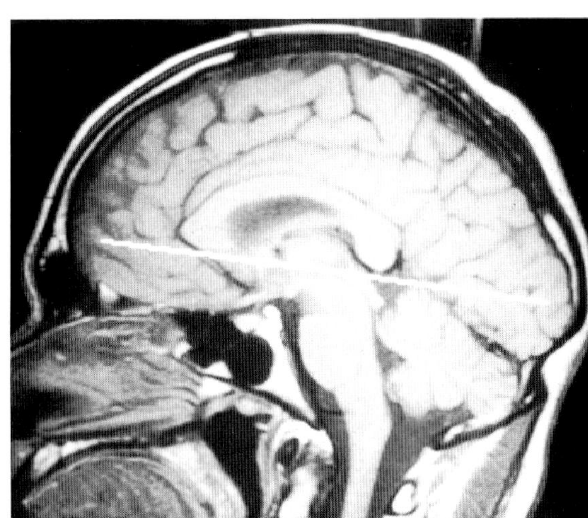

Fig. 6. Systematic sampling and analysis of PET, MRI, and SPECT brain images require a method for locating each region in three-dimensional space. By using the midpoint of the AC-PC distance, in the midsagittal plane, as the zero point in an x, y, z coordinate system, we are able to generate a normalized coordinate geometry; each measurement will be characterized by its location in this system

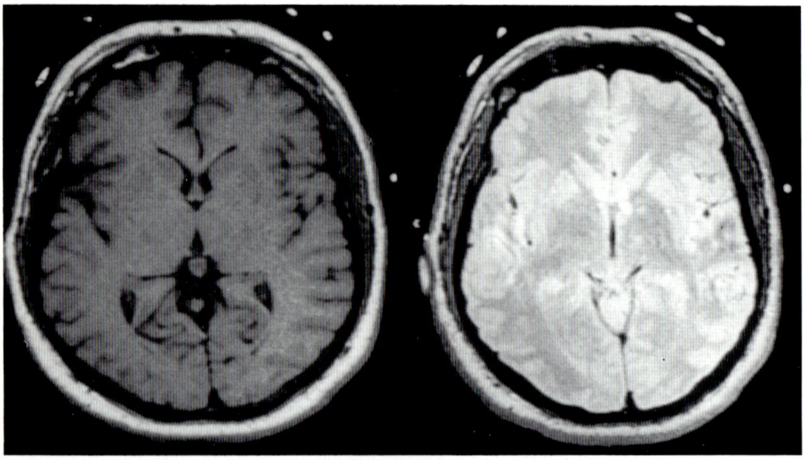

7

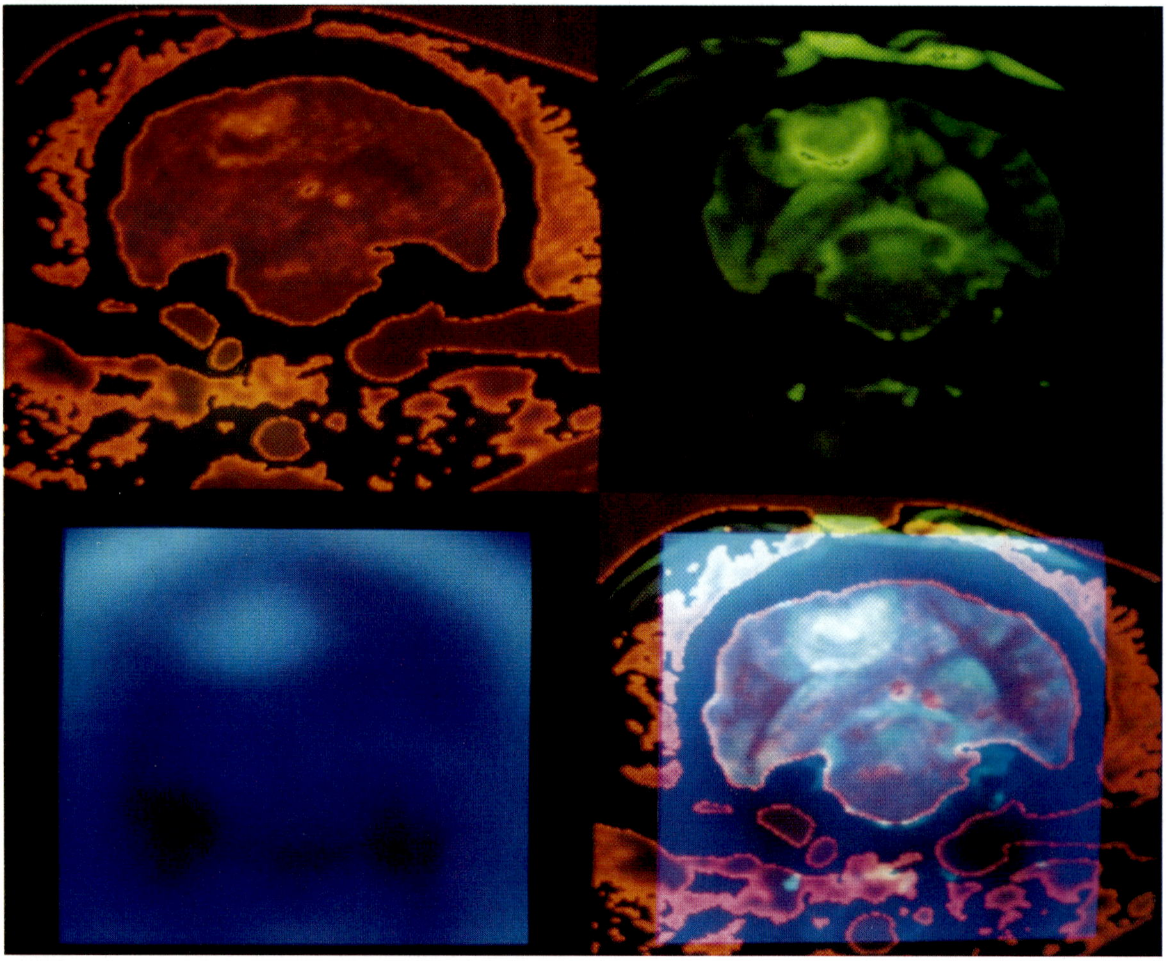

8

Fig. 7. Transaxial T_1 *(left)* and T_2 *(right)* MR images illustrate the use of a unique, mask-based reference system. Each point around the perimeter of the images is a 3 mm thick cross-section of a plastic tube containing vegetable oil. These particular images were acquired from a subject wearing a mask reference system different from that illustrated in Fig. 5

Fig. 8. Three registered images of an implanted canine glioblastoma are shown in this panel. *Top left:* XCT; *top right:* MRI; *bottom left:* [^{11}C]thymidine PET (courtesy of the Johns Hopkins PET Research Facility); *bottom right:* composite registered overlay image of the three principal images. Registration and superimposition of multimodal images permit parametric characterization of a tissue's biology. In this case, the registration system was implanted to provide exact localization of the tumor

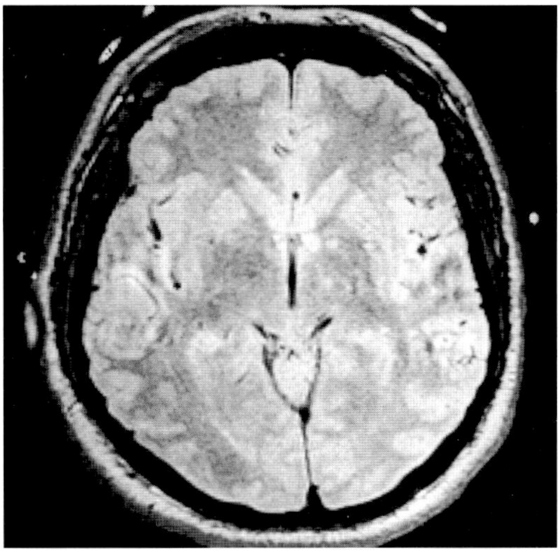

9

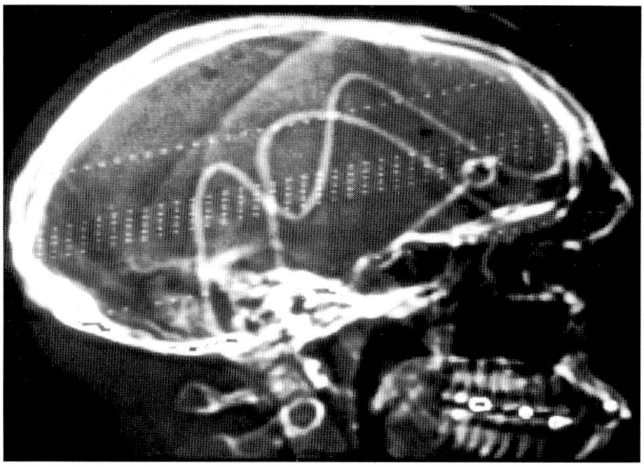

10

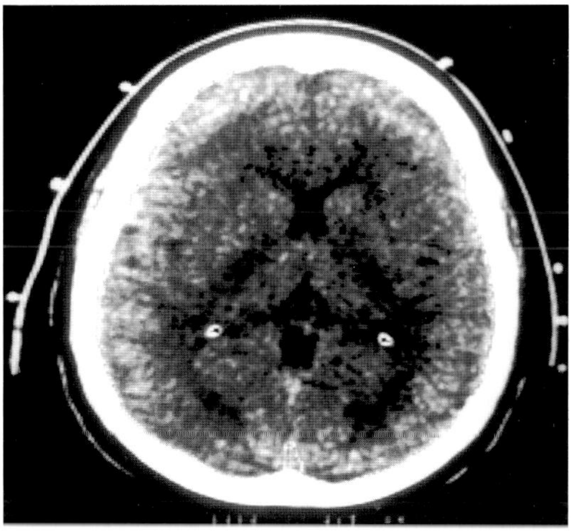

11

Fig. 9. Enlarged illustration of fiducial system relative to an MR image

Fig. 10. X-ray computer-assisted tomography image showing a system of reference tubes filled with a radiopaque substance

Fig. 11. X-ray tomogram illustrating a reference tube system taped to a mask. Each image plane will capture a unique geometry of points similar to those shown in Fig. 10

Fig. 12. Midsagittal MR images usually permit the investigator to directly identify the anterior and posterior commissures. Having determined the midpoint of the AC-PC segment, in the midsagittal plane, the zero x, y, z coordinate point is established. The location of all planes captured is then known absolutely. *Left*, an MR scout image showing the location of all 3-mm images relative to one another. *Right*, a horizontal scout image indicating the relative positions of sagittal images

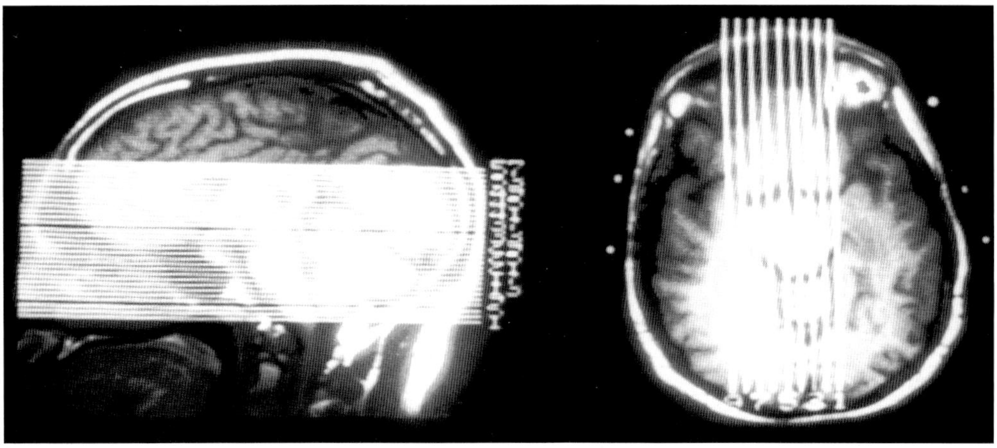

12

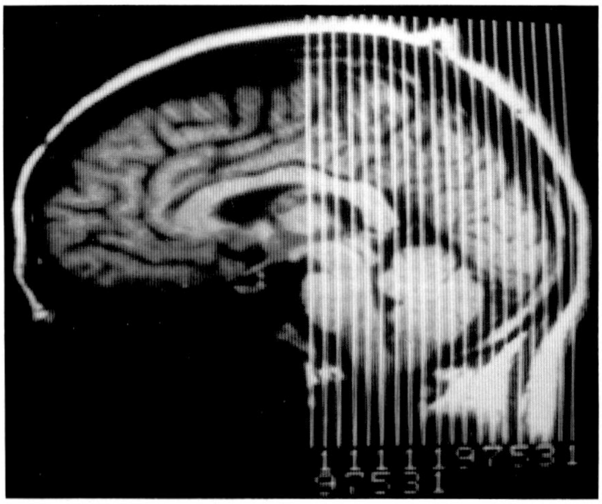

Fig. 13. Coronal MR images, displayed on this sagittal scout, are also amenable to triaxial stereotaxic geometry. In this case one must know the angle of the image relative to the AC-PC axis

structure's location, volume, shape, and gray-white ratio, the investigator gains important knowledge regarding pathological and normal processes.

For example, in an ongoing research application, stained histologic and autoradiographic serial sections were registered by alignment with fiducials in a fixed geometric relationship with the MRI/CT registration tubes for animal imaging (Fig. 16). The ability to match and register images will also be extremely important in stereotaxic surgery.

Significant benefits will also accrue in the use of image matching and ROI templating features. For example, CT or MRI images entered via video digitization or magnetic tape are scaled and registered to the size and location of the corresponding functional nuclear medicine images. ROIs would then be generated either automatically or under operator control on the anatomic images and automatically "redirected" to the registered functional images. Automated storage of the ROI templates would allow them to be superimposed on subsequent studies.

Brain tumors exhibit marked tissue heterogeneity. The tissue characteristics of various tumor regions are particularly important to the neuro-oncologist. Neither MR nor XCT can reliably differentiate between edematous tissue, necrotic tissue, and aggressive tumor. Each of these "compartments" has unique metabolic characteristics. Glucose and amino acid metabolism will both exhibit different profiles in these three regions. By registering the MR and PET images the radiologist is in a position to characterize the metabolic behavior of various brain regions emitting distinctive MR signals. This alignment is accomplished by using the thermoplastic mask coupled with a rigid set of tubes containing vegetable oil (easily detected on MRI). Using the registered image sets, the radiologist/image analyst resamples MR images using major and minor axes of the image, to conform to the companion PET image (Figs. 17–19). Once companion images have been connected, pixel-for-pixel, the analyst specifies ROIs on the MR or PET image set and, through redirected sampling, obtains metabolic or MR information from corresponding spatial areas.

Images presented in Fig. 20 illustrate registered MR and PET data from a patient with a brain tumor. These data permit one to easily assess the metabolic and, by inference, pathologic characteristics of regions emitting different MR signals. By competitively blocking transport of [^{11}C]methionine into the tumor with phenylalanine administered prior to the second PET study, we have provided additional metabolic information regarding the integrity of amino acid transport in these various compartments (O'Tuama et al. 1988).

This combination, MRI/PET with or without perturbation, is uniquely suited for the clinician who wants to assess the effects of radiation or antineoplastic treatment. Serial studies of this kind will permit more rational dosing of potentially harmful agents such as ionizing radiation and neurotoxic antitumor agents.

3.5.3 Image Overlay, Rescaling-Resampling

Image registration generally requires some form of multi-image overlay and often requires that the images be rescaled. Rescaling can also require digital resampling. Image overlay is then accomplished either by analog or digital techniques.

A very rapid and inexpensive method for registering images involves the use of an intermediate video image. The analog technique involves electronic superimposition of the video signals using film image as the base. The digital technique involves computer-related movement of images located in different regions of the display memory.

Both techniques have been successfully demonstrated. Video signal mixing provides a rapid means of superimposing film products such as a receptor autoradiograph directly onto the graphic display of PET images. This feature is useful for rapid direct

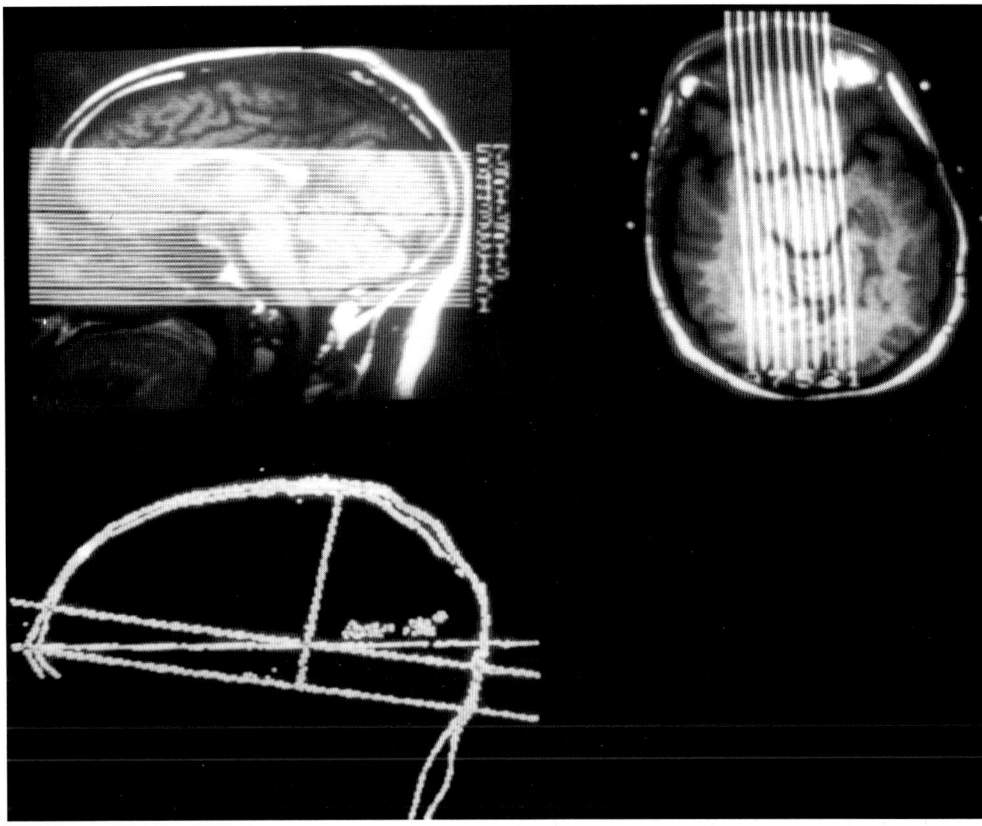

14

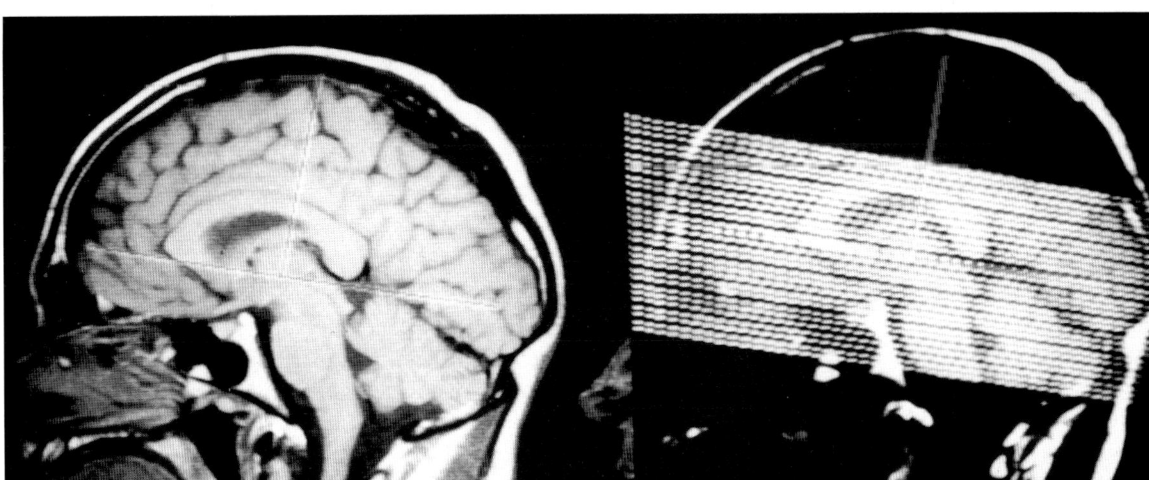

15

Fig. 14. If the anterior and posterior commissures cannot be located reliably on the sagittal image, the axis passing through those points can be estimated by locating a plane parallel to the GI line, offset by 20% of the perpendicular distance from the GI line to the vertex. *Top left:* Transaxial MR images parallel to the AC-PC axis. The 0 point for the y (anteroposterior) and z (dorsoventral) axes is located midway between the anterior and posterior commissures. *Top right:* Sagittal MR images orthogonal to a transaxial scout image. The midsagittal plane defines the 0 point in the x (mediolateral) axis. *Bottom:* Because images are frequently acquired oblique to the AC-PC plane, it is necessary to determine pixel location using an angle correction calculation. This is easily done once the angle is determined either from the MR monitor or the film image

Fig. 15. Normalized geometry is generated by expressing location as a percentage of the distance from the triaxial origin to the lateral border the cortical surface (x axis), to the frontal cortical surface (y axis), and to the cortical vertex (z axis). *Left:* The anteroposterior line segment is the AC-PC, or y axis, and the line perpendicular to it is the z axis. *Right:* The image set is parallel to the AC-PC plane. This eliminates the need for angle correction

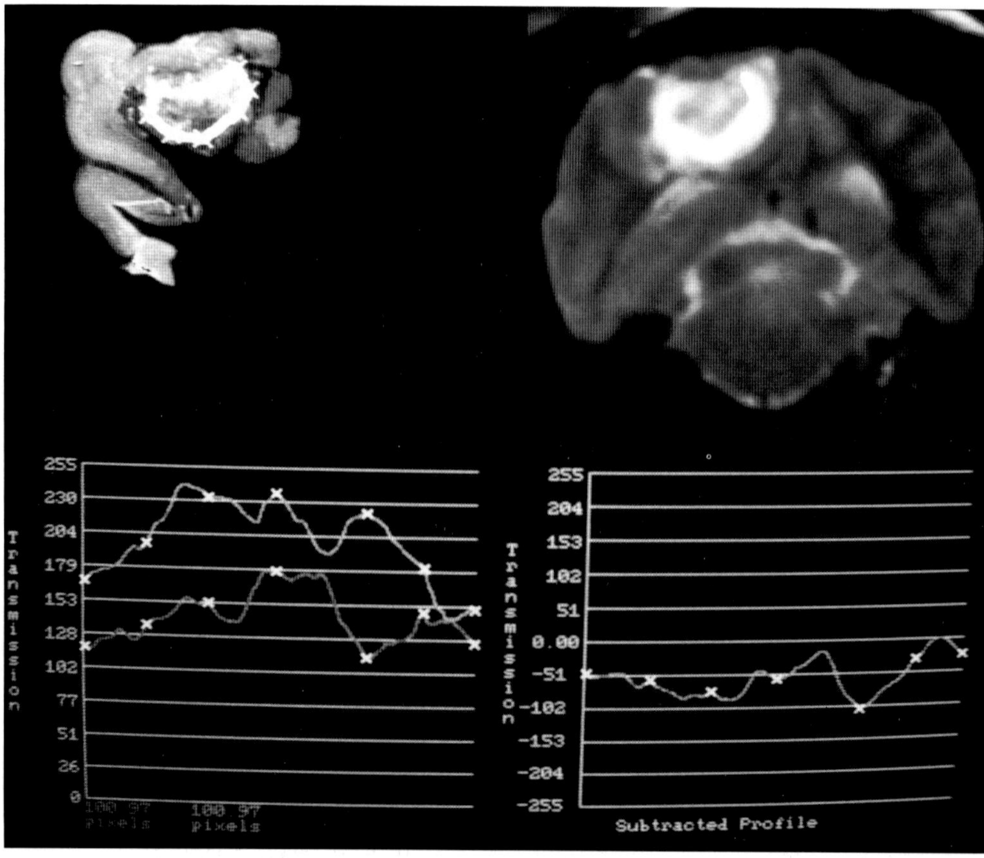

Fig. 16. Registration of a stained histologic section *(left)* and an MR image *(right)* of the same region permits systematic biochemical and morphologic correlation between tissue and image. This provides a rational approach for image interpretation

qualitative visual alignment and comparison of features of interest.

Rescaling of images is required to accommodate the different resolutions of the various imaging modalities. Rescaling will be accomplished for film images by anamorphically stretching the film images onto predigitized base images and stretching in the x, y dimensions to fit. Anamorphic transformations can be accomplished by automatically altering the x and y scan characteristics of the video scanner for film images.

Rescaling, translation, and rotation can also be accomplished by digital resampling techniques: bicubic or biquadratic resampling, simple pixel replication, or linear pixel translation. Menu-driven software utilities for rescaling and resampling from one image base to the reference image base have been developed and tested.

3.6 Statistical Pattern Recognition, Feature Recognition, and Signature Analysis

While it has been generally accepted that statistical pattern recognition is important to image analysis and understanding in many fields such as satellite remote sensing and character recognition, it has been significantly underutilized in radiology. The purpose of image analysis is to provide a contextually useful description of the displayed image scene. For example, in human lung imaging the context might be the detection of malignant lesions. There are various hierarchical levels of discrimination in the image. On the one hand one could describe each lesion in the image as a convex region with pixel intensity values or group intensity texture levels distinct from the surrounding background. Or the image description could be more simply defined as being a tumor. The classification or labeling of the object is perhaps the most concise method of description.

Multidimensional discrimination based on spatial statistical principles has been identified as a

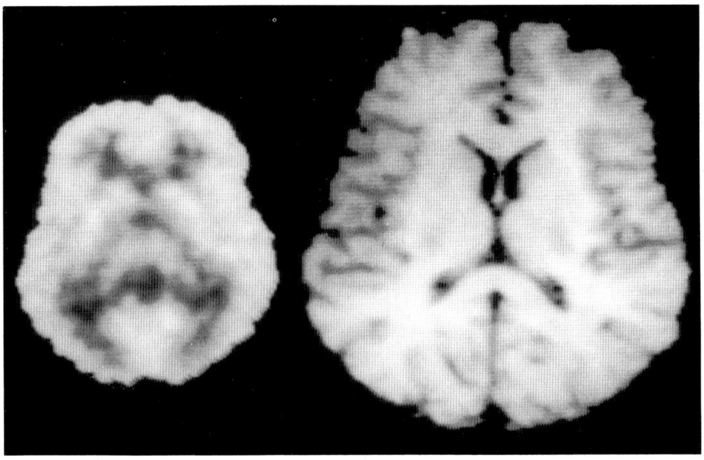

17

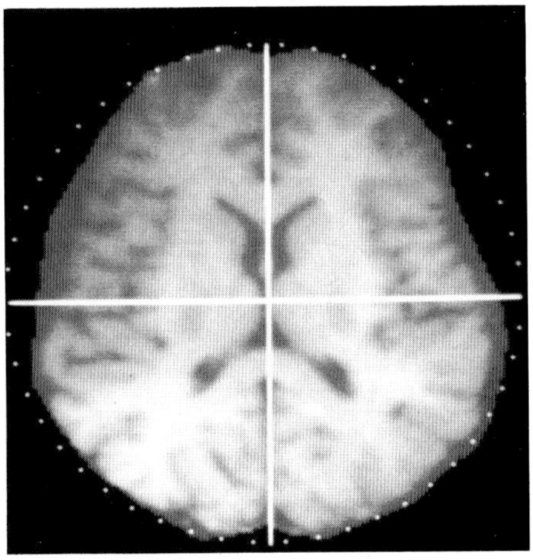

18

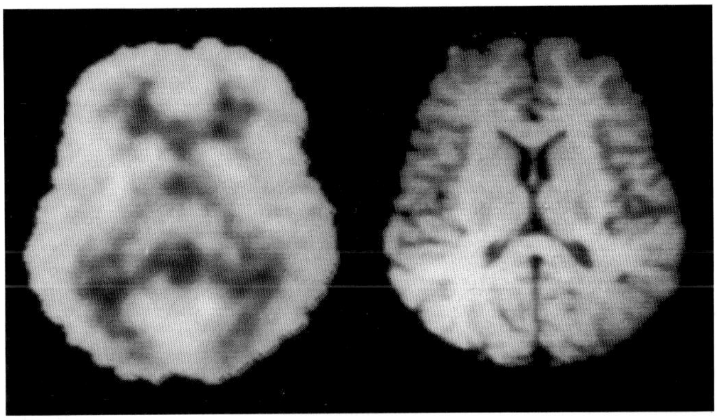

19

Fig. 17. In their original digital environments, PET images *(left)* and MR images *(right)* are mismatched with respect to size and orientation

Fig. 18. This MR image is resampled and rotated to match its companion PET image

Fig. 19. Rotated and resized, the MR image is now ready for interimage registration. This will allow redirected sampling from one image to another

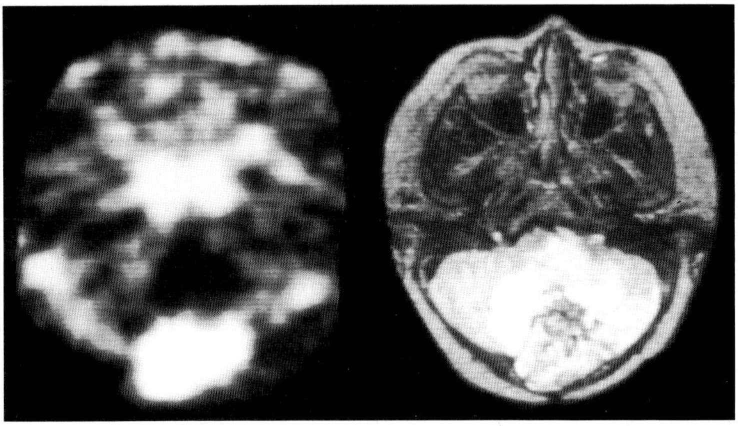

Fig. 20. Matched and registered PET-MR images are particularly important for neuro-oncology. This [^{11}C]methionine PET study *(left)* and its matched MR image *(right)* can now be used cooperatively to assess "tumor" volume and distribution. The composite PET-MR image now permits accurate anatomic characterization in association with essential biochemical data

possible approach. The fundamental purpose of image processing of radiologic images is to enhance the detection of signals in the images. The basic postulation of this problem is known as SKE (*s*ignal and its parameters *k*nown *e*xactly). In this postulate the signal is characterized relative to the standard deviation of its noise. (SNR = Signal to Noise Ratio)

For photon images this can be related to the product of contrast (C) and the square root of the counts (N) in the target region.

$$SNR = C\sqrt{N} \quad (2)$$

In more general terms

$$SNR^2 = \int |\Delta S|^2 \, NEQ(f) \, df \quad (3)$$

where ΔS is a measure of the spectrum of the discrimination and NEQ(f) is the spectrum of the noise equivalent quanta. Most radiologic applications also have significant edge detection and enhancement requirements. Edge detection and enhancement routines typically de-emphasize the low frequency components of the image and emphasize the mid and high frequencies. The high frequency components tend to contain major fractions of the noise contained in the image.

Radiologists typically act as ideal Bayesian observers (IBOs). For example, for two-dimensional measures, with Gaussian error distributions, an IBO weights his decision based on the separation of the error centroid and inversely to the individual noise (error variance). Image processing variously defines the direct weighting (separation of mass centroids) as template matching, cross-correlation, or matched filtering. The term prewhitening is sometimes used to characterize weightings which are inverse to the error variance.

A number of different strategies exist for isolating and separating normal and abnormal features within the images. Most strategies adopt so-called symmetrical cost paradigms in which the intersection of isocontours of constant probability define the threshold. The use of digital images permits statistical approaches to image segmentation and pattern recognition.

Approaches which assume that the "signal" is specified only in a statistical sense are being developed. This approach is optimal for the class of problems in which the target phenomena are due to the implicit structural or anatomic feature variability, indicative of a broad class of radiologic imaging problems. This requires intensive use of spatial statistical pattern recognition techniques both to address the problem of the cross-correlation of multiple internal structures in single mode image and to accommodate multimodal images.

Statistical pattern recognition generalizes the signal/background contrast analysis to discrimination tasks where the noise is characterized by interclass scatter which includes both measurement errors, patient variability and intramode image correlation. For this class of problems, a Bayesian observer using linear features is modeled in terms of the Hotelling trace of the quotient of these matrices. Other embodiments of these approaches can be classed as maximum a posteriori classifications which maximize the a posteriori probability of a solution s from a given image data set (i) based upon the Bayes rule:

$$P(s \mid i) = P(i \mid s)\, P(s)/P(i) \tag{4}$$

that is, the posterior probability (P) of a solution (s) given a specific image (i) is determined by the conditional probability of (i) given (s) and the prior probabilities of (i) and (s). The goodness-of-fit depends on the nature of the prior model, e.g., organ or lesion shape, metabolic distribution, locus of organ or lesion centroid, etc.

Classification is the process of naming or labeling objects within the image. In this process the pattern that is characteristic of the object is assigned to one of a class of patterns. When this is accomplished by deriving a statistic for the pattern and assigning this pattern to a class based on its statistical closeness this process is termed statistical pattern recognition.

In many cases this classification is a binary process, i.e., determination of the presence or absence of tumor. However, in most cases more information is required – tumors classified by number, size, and grade. Various levels of attributive and relational information are required; therefore a hierarchical set of descriptive levels exist and characterize the classification procedures and techniques required. When the process is dominated by mainly attributive information and/or the classification is done at the pixel level the procedures are termed low level classifications. When the process is accomplished at the object level and is dominated by relational information the term high level classification is used. At the higher classification levels the decision making process requires the implicit or explicit definition of the rules which define the relationship between image entities (objects). Figure 21 illustrates the analysis stages.

Alzheimer's disease and Parkinsonian dementia often have overlapping cognitive characteristics and illustrate the utility of statistical pattern recognition techniques. Word finding difficulty and visuospatial recall may be prominent in both. Brain image data may help the clinician classify patients who have partial membership in both diagnostic groups. Image classification routines developed for satellite surveillance depend on multispectral measurements. Whereas MRI provides multiple image sets (multiecho, multiple inversion, and spin-spin protocols) only dynamic cerebral blood flow (Phelps et al. 1982) permits the large number of PET studies needed for multispectral analysis. Nonetheless, by using a large number of reference cases, one may generate rules of classification.

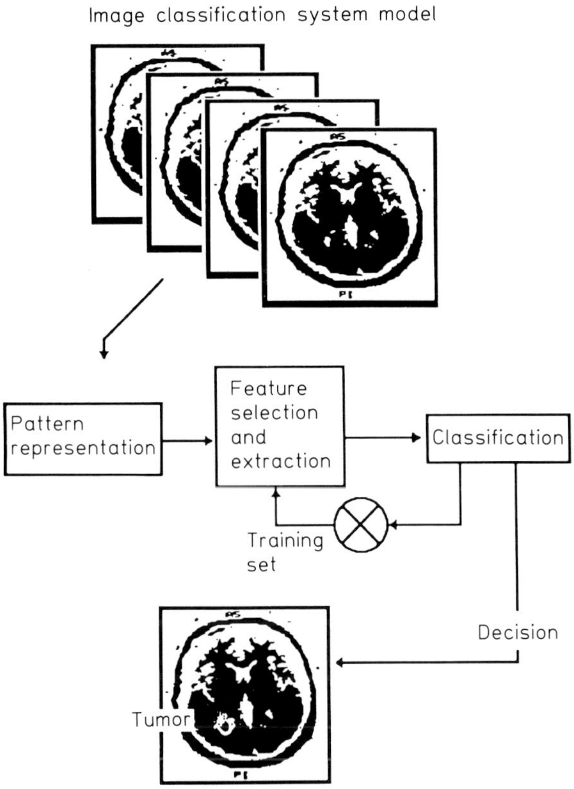

Fig. 21. The recent (5 years) arrival of dynamic, [^{15}O]labeled water, cerebral blood flow studies, multispectral MR imaging, and a growing armamentarium of radiolabeled PET and SPECT tracers now makes pattern detection/classification research highly relevant to radiology. Tumor biology may become one of the first targets of this approach. Amino acid transport, glucose metabolism, blood flow, blood volume, oxidative metabolism, and water content (MRI) can each be assessed using registered cross-correlated images. The classification of that tumor, or signature, will emerge from the composite profile generated by these various image modalities

3.6.1 Tissue Segmentation

Accurate discrimination and identification of tissue types within the image are prerequisites for accurate volume measurement. The development of accurate and objective tissue segmentation and volume mensuration is significant in diagnosis, disease staging, treatment evaluation, and surgical and radiation therapy planning. This is particularly important in tumor treatment, where the tumor volume and its recession/growth are the primary measures of action. Radiologists often determine soft tissue boundaries from slice to slice by visual comparison and mental integration of the relationship of a structure in individual slices. Another technique which is used with digital imagery is to identify tissue contours on individual image planes.

WINDHAM et al. (1988) have used techniques of linear filtering (eigenimaging) to produce a single composite image from a sequence of spin echo images of the same individual at a single repetition time with a series of increasing echo times. In these techniques the characteristic pattern for a specific tissue is described as a weighted vector of contributions from the different images. The n-dimensional vector space formed from the image data set is transformed by rotation into a new set of basis functions which maximize the statistical separation between the individual tissue types.

Statistical classification techniques patterned after those developed for satellite classification of earth resources were used by VANNIER et al. (1987). A multiecho MRI data set is formed and signatures of a number of tissue classes are developed by supervised and unsupervised classification techniques. A set of distinct signatures based on the different MR pulse sequences can be obtained. Theme maps can then be produced for characteristic classes such as CSF, brain parenchyma, bone, skin, etc. Supervised classification is performed by using the observer to identify ROIs for the various classes, thus providing training classes for subsequent computer classification. Class separation can be accomplished by linear or nonlinear discriminant analysis or with more simple parallel-piped classification which is easier to implement. Unsupervised classification can be performed by bootstrap clustering algorithms which links pixels in the image based on their class assignments.

HOLCOMB et al. (1988b) developed a computer program for producing weighted composite images from multiecho MRI images in order to isolate gray matter from white matter and to "feature enhance" small structures like the globus pallidus. Figure 22 shows a series of images built from weighted MR images with a common TR of 2700. The first image in the sequence used only the information from the TE=50 image. The second image added information from the TE=75 image. The third used the TE=100 image. The full combination image (TE=25, TE=50, TE=75, + TE=100) in the lower right quadrant clearly shows significant enhancement of the globus pallidus.

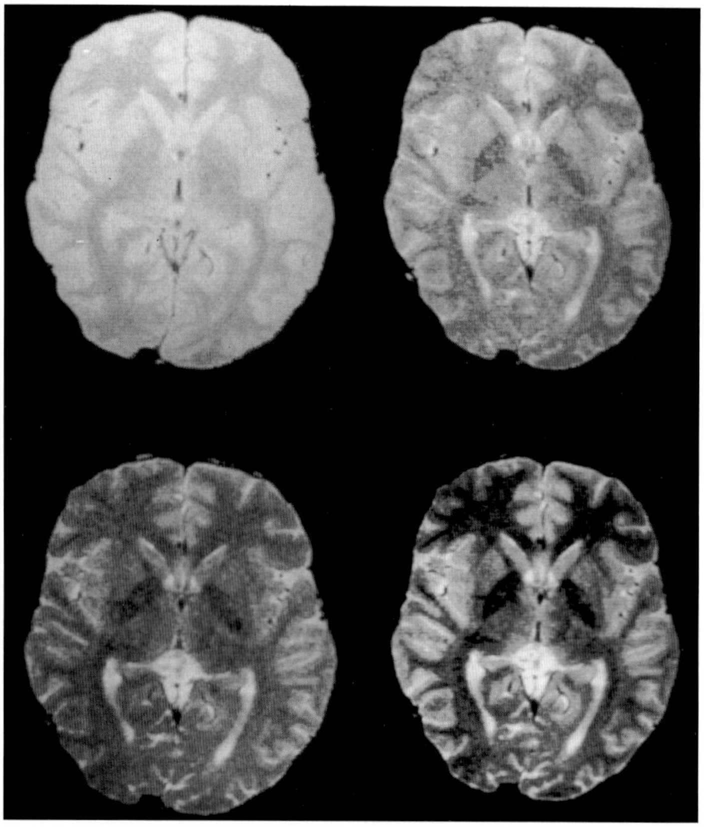

Fig. 22. Multispectral MR image generation is a powerful tool for selective feature enhancement. By measuring the gray level intensity of a target feature and its surrounding regions over a series of MR images, one can determine which image, or image combination, provides the best separation, or discrimination, between various combinations of features. Bordered by the internal capsule and putamen, the globus pallidus (internal and external segments combined) is a particularly subtle feature in some MR images, but clearly delineated in others. *Top left:* TR 2700, TE 50; *top right:* TR 2700, TE 75; *bottom left:* TR 2700, TE 100; *bottom right:* weighted composite image of TE 25, 50, 75, and 100. This composite image markedly enhances pallidal contrast

3.6.2 Corrections for Feature Contamination (CSF Pixel Deletion)

T_2 images obtained at multiple echo time points can be used together to generate composite, tissue-partitioned pictures with marked reductions in signal overlap. Briefly, echoes at 30 ms (TR 2700 ms) generate pictures with good gray-white definition and poor CSF contrast, whereas 80-ms echoes provide fair to poor gray-white definition but good CSF contrast. In TE = 80 pictures, sampling (from magnetic tape MRI data) the CSF in the ventricles provides, through histogram analysis, a good approximation of pure and mixed CSF pixel MRI transmission values. A threshold is chosen which best partitions CSF from gray or white tissue; the inflection point on the histogram is a good estimator. Using this threshold we generate a binary mask that represents all pixels above that partition as 0 values, and all pixels below that value as 1. Putative CSF pixels are then subtracted from the TE = 30 image. This provides a new image with high contrast between gray, white, and CSF spaces.

Using this method of generating CSF-free TE = 30 pictures we then further partition gray and white tissues based on transmission histograms. Gray tissue exhibits a higher pixel value than white matter in these images. Because many pixels are mixed it is useful to express gray-white values along a continuum rather than as strict thresholds. This is effectively facilitated using Z score pixel values; means and standard deviations for the entire CSF-free brain are readily computed. Transformation by gray/white Z score permits consistent and rational choices regarding ROI size and location.

3.6.3 Hybrid Color Display

There are two basic types of color scale used in radiologic imaging: pseudocolor and color composite. In the pseudocolor technique, the monochrome intensity values in an image are mapped into a three-dimensional color space (RGB). Various subranges of the intensities are mapped into separate colors. The use of pseudocolor is somewhat controversial in radiology since its detractors posit that the pseudocoloring does not add information and may exaggerate insignificant gray scale differences.

On the other hand its proponents suggest that the value of pseudocoloring comes from its capacity to separate features.

The color compositing technique is used to map separate images into a three-dimensional color space. This obviously increases the capability to present more information and yields both aesthetic and quantitative benefits. One important benefit of color compositing is the capability of combining tissue differentiation with tissue identification. Color compositing has been used to separate neoplastic lesions or hemorrhage from surrounding edema, to provide enhanced demarcation of tumors, and as an aid in tumor grading.

Current image processing is accomplished mainly on monochrome images. Color images produced using this monochrome data are in reality pseudocolor or red, green, and blue (RGB). Color values are arbitrarily selected and mapped into distinct gray scale ranges. This leads to large and sometimes unwanted differentiation between associated tissue and anatomic structures. The pseudocolor approach is, however, very useful in isolating features. For example, if a tumor exists in an image within a distinct gray scale region, heightened visibility is achieved by simply assigning a distinct color for that region, i.e., red, vis-à-vis the normal gray scale black and white background.

Alternatively, multimode images such as MRI/PET, CT/PET, or multiecho MRI combinations are simultaneously reviewed by the diagnostician who must mentally integrate the separate unidimensional images. This often leads to the inability to ascertain subtle effects and gradations in lesions, edemic regions, etc.

Displays incorporating natural three-dimensional contrast scales based on hue, saturation, and intensity (HSI) scales have been proposed and are currently being implemented. The conversion from RGB to HSI has significant hardware and software consequences. Hue is the color attribute which describes pure color; i.e., pure red, etc. Saturation is the attribute which describes the dilution of the color with white. Intensity is a color neutral attribute which describes the level of brightness. The primary advantage of the HSI color space lies in the fact that the HSI image buffers are relatively uncorrelated with one another as distinct from the high correlation in the RGB color space. Humans have a significantly higher power to discriminate in color space compared to black and white. The conversion of black and white images relative to a rational color assignment based on tissue and anatomic feature discrimination will become more prevalent, particularly as greater reliance is placed on the newer imaging modalities such as MRI.

Both for the discrimination, identification, and isolation of target structures in the image and to fully utilize the extra information from multi-images, present "black and white" thinking will give way to analysis based upon meaningful hybrid color displays.

The use of artificial intelligence is more and more frequently being suggested for image analysis but has not yet been adapted to any significant radiologic applications. These techniques tend to be very enticing since they have the potential to capture expert knowledge acquired from long years of experience by recognized radiology experts and to thus transfer this knowledge to large numbers of recipients. Another important application of artificial intelligence or perhaps of neural network concepts is in the comparison of images from one individual against a collection or synthesis of other, or the same, individual(s).

3.7 Three-dimensional Reconstruction, Display, and Measurements

While the advent of 3-D digital display has brought a new visual perspective, it has not substantially altered the level of image quantitation. Direct measurements on 3-D displays will require significant alterations in the way radiologists interact with images.

Radiologists usually need to view the interior of organs and are not directly affected by the current developments in surface modeling approaches which display 3-D surface rendered views of bony structures. The eye of the radiologist is basically a 2-D receptor and the analysis capability of most display utilities is highly restricted to planar data. The goal of 3-D diagnostics can be met by meaningful displays of single or multiple slices through the 3-D imaging space. These can be assisted by the transparent rendering of the 3-D volume if appropriate tissue segmentation and discrimination can be provided. The 3-D analysis capability would provide rapid access, throughout the body elements imaged, to slices of variable thickness and orientation that are centered on the plane of interest. The capability should have orthogonal display, rotation for perspective, and 3-D volume reconstruction and measurement capability by keystroke demand.

MRI imaging has the capability of supplying 3-D anatomic information given that the appropriate corrections can be made to compensate for spatial inhomogeneity in the imaging process.

Microcomputer software programs for 2-D and 3-D quantitative analysis and display of CT, MRI, and ECT images of the brain are undergoing significant and rapidly accelerating development. Software programs centered on quantitative analysis do not currently exist as an integrated, comprehensive approach capable of utilizing and accessing the multiple images required for precise quantitation. As ECT becomes more widespread in both research and clinical uses, multi-imaging systems will gain increasing importance.

Fig. 23. Thresholding the gray scale of an image, in combination with color enhancement, permits rapid area measurements of tissue/fluid regions. *Top left:* red indicates gray matter and yellow indicates white matter, green corresponds to a mixed tissue type. *Top right:* red indicates gray matter. *Bottom left:* dark blue and white indicate cerebrospinal fluid, green indicates mixed white and gray matter. *Bottom right:* dark blue and white indicate CSF, grayish white indicates white matter and mixed gray-white tissue

3.7.1 Areas and Volumes by Thresholding

Once transmission thresholds have been chosen for a given set of pixels, using the image histogram, the number of pixels in each partition can be easily computed. Using simple calibration this number can easily convert from those pixels into units of surface area or volume. One method for segmenting the image is to partition the image based on gray scale values related to the boundaries of observed anatomic features (Fig. 23). An alternate technique uses automated edge finding routines which search near-neighborhood regions for similar contiguous pixel values and constrains the boundary set to conform to the natural edges of the features (Fig. 24). Once the boundaries and enclosed area of the target features are defined the computer simply counts the number of pixels in the contained area. Using the multimode registration techniques previously described, higher precision boundaries can be isolated on the highest resolution or highest contrast image and projected onto the lower contrast or resolution target images (Fig. 25).

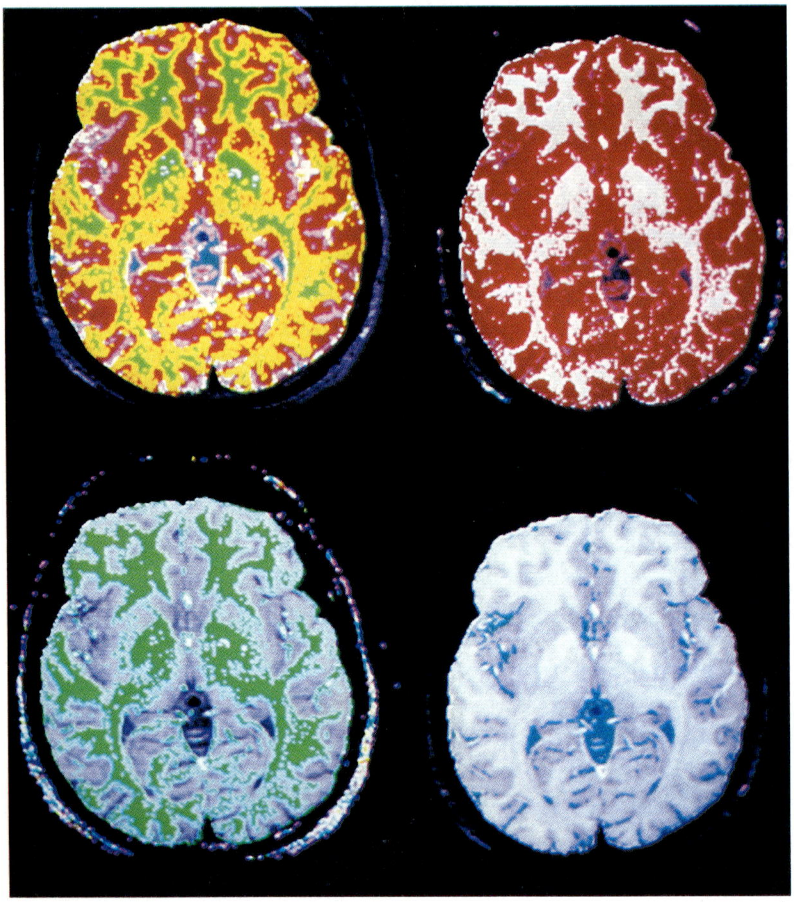

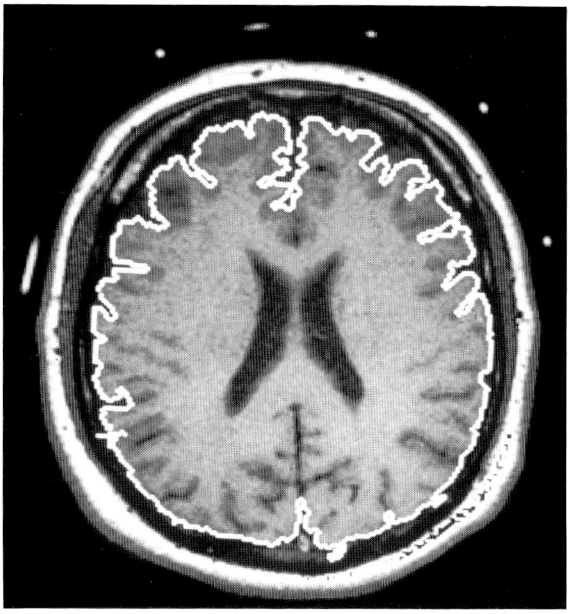

24

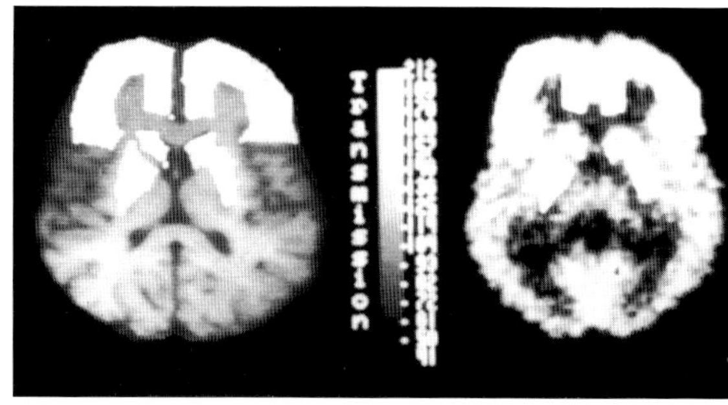

25

Fig. 24. Automated edge routines help to standardize boundary identification. This is particularly helpful when measuring sulcal or ventricular volume

Fig. 25. Thresholding and edge detection facilitate feature segmentation in images with high resolution and contrast characteristics. Registration and redirected sampling are then used to transfer those boundaries from one, high resolution, image to another, low resolution image. *Left:* MRI with cortical gray matter, caudate, and putamen outlined. *Right:* PET FDG scan sampled through redirection

3.8 The Impact of Future Image Analysis Hardware Developments on Radiology

The future development of image processing and analysis in radiology operations is equally dependent on hardware and software developments. The advent of high performance microcomputers with the memory and speed capability to accommodate large image data sets has fostered a revolution in the way image analysis is applied to radiologic applications. This chapter projects future developments of computer-based image analysis techniques as they affect radiology applications. Of particular importance in projecting future image processing development in radiology is the rapid and significant state of development of computer imaging hardware. Figure 26 is a performance/price plot showing that the mini- and microcomputer imaging workstations such as the SUN2/360, the COMPAQ 386/20-1167, and the Microway Quadputer have higher performance/price ratios than the larger VAX and IBM series computers.

For example, an AT or XT microcomputer provided with a single parallel transputer coprocessor can equal the numeric processing power of a VAX 8600. When provided with four transputers (Quadputer) the system has the processing power equivalent to 16% that of the Cray supercomputer. Multiple quadputer boards can yield the power of a Cray at approximately 90% cost reduction, thus promising major image processing capability enhancements.

In addition, the price and performance of RAM (random access memory) chips are continuing to improve. Quarter megabit (256 K) DRAM chips are conventionally employed in current micro/mini and super micro-workstations. Megabit (1000 Kbit) DRAMs are in advanced development and are reaching the market. The speed of these chips is below 100 ns and provide low-cost high speed on-line memory. Currently on the horizon are megabit dual ported VRAMS (video rams) which permit display resolutions of 1024^2 to 2048^2 at near video refresh rates.

Standard image processing techniques implemented on low-cost mini- and microcomputers are currently finding their way into radiology and should result in significant improvements in the near future.

3.9 Prospects for the Future

Image analysis can be thought of as the central synthesizing component of future radiology operations. By converting conventional visual analysis to reproducible quantitation the prospect is for better decision management, and therefore improved patient care. This improvement will naturally foster a better foundation for controlling and justifying medical

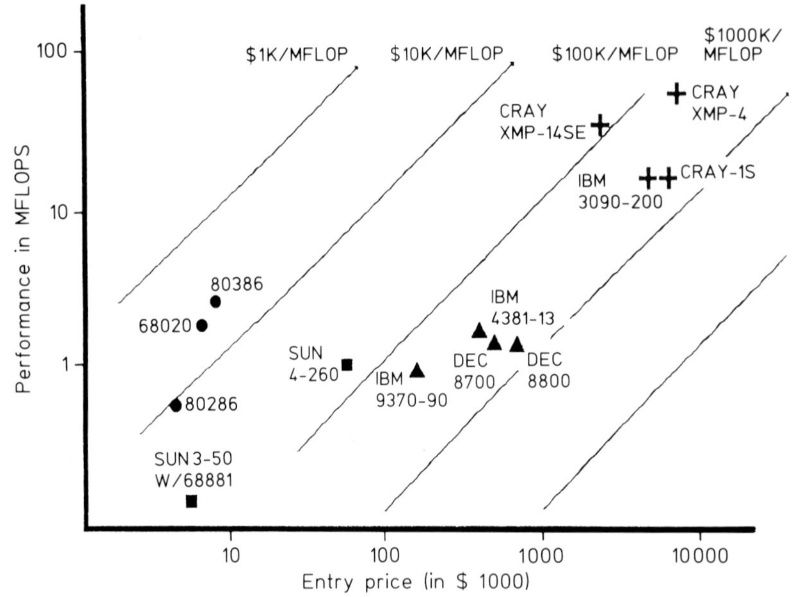

Fig. 26. This performance/price plot indicates that the mini- and microcomputer imaging work stations (SUN2/360, COMPAQ 386/20-1167, and Microway Quadputer) have higher performance/price ratios than the larger VAX and IBM series computers. It is this technological shift that has made affordable, state of the art image processing possible

costs. The prospect that the patient population base is gradually increasing in age will cause the analyses to shift to the identification and quantitation of more subtle and to some extent less pathologic modes. This is also true of the current diseases and conditions such as AIDS.

Future developments in radiology will strongly depend on the large-scale adaptation of image analysis techniques and hardware. In the near future cost reductions in digital processing hardware will foster the conversion to an increasingly digital image environment. The increased discrimination afforded by color versus black and white and the advent of mixed functional and structural images will almost certainly lead to significant advances and changes in the practice of radiology.

If these new advances are not readily adopted by radiologists then the automated analysis capabilities inherent in digital images coupled with the ever lowering costs, ease of use, and rapidly increasing performance capacity of stand-alone digital imaging systems could and probably will engender a transition and translation of image analysis function directly to non-radiology-based clinical specialists.

The current and projected costs of image analysis, dominated as it is by low-cost stand-alone workstation technology, offer the best bet for return on investment.

References

Bartoo GT, Kim Y, Haralick RM, Nochlin D, Sumi SM (1988) Mathematical morphology techniques for image processing applications in biomedical imaging. Medical Imaging II SPIE 914: 466–475

Fox PT, Perlmutter JS, Raichle ME (1985) A stereotaxic method of anatomical localization for positron emission tomography. J Comput Assist Tomogr 9: 141–153

Holcomb HH, Loats HL, Tamminga C, et al. (1988a) Registration of MRI-PET images, procedure and validation. J Nucl Med 29: 853

Holcomb HH, Loats HL, Tamminga CA, Summerfelt A, Slusarcick A (1988b) Volume, shape, location and gray/white tissue analysis of brain magnetic resonance images. CINP Congress, Munich

Kandel A (1986) Fuzzy mathematical techniques with applications. Addison-Wesley, London

Kundel H, Nodine C (1987) Report to the special imaging forum of the American Association for the Advancement of Science, Chicago, Illinois

LeBihan D, Breton E, Lallemand D, Aubin M, Vignaud J, Lavol-Jeantet M (1988) Separation of diffusion and perfusion in intravoxel incoherent motion MR imaging. Radiology 168: 497–505

Lodwick GS (1983) Expanding the computer's gunbarrel vision. Diagn Imag 5: 159–167

Matsui T, Hirano A (1978) An atlas of the human brain for computerized tomography. Igaku-Shoin, Tokyo

Nguyen PT, Quinqueton J (1982) Shape filling curves and texture analysis. IEEE CH 1801-0/82/0282

O'Tuama LA, Guilarte TR, Douglass KH, et al. (1988) Assessment of [11-C] methionine transport into the human brain. J Cereb Blood Flow Metab 8: 341–345

Pearce RB (1987) Expert systems enable computers to share in imaging decisions. Diagn Imag 9: 146–152

Phelps ME, Mazziotta JC, Huang SC (1982) Study of cerebral function with positron computed tomography. J Cereb Blood Flow Metab 2: 113–162

Pictikainen M, Rosenfeld A (1982) Edge based texture measures. IEEE CH 1801-0/92/0298

Ratib, et al. (1988) A new technique for elastic registration of tomographic images. Medical Imaging II SPIE 914: 452–461

Schaltenbrand G, Wahren W (1977) Atlas for stereotaxy of the human brain. Tear Book Medical Publ, Chicago

Schnitzlein HN, et al. (1985) Imaging anatomy of the head and spine. Urban & Schwarzenberg, Baltimore

Talairach J, Szikla G, Tournoux P, Prossalentis A, Bordas-Ferrer M, Covello L, Jacob M, Mempel E (1967) Atlas d'anatomie stereotaxique du telencephale. Masson, Paris

Vannier M, Butterfield R, Rickman D, Jordan D, Murphy W, Biondett P (1987) Multispectral magnetic resonance image analysis. CRC Crit Rev Biomed Eng 15: 117–144

Windham JP, et al. (1988) Eigenimage filtering in MR imaging. J Comput Assist Tomogr 12: 1–9

4 Three-Dimensional Imaging: Advanced Medical Applications

ELLIOT K. FISHMAN, DONNA MAGID, DEREK R. NEY, KENNETH I. MACRAE, JANET E. KUHLMAN, and DOUGLAS D. ROBERTSON

CONTENTS

4.1 Introduction 47
4.2 Overview and History 48
4.3 Standard Imaging Technique 49
4.4 Clinical Applications in Orthopedics 50
4.4.1 Evaluation of the Hip and Acetabulum 50
4.4.2 Evaluation of the Shoulder 54
4.4.3 Evaluation of the Sacrum und Spine 55
4.4.4 Evaluation of Muscle and the Soft Tissue 56
4.5 Custom Orthopedic Prosthetic Design 57
4.6 Radiation Therapy Simulation and Planning 62
4.7 Other Clinical Applications of Three-dimensional Imaging 63
4.8 Tumor Volumetrics 65
4.9 Three-dimensional Database and Combining Images 66
4.10 Pattern Recognition and Artificial Intelligence . . . 67
4.11 Conclusion 67
References 68

4.1 Introduction

The past decade has been witness to a technological revolution in diagnostic radiology with the introduction and rapid acceptance of computed tomography (CT) and magnetic resonance imaging (MRI). The development of these new technologies provided the clinician with diagnostic tools unsurpassed for the evaluation of the inner structures of the human body. Diagnoses previously reserved for laparotomy could now be made accurately in a noninvasive fashion. Definition of normal and abnormal anatomic structures could be displayed in detail usually reserved for schematic diagrams in textbooks.

ELLIOT K. FISHMAN, M.D., DONNA MAGID, M.D., DEREK R. NEY, B.S., KENNETH I. MACRAE, M.D., Ph.D. JANET E. KUHLMAN, M.D., Dept. of Radiology and Radiological Science, The Johns Hopkins University, School of Medicine, 600 North Wolfe Street, Baltimore, MD 21205, USA
DOUGLAS D. ROBERTSON, M.D., Ph.D., Department of Orthopedic Surgery, Brigham and Women's Hospital, Harvard Medical School, Boston, MA 02115, USA

Yet, the need for this information was always present. What was the driving force behind the development of CT and MRI? The answer can be found in the computer revolution which has occurred over the past 15 years. The development of smaller and cheaper computer systems, each with increased speed, memory, and functionality, has been the dominant force of the computer industry. It is these advances which have in part driven the progress in medical imaging. For example, computer workstations by leading manufacturers such as Sun Microsystems (Mountain View, California) which cost in the range of $ 100000 just 2 years ago are now in the $ 20000 range. In addition to the precipitous price drop the machine has more speed, memory, and functionality. Newer systems such as the Sun Microsystems 386i will drive prices even lower. These systems can also be easily upgraded by "accelerator" boards such as the TAAC-1 (Trancept Systems). Development of accelerator boards will be critical in the delivery of low-priced medical workstations.

Another example of a technological breakthrough is the emergence of the Apple Macintosh as a low-priced alternative for image processing. At the Siggraph meeting in Atlanta in 1988 a Macintosh II driving a Pixar Imaging Computer was introduced. Other sophisticated graphics and image processing tools are now being introduced on a system that many considered but a "word processor." It looks more and more that Steve Jobs' prophecy of a "Mac" on every desk may prove true. Yet, these innovations are but the beginning of a new computer revolution that will change the way we practice radiology today.

The standard display of CT images is a transaxial view. These images provide fine detail of anatomic structures and their relationship to adjacent organs, muscles, and bone. The integration of multiple CT slices into a true three-dimensional (3D) model is usually done intuitively by the radiologist and nonradiologist alike. Radiologists, due to their extensive training in multiple imaging modalities, usually have a better understanding of 3D anatomy based simply on reviewing transaxial imaging. Other physicians may not have similar capabilities. Yet decisions as to operability, surgical planning, and therapy are not usually in the hands of the radiologists. There is therefore the need, for both the radiologist and nonradiologist, for the display of data in a form which provide the most information from a standard image set. This has been the impetus for 3D imaging – the need to provide a more thorough understanding of a dataset in three planes. This chapter will review the rapid development in the exciting field of 3D imaging as well as define some of the applications which have proven successful at the present time. We will explore the future of 3D imaging based on the technology available today and the technology being developed at major computer graphics companies in the United States.

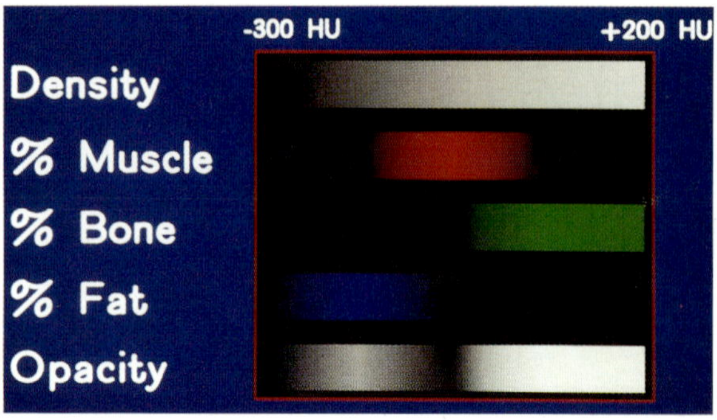

Fig. 1. Schematic diagram defining how volumetric technique is used for definition of CT data. The CT density in Hounsfield units is looked at and a different percentage classification is given for structures of muscle, bone, and fat. Notice there is some overlap an each of these densities, which is the advantage of volumetric rendering as opposed to thresholding. A degree of opacity or transparency is assigned. This is the key parameter in the recontruction of high quality 3D images

4.2 Overview and History

Soon after high quality transaxial images were being routinely generated by CT scanners it became apparent that a reformatting of the basic digital information was necessary to provide the maximum information to both the radiologist and nonradiologist alike. The major computer vendors soon provided basic software which allowed the creation and reformatting of routine sagittal, coronal, or paraaxial image reconstructions. Several of the vendors, the most prominent being Siemens Medical Systems, developed dedicated software packages offering automated display of transaxial, coronal, and sagittal data. This multiplanar display and reconstruction package has proven very valuable, particularly in orthopedic applications (FISHMAN et al. 1986). At the Johns Hopkins Hospital we have examined well over 2000 patients using this software package and have found wide acceptance with both radiologist and clinicians alike. With the experience gained from the multiplanar imaging it soon became apparent that the optimal display would be a 3D one created from routine transaxial images. Ideally, the system to produce this should be easily used, provide high quality images, and be inexpensive. The initial attempts at 3D imaging were done by the research and development software groups of the major CT vendors. The two most successful vendors were Siemens Medical Systems with a package developed in cooperation with Michael Vannier of Mallinckrodt Institute of Radiology, and the General Electric 3D83 and 3D98 package developed with Gabor Herman and his associates at the University of Pennsylvania (HERMAN et al. 1985).

Freestanding 3D imaging systems were developed by a variety of companies such as Phoenix Medical Systems (Albany, New York), Cemax (formerly Contour Medical Systems, formerly Cemax Medical Systems, Santa Clara, California), and Dimensional Medicine (Minneapolis, Minnesota). These systems cost in the range of $ 200000–$ 250000 and were never widely accepted or used. This was due to a variety of causes including:

1. Poor image quality with many artifacts
2. Long reconstruction times
3. Limited display formats
4. Lack of satisfactory user interface
5. High cost (freestanding systems)

One of the major limitations of both scanner-based and freestanding 3D image systems was their use of edge detection thresholding technique (Figs. 1, 2). Thresholding provides a surface reconstruction based on a preset CT Hounsfield level. The level chosen tries to distinguish between the structures of interest and other background structures. However, because all structures have a wide range of attenuation values, the technique results in data loss to a variable degree. This causes the final image set to be of limited quality with often inaccurate representation of edges, surfaces, and articulations.

With the recent advances in computer technology in both hardware and software it became obvious that this evolving technology could have an impact on medical imaging. During the past 3 years we

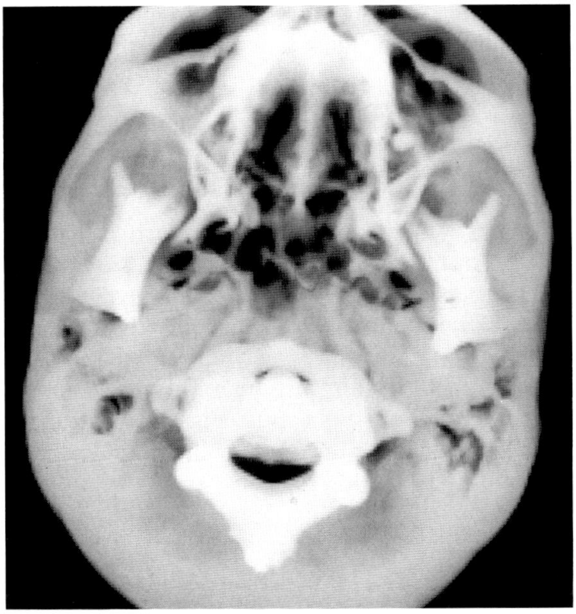

Fig. 2. 3D reconstruction of the base of the skull demonstrating detailed definition of basilar foramen. Notice fine detail around area of orbital rim and zygoma

have worked with one of the primary companies in the field of advanced computer technology, Pixar (FISHMAN et al. 1987). Originally the research and development arm of Lucasfilms Ltd., Pixar has developed a computer which in its simplest form can process up to 40 million instructions per second (MIPS). The problem of an accurate 3D display of a typical CT or MRI volumnal dataset posed a situation where cutting edge computer graphic technology could be applied. The leader in volume graphics and volume visualization is Pixar (San Rafael, California). Exploiting technology originally perfected for the movie and graphics industry, Pixar is presently addressing problems in such varied disciplines as medicine, astronomy, fluid dynamics, nondestructive testing, and landsat satellite data.

Volume visualization is the technique of displaying a volume of data rather than its surfaces or edges. Traditionally, datasets were rendered with traditional technique involving thresholding, or other highly nonlinear approximations. This introduced inaccuracies into the representation which were not present in the original data. Problems with aliasing and quantization would arise in a new guise, interfering with an accurate representation and hence interpretation of the data.

Volume visualization (volumetric rendering technique) displays every point in a 3D volume, with no surface or edge approximation. Each point in a volume is called a volume element or voxel for short. The voxel is displayed in an arbitrary color and partial transparency. The color displayed on a display screen is the combination at that point of all voxels lying along the line of sight to that point.

4.3 Standard Imaging Technique

The patient is positioned in the scanner in the supine position. Paper tape is used around the hips, knees, and ankles to keep the patient from inadvertently moving during the examination. Patients are scanned on either a Siemens Somatom DR-3 or DRH scanner using parameters of 3 s, 230 mAs, 125 kVp, and 4 mm collimation. Scans are obtained at 3-mm intervals allowing 1 mm of overlap. An average of 35–40 scans are obtained in each patient. Following acquisition, the images are recorded on nine track magnetic tape and transferred to the Pixar Image Computer.

The Pixar system consits of a Sun Workstation host with a slave Pixar computer. The host is either a Sun 3/160 with 380 Mbytes of hard disk storage and 4 Mbytes of system RAM or a Sun 3/280 with 950 Mbytes of hard disk storage and 8 Mbytes of system RAM. The imaging computer is a Pixar. It has 24 Mbytes of video RAM configured as 4 Megapixels, each pixel consisting of four 12-bit channels [red, green, blue, and opacity (alpha)]. It has 64 K of high speed scratchpad ram which is 16 bits wide. The Pixar is conceptually a single instruction multiple dataset (SIMD) parallel architecture. It has four channels which each have dedicated AMD (advanced micro devices) 16-bit processors. Each processor runs at 10 MIPS for a total of 40 MIPS in four channels. The video output is to either a 1024 by 768 resolution Barco monitor or to a ¾″ Sony NTSC monitor/recorder combination. Static images can be generated on a Matrix 3000 camera (Matrix, Orangeberg, New York).

The images are read into the video ram. These are gray scale images (intensity only) and so one of them is put into the red, then one to the blue, then the green, then alpha channels. Then the next region of memory gets four images, etc. This allows the four parallel processors to act simultaneously on these images (one channel per cpu) doing some initial processing such as slice interpolation to give the same longitudinal and transverse scales or removing unwanted background. These preprocessed images are stored to disk. The large size of the video ram means that up to 84 256 × 192 full color 48-bit images or 256 256 × 256 single color 12-bit images can be held in the video memory at once. They can then be displayed in rapid succession on one of the monitors at selectable speed, giving a motion picture effect (Fig. 1).

To optimize the efficient use of this system, a simple operating system was developed on the Sun 3/160 workstation at Johns Hopkins Hospital. Under the guidance of Derek Ney, the "Doctor Program" was developed as an interface to the Pixar. In its basic form the progress consisted of three subsections: image creation and display, archival, and image review.

4.4 Clinical Applications in Orthopedics

Over the past year we have moved from evaluating a revolutionary reconstruction algorithm (volumetric rendering) on a state of the art computer (Pixar Image Computer) to the day-to-day application of this technology to patient care. We are presently using the Pixar for the evaluation of complex orthopedic problems involving the hip, shoulder, knee, and pelvis. Additionally, we are using its soft tissue capabilities for imaging tumors and for plastic surgery planning.

4.4.1 Evaluation of the Hip and Acetabulum

Computed tomography has become the study of choice for the evaluation of the traumatized patient (Scott et al. 1988a,b) (Figs. 3–7). It permits rapid and relatively noninvasive imaging of the full spectrum of traumatic injury, including multiple body parts and multiple organ systems. In the evaluation of pelvic and acetabular fractures, CT has become the study of choice due to its ability to detect fractures missed or underestimated on plain films, to define the true extent of complex fractures, and to examine the joint space for detection of intraarticular foreign matter or bone fragments. Despite the

Fig. 3. Sequence of images showing bone and muscle reconstructions. The *upper half* of each image is bone opaque, muscle transparent with *bottom half* muscle opaque, bone transparent. Notice the left acetabular fracture

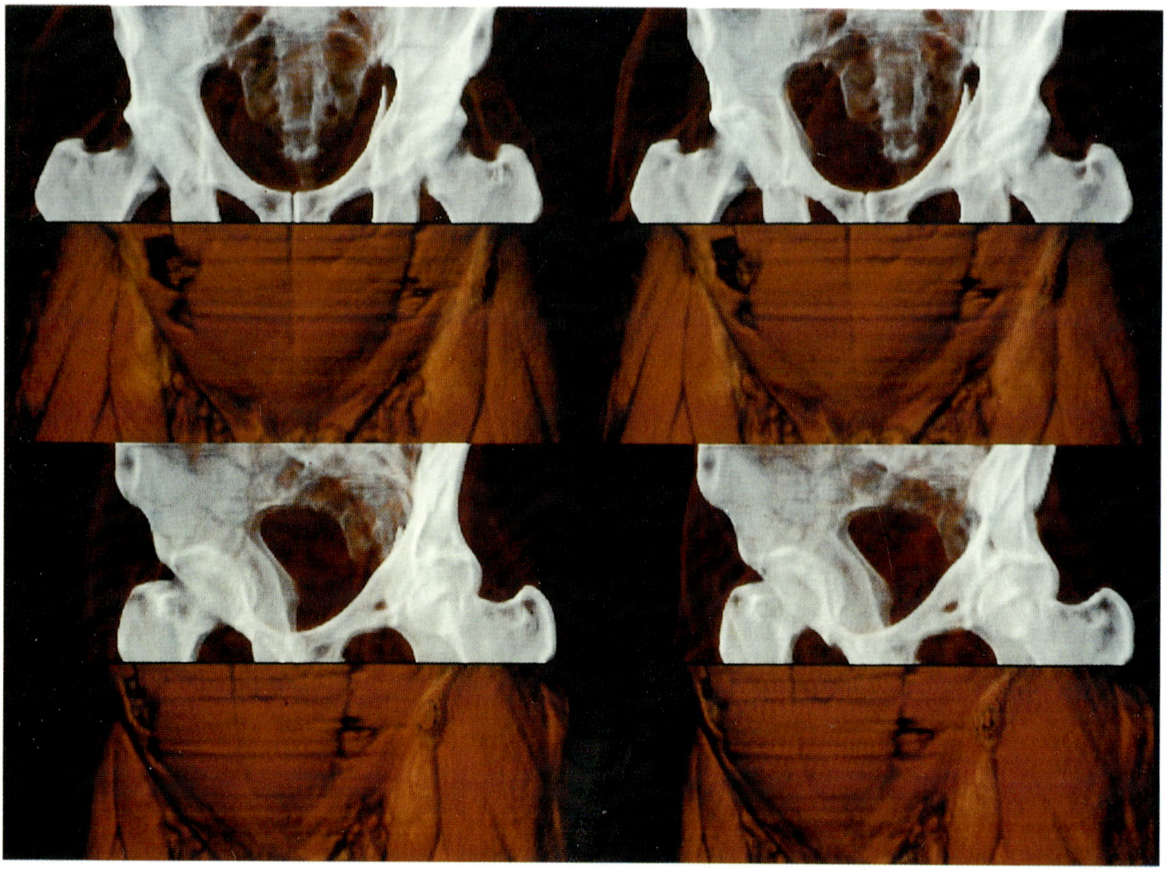

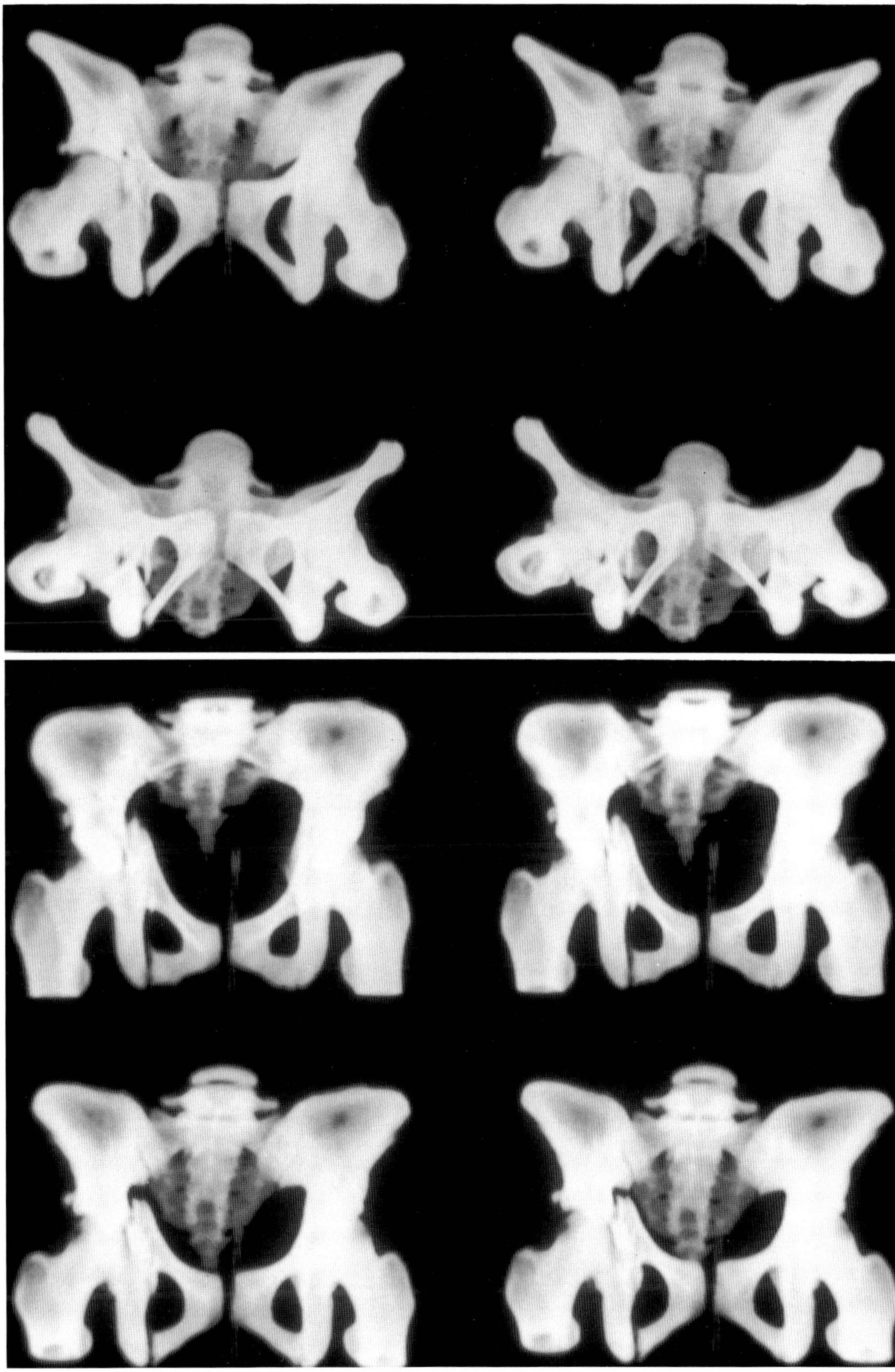

a

b

Fig. 4a–c. Sequence of images in somersaulting axis in patient with right acetabular fracture. Notice the ability to rotate provides maximum definition of the full extent of the fracture. Diastasis of right sacroiliac joint best seen on views directly from above

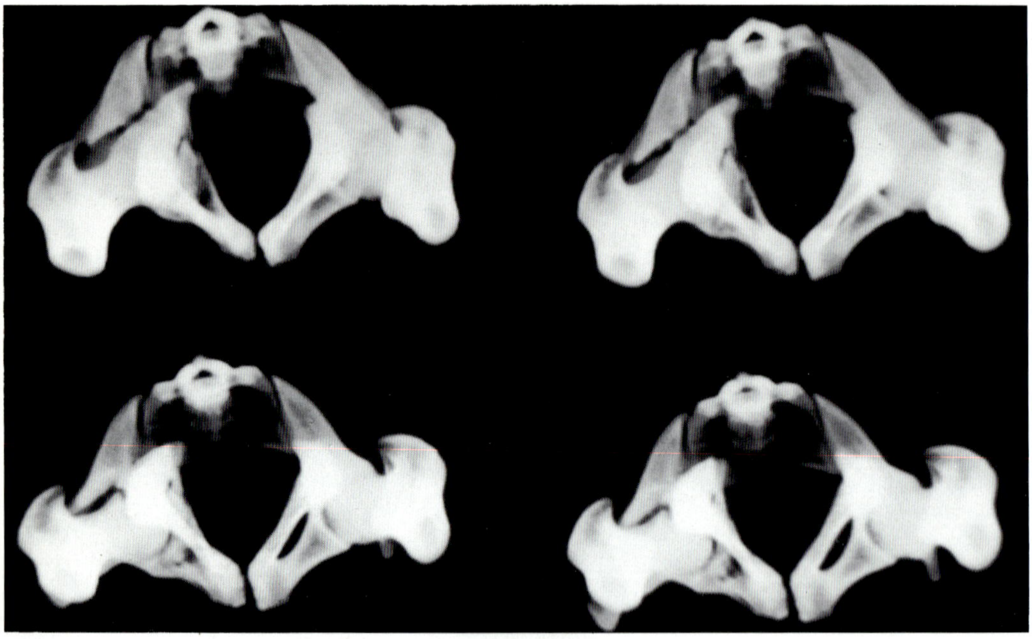

Fig. 4c. Text see p. 51

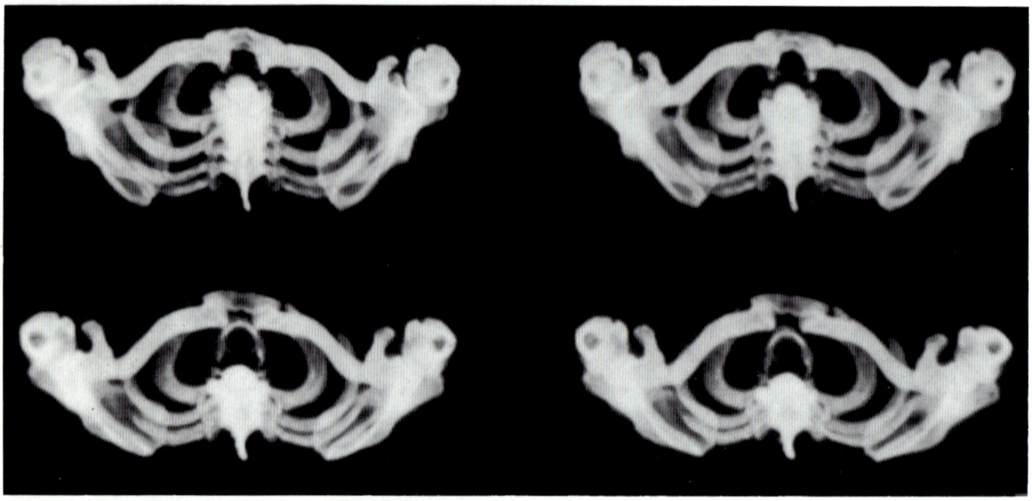

5

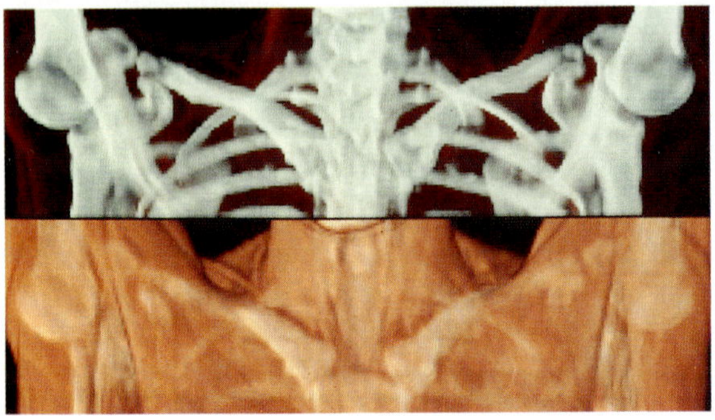

6

Fig. 5. Sequence of CT scans of normal shoulder. The view is from the lower thoracic cage looking upward. The usefulness of these images is best understood by reviewing the video sequence

Fig. 6. 3D reconstruction of shoulder with *upper half* of image showing muscle opaque and *lower half* bone opaque. Notice fine vascular detail seen in lower image. (Fishman et al. 1988 a)

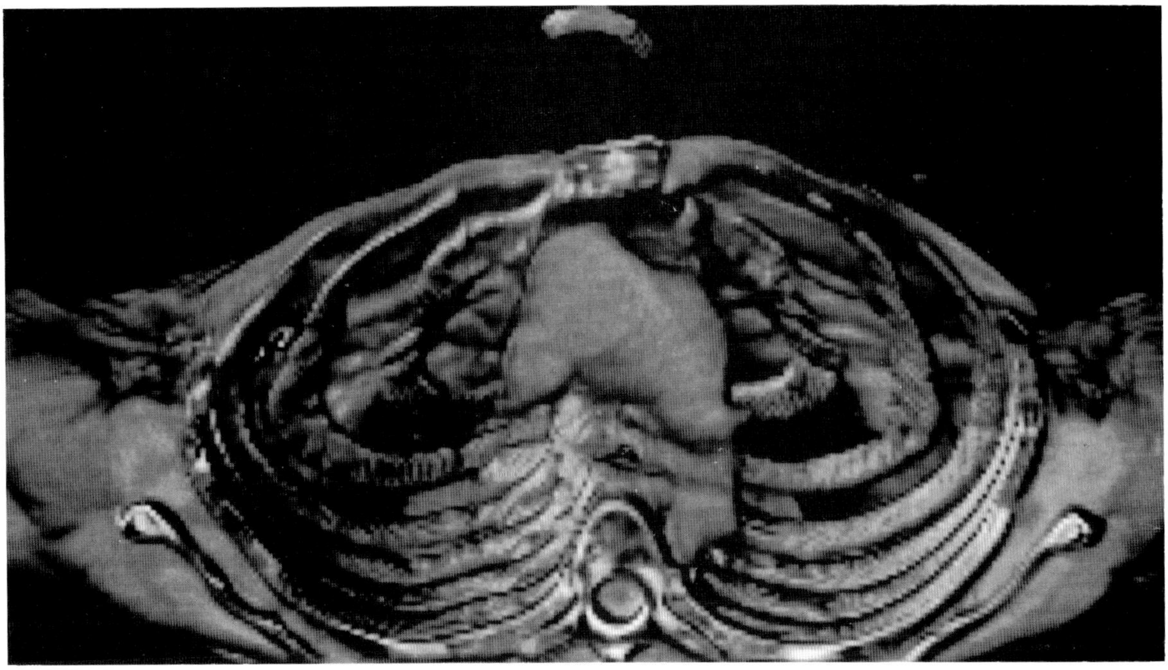

Fig. 7. CT scan of the chest looking from base of heart upward into apex of thoracic cage. Notice cardiac structures, including aorta and pulmonary arteries, clearly defined

success of routine transaxial imaging in the evaluation of pelvic fractures, there are still distinct limitations to this technique, including partial volume effect compromising assessment of the superior pole of the femur and the superior portion of the acetabular joint, and difficulty in conveying a true understanding of the relationships of fracture fragments in cases of complex pelvic trauma.

The addition of coronal and sagittal reformations provides superior visualization of the key weight-bearing structures: the superior pole of femur, the acetabular dome, and the articular surfaces (MAGID et al. 1986a,b). The continuity (fragment distraction) and the congruity (surface step-off) of the acetabular side of the joint are best displayed on these reformatted images. In our initial series of 40 patients we found that in four patients the CT/MPR allowed fractures to be detected that had either been missed (three) or questionable (one) on plain film. Equally important was the effect on patient management. Five patients with planned closed management by traction subsequently underwent open reduction and internal fixation as direct results of CT/MPR. Three patients who had been scheduled for surgery prior to CP/MPR were instead treated more conservatively, without surgical intervention. Historically, there is a high morbidity rate associated with acetabular fractures; we anticipate that increased diagnostic accuracy and detail will contribute to improved clinical outcomes. Although the coronal and sagittal images do provide additional information and do localize the abnormality, these image sequences still require mental integration of individual slices. This requires experience and familiarity with these imaging planes, and it can be very difficult.

Three-dimensional imaging helps to overcome this limitation (BURKS et al. 1985). We routinely create three sequences of images on the Pixar Image Computer. They are the spinal (or pelvic axis) rotation, the somersaulting axis rotation, and the edited spinal rotation, for which part of the initial CT data is removed for an unimpeded view of the part of interest. In patients with a fracture this usually means removal of the contralateral hip. The 3D images created can be viewed as either a simulated real-time video or as serial static images. We found that the 3D real-time rotating image is optimal for both the surgeon and radiologist for a total overview of the abnormality. The ability to rotate the image in 360° in real time is crucial in determining the optimal views for fracture analysis. In patients with complex fractures, this approach allows better preoperative assessment and surgical planning. This 2D and 3D approach has been well received by the orthopedic surgeons in our institutions and is now the central part of any fracture evaluation.

Although three series of view are created, the most important ones in evaluation of acetabular trauma are the edited spinal and somersaulting rotations. The edited spinal axis views tend to be most important for determination of the involvement of the medial wall of the acetabulum and the extent of cephalad extension of fracture line. Fracture mapping clarifies the forces acting on the pelvis during the initial injury, which will influence the approach to reconstruction. The unimpeded view of the inner pelvic wall is particularly unique and is very helpful in orienting to and understanding the exact configuration of the fracture. The somersaulting rotation also provides unique views from a perspective otherwise impossible to obtain. The somersaulting encompasses a series of inlet-outlet views, with the most helpful views often being the direct overhead "bird's eye" view of the pelvic ring. On these views one can best ascertain the integrity of the pelvic ring and its involvement in the fracture, with displacement of medial wall or extension into the ilium clearly defined. Orientation of the femoral heads is particularly helpful in patients with subtle posterior hip dislocation.

With CT being accepted as the study of choice in the evaluation of complex pelvic fractures, essentially little or no additional radiation is required to acquire sufficient data for the 2D and 3D sequences. The main additional requirement is simple computer time on the satellite console of the main CT scanner or on freestanding imaging systems such as the Pixar Image Computer. We feel that the additional information obtained and its effect in clinical management justifies the small additional cost to the patient and time and effort on radiologist's part. We believe that 2D and 3D imaging should be routinely obtained in this group of patients. To evaluate the potential impact of the Pixar 3D images, we reviewed the 3D studies in 19 patients and compared them with conventional X-ray views (Scott et al. 1988a). The purpose of the study was to determine whether the 3D studies added any information to the standard views. The conventional roentgenogram study consisted of between two and five views (AP, oblique, inlet tangential) depending on the individual patient. All 3D studies consisted of spinal (or pelvic) and somersaulting axis rotations. We found that in 10 of 19 cases a nonconventional oblique view (from the spinal series) and in 13 of 19 cases cephalocaudal angulation (from the somersaulting series) other than the inlet, tangential, or AP view best demonstrated the fracture (Table 1). The potential impact of cost of the 3D study was also evaluated and found to be only slightly more than a standard film study (Table 1, 2). The standard imaging technique now employed at Johns Hopkins for suspected pelvic trauma is a routine AP view for detection of the fracture followed by a CT with 2D and 3D imaging.

Table 1. Projection for best fracture visualization

Rotation about	Number of cases	Best projection
Vertical axis	9	45 degree oblique +/− degree or AP
	10	Other obliquity
Horizontal axis	13	Straight above or straight below
	4	Tangential or slightly modified tangential
	1	Inlet
	1	AP

Table 2. Costs for Conventional and Pixar 3D examinations

Examination	Charge
AP pelvis Oblique Inlet Tangential	\$40.50 each
3D Pixar Study	\$250.00 (in addition to modified CT exam charge)
Average conventional film study (2.5 views)	\$101.25
Maximum conventional film study (5 views)	\$202.50

4.4.2 Evaluation of the Shoulder

The shoulder and shoulder joint can often be optimally evaluated using a 3D technique (Figs. 5, 6). In our experience, the most helpful applications include evaluation of fracture and/or dislocation of the humerus, fracture and/or dislocation of the sternoclavicular joint, and evaluation of the thoracic inlet. The key rotational views in these cases are the somersaulting rotation and the edited spinal rotation. In the edited spinal rotation the contralateral shoulder is made totally transparent so as not to mask the abnormal anatomy. The specific advantages include:

1. Definition of sternoclavicular joint is best on the somersaulting view. The best angle presentation has proven to be $-10°$ to $+20°$ in these cases. Orientation of clavicular fracture fragments is best seen on this view as well.
2. Definition of shoulder joint articulation and acromioclavicular joint is best seen on the spinal axis. Any narrowing of joint space or dislocation of joint is best seen on the somersaulting axis. Any narrowing of joint space or dislocation of joint is clearly appreciated on this view.
3. The somersaulting views at 0° and 180° are the optimal viewing angle for evaluating thoracic outlet syndrome due to skeletal causes.
4. The spinal and somersaulting axes rotation with muscle - only views are excellent for evaluating the axillary compartment. With the use of intravenous contrast (Hypaque-60) via the antecubital vein one can clearly outline the individual vascular structures (especially the axillary vein). This is particularly helpful in definition of the relationship of nodes or tumor to the vessels and brachial plexus (the brachial plexus is not defined as a discrete structure but runs in a neurovascular bundle with the axillary artery and vein).

4.4.3 Evaluation of the Sacrum and Spine

The use of volumetric rendering technique is especially valuable in evaluating the lower spine, sacrum, and sacroiliac joints (Figs. 8, 9). The ability to make bone translucent is particularly valuable in looking at the sacroiliac joints, sacral foramina, and articular facets of the lower spine. The somersaulting view is excellent at displaying subtle abnormalities of the sacroiliac joints, including fracture/dislocation and sacroiliitis, and in documenting extension of tumor across the joint space.

With the continuing evolution of these imaging techniques the optimal opacity of bone for individual anatomic zones is undergoing continuous review. The use of increased opacity for bone may prove more useful in imaging the spine, especially the vertebral bodies; Fig. 8 shows the spine visualized with more "opaque" bone. The area of involvement is clearly defined, with excellent definition of the posterior column and adjacent ribs. As mentioned previously, one of the significant advantages

Fig. 8. 3D reconstructions of spine in patient with tubercular osteomyelitis of the spine

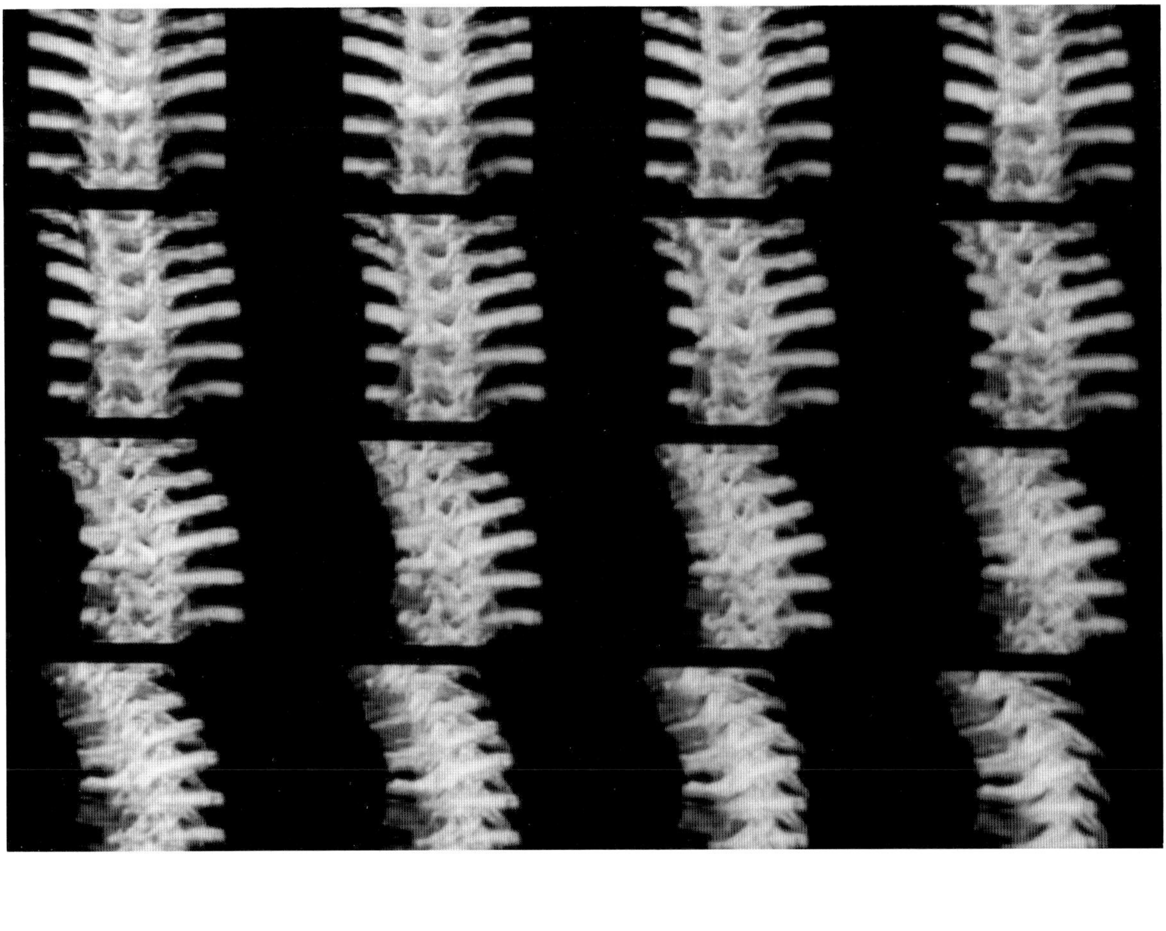

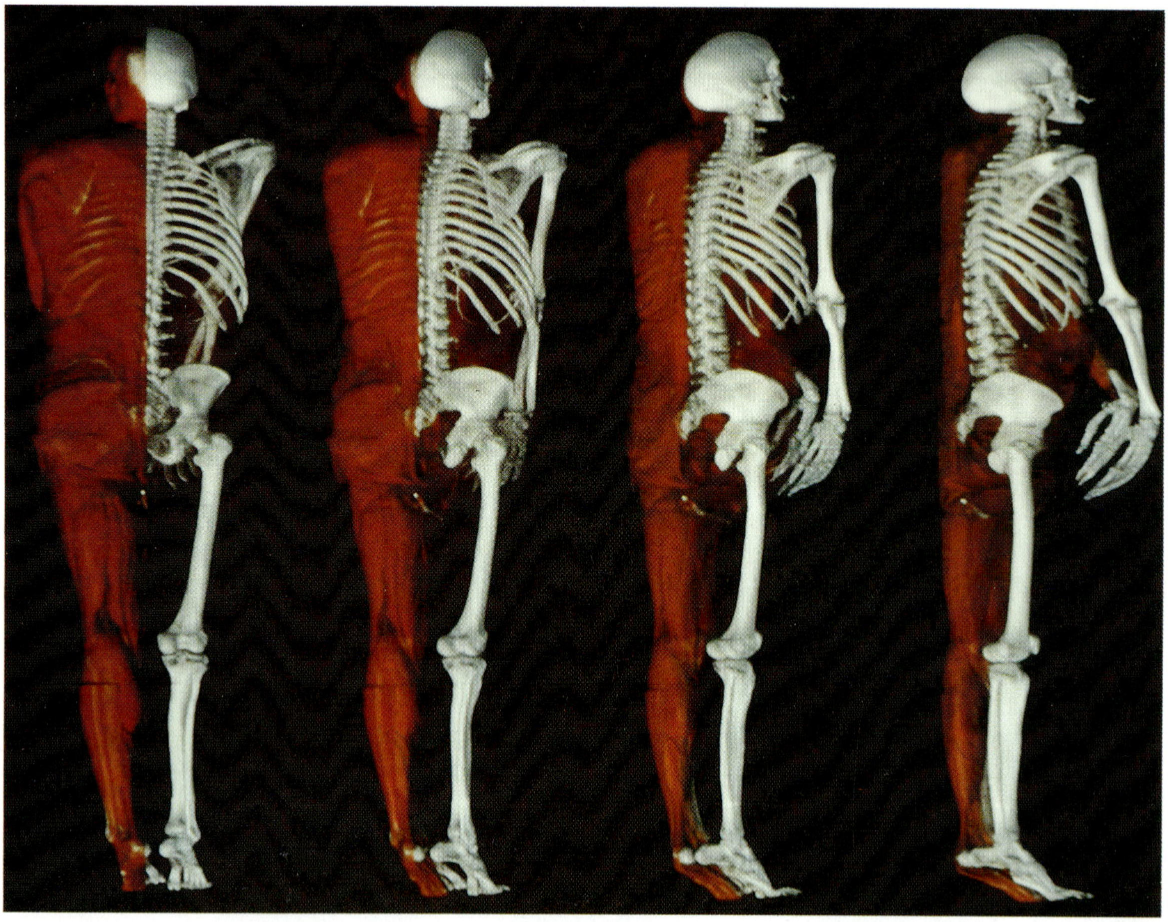

Fig. 9. CT scan of cadaver with half image showing bone opaque and half muscle opaque. Notice detail of structure and muscular definition. (Fishman et al. 1988b)

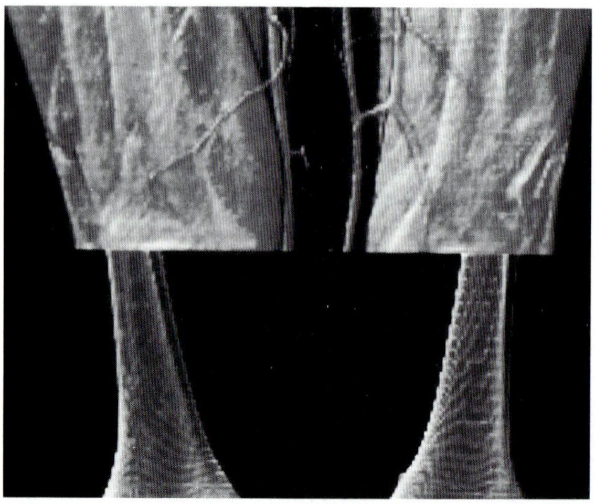

Fig. 10. 3D reconstruction through thigh demonstrating fine vascular detail typically obtained. Vessels with 2 mm thickness in transaxial images can be clearly defined

of volume rendering technique (VRT) is the ability to vary the image parameters to suit the needs of the clinician.

4.4.4 Evaluation of Muscle and the Soft Tissue

The ability to image muscle and soft tissue structures was essentially impossible with classic thresholding techniques. Representation of the subtle attenuation differences between adjacent muscle groups, vascular structures, and tumors was limited with these technologies. With VRT one can display images with bone transparent and muscle opaque. In these images individual muscle bundles as well as vascular structures in the range of 2–3 mm can be displayed with detail approaching anatomic dissection (Figs. 10, 11).

The clinical applications of soft tissue imaging are numerous. To date, they have included:

1. Surgical Planning. Intricate plastic surgery requires understanding the underlying muscle bun-

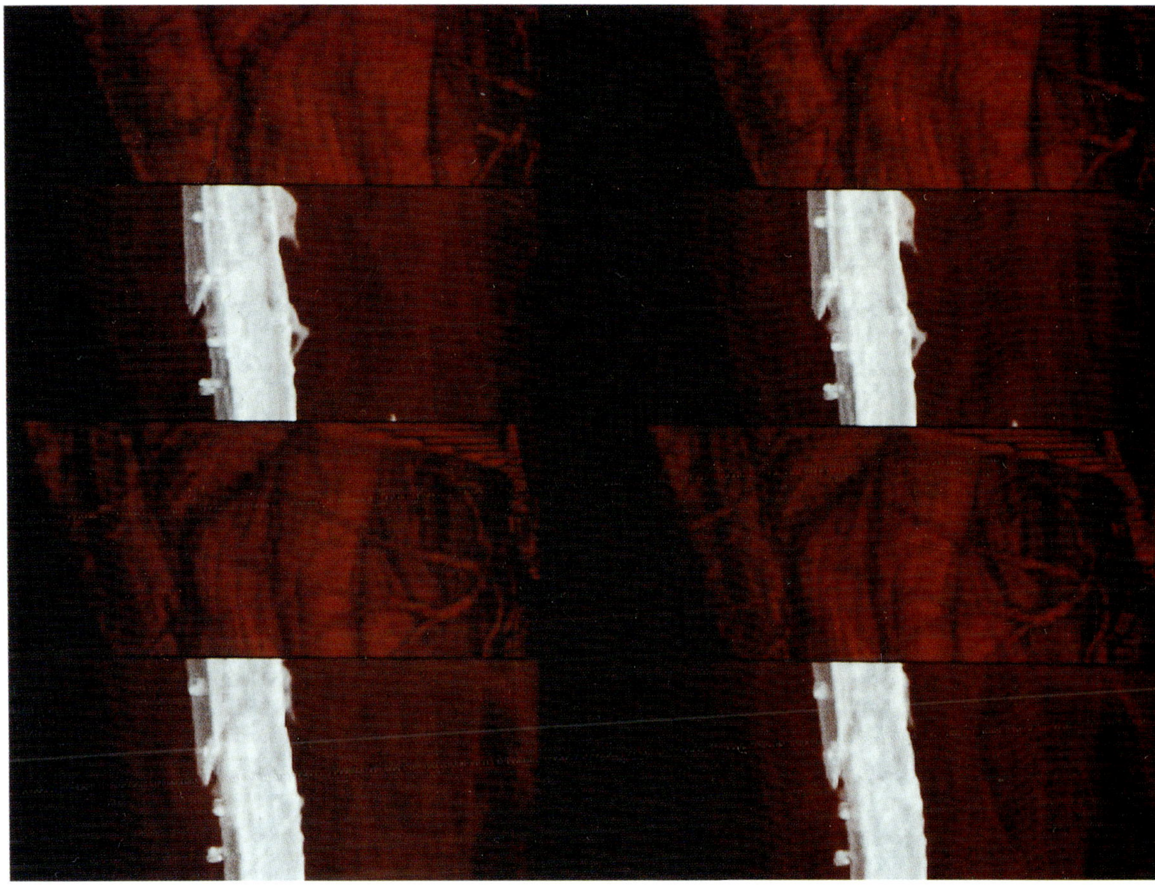

Fig. 11. CT scan of suspected nonunion of femur. Notice evidence of prior pinning with area of nonunion present. Muscle views demonstrate exquisite detail of fine vascular structures of thigh

dles, structures often distorted by prior injury or congential malformation. The 3D representation of such data can be used for deciding on a surgical approach. One limitation of techniques for cosmetic plastic surgery is the use of ionizing radiation for the acquisition of the original dataset. A novel approach to solving this problem is the use of a 3D digitizing system developed by Cyberware Laboratory, Inc. (Pacific Grove, California (Fig. 12). Using a low power laser, the 4020/PS Digitizer rotates around the subject and takes over 250000 3D measurements. The resultant dataset represents the surface of the skin. The data can be represented as a computer-generated image or as a model which can be milled from the 3D information. This technique is new, and more clinical experience will be necessary to determine its accuracy and clinical applicability.

2. Evaluation of Soft Tissue Masses. The use of volumetric rendering technique allows the 3D reconstruction of muscle and soft tissue. Individual muscles and vessels can be defined with fine detail. This provides for the use of 3D CT for localizing soft tissue masses and tumors. At present this information is used for surgical planning. In the future, the information will be used for radiation therapy (Figs. 13, 14).

4.5 Custom Orthopedic Prosthetic Design

Advanced 3D imaging provides far more potential than the simple display of image datasets (Figs. 15-19). The ability to interactively manipulate the data is one of the potentially important advantages of these techniques. Orthopedic prosthetic design can now be done with an increased accuracy and precision (NERUBAY et al. 1981; PELLICCI et al. 1982).

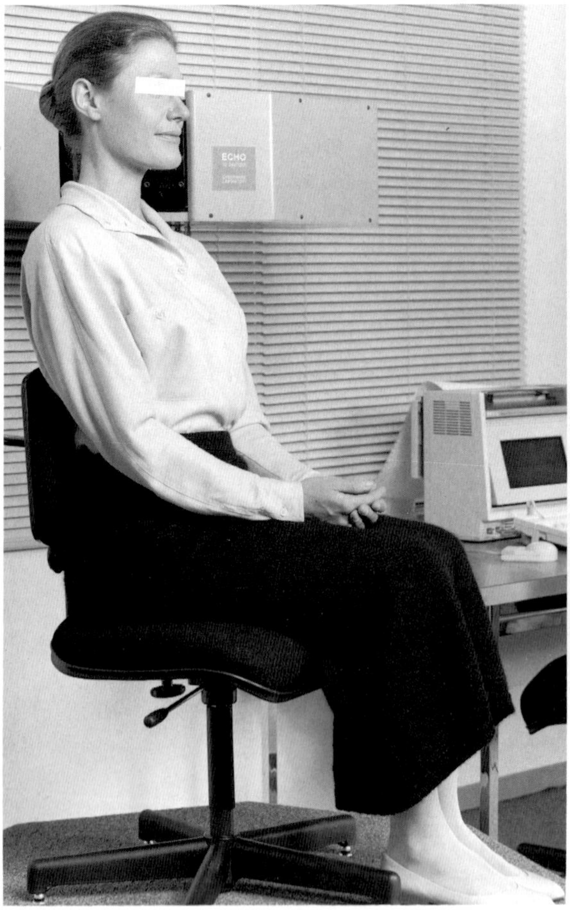

a

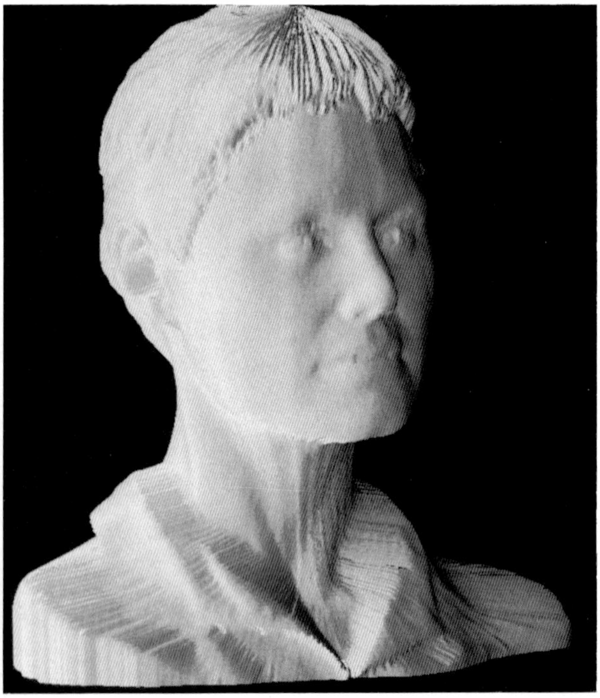

b

Fig. 12. **a** Patient being scanned using Cyberware digitizing system. The chamber will rotate around the patient. **b** Model of patient created seconds after the patient was imaged. No ionizing radiation used in this technique. (Images courtesy of Cyberware Laboratory, Inc.)

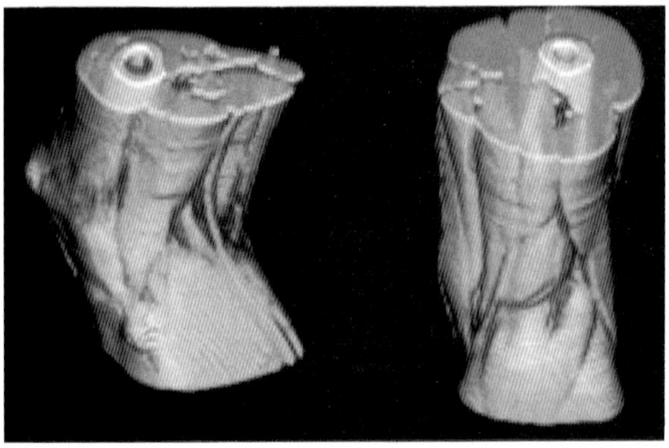

Fig. 13. CT 3D reconstruction of popliteal fossa of both lower extremities. Notice fine detail of muscle and vascular structures

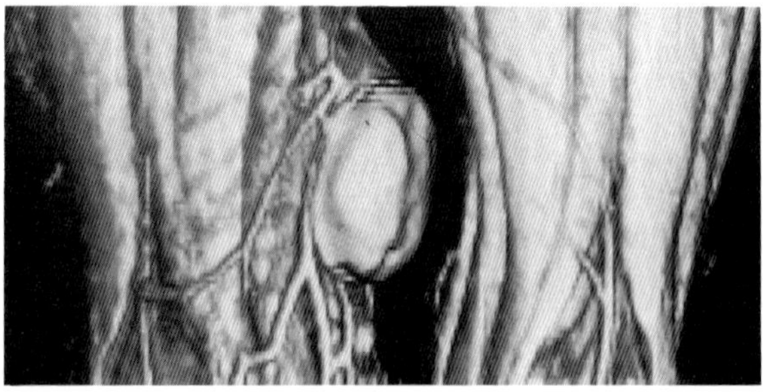

Fig. 14. 3D CT scan reconstruction of mass in right midthigh. Notice the location of tumor as well as the extent of hypervascularity of the mass. Notice the fine detail of vascular as well as muscular structure in this reconstruction

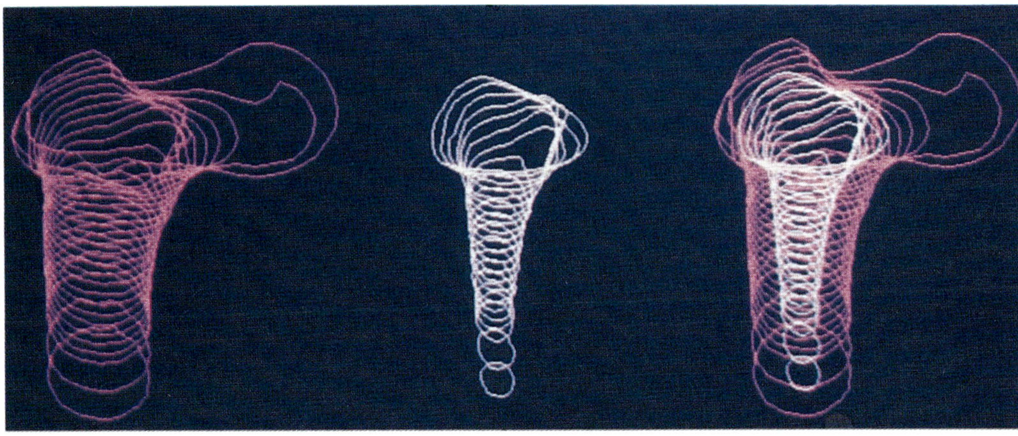

Fig. 15. Stacked transaxial cortical contours. The outer cortical surface is shown in pink and the endosteal or inner cortical surface in white, with these surfaces shown independently (*left* and *center*) and superimposed (*right*)

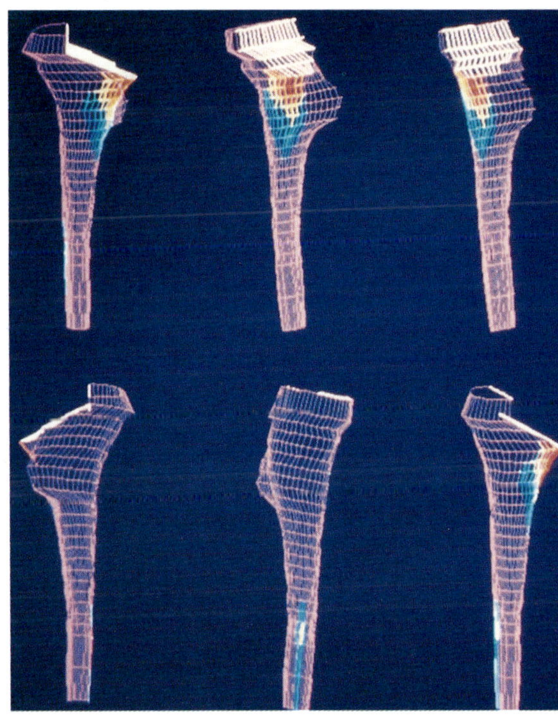

Fig. 16. A "wire-frame" display model of the inner cortex has been scored to designate high priority contact zones: the proximal medial region (approximating the native calcar) and the distal lateral region

The normal and abnormal hip can be used to illustrate many general orthopedic principles, problems, and techniques. The hip arthroplasty, for example, has drawn the interest and attention of researchers in biomechanics, orthopedics, and diagnostic imaging for many years. The hip is the largest weight-bearing joint in the body; the goal of arthroplasty is the recovery of a pain-free range of motion and maintenance of biomechanical integrity under full weight-bearing conditions. With increasing life expectancies, a more active older population, and the increasing survival of younger patients with such problems as organ transplants, severe trauma, or collagen vascular disease, it is of little surprise that hip arthroplasty is an increasingly common procedure. One drawback to this procedure has been its predictably limited life span; the 35 year old renal transplant with steroid-induced avascular necrosis and the active 60 year old with a femoral neck fracture must both be advised of the possibility of a revision procedure at a later date (Chandler et al. 1981).

Improvements in prosthetic design, implant technique, metallurgy, and other technologies have extended the expected functional life of the hip arthroplasty. It is anticipated that the applications of current and emerging 3D CT technology will allow still further improvements in this area. This can be illustrated by a closer look at one application, the design of custom optimal-fit femoral components (Poss et al. 1987).

The expanded prosthetic inventory now includes bipolar, threaded ingrowth cemented, and various custom designs, each appropriate to certain situations or addressing certain shortcomings in earlier designs, and each requiring certain specialized tools and surgical experience for implantation. Conventionally, the custom-designed component has been sized and designed using either 2D radiographs (AP and lateral views) or transaxial CT. The latter has provided more accurate measurements of the area of interest, but in most cases the actual process of design remains a manual function (Poss et al.

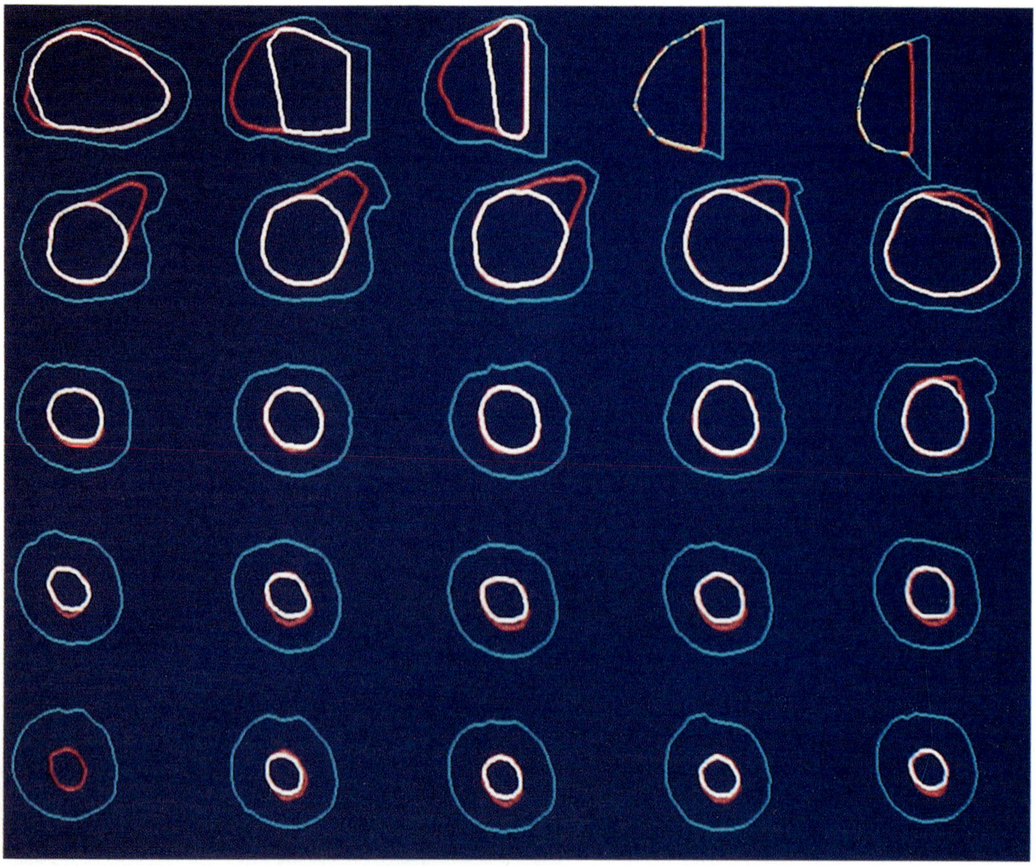

Fig. 17. Transaxial sectioning of the optimal-fit stem-bone computer model maps the outer cortex in blue, the endosteal surface in red, and the stem in white. Gaps between the inner surface and stem are necessary to satisfy the geometry of insertion. Areas of high priority contact show overlap of red and white, indicating optimal canal filling at those points. (Proximal to distal, from *top row* to *bottom left*)

1987). The potentially conflicting goals of the final design include maximizing internal cortical contact with metal and reasonably easy surgical insertion through the proximal femoral exposure. In the uncemented prosthesis, maximum endosteal contact improves distribution of stress, resists axial torque, reduces bone resorption and sinkage, and restricts micromotion. An exact-fit stem, which would in fact be precisely canal shaped, would be the biomechanical ideal; unfortunately, such a component could not be inserted through the proximal femoral exposure. The complex geometry of the proximal femoral shaft, which curves in three planes, requires that portions of the exact-fit stem be reduced or removed to allow insertion. An optimal-fit stem must be designed, therefore, which can be surgically inserted while retaining as much cortical-stem contact and as many biomechanically desirable properties as possible.

This can be done with 3D CT (Poss et al. 1987). The transaxial CT data are transferred to an image processor. Edge detection algorithms with dimensional corrections increase the accuracy of measurements of the periosteal (outer) and endosteal (inner) aspects of canal geometry. Bone specimen and bone phantom tests correlate sizing accuracy; our bone geometry measurements display less than 1% (or less than 1 mm) inaccuracy at the periosteal cortical surface and less than 5% (still less than 1 mm) at the endosteal cortical surface (Robertson and Huang 1986). Three interactive software modules (preprocessing, stem design, and post-processing) are applied. The preprocessing module will simulate bone preparation (head and neck resection, and canal reaming and rasping) prior to stem insertion. Critical endosteal surface for stem-bone load transfer and for stem immobility are identified and assigned a high priority score; high score regions (for example, the contact at the medial wall and calcar, and at the distal lateral wall, to control load transfer

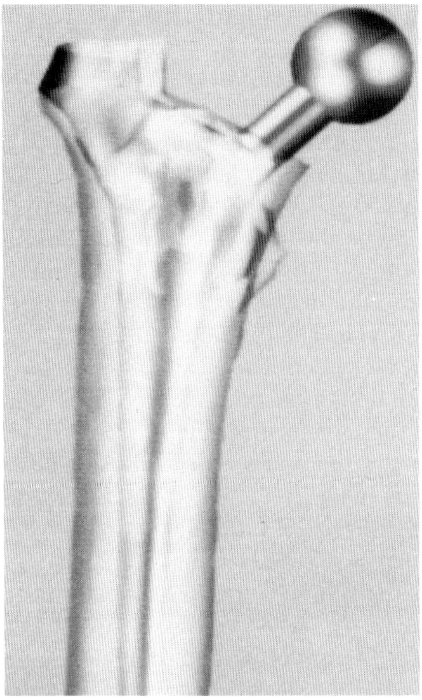

18

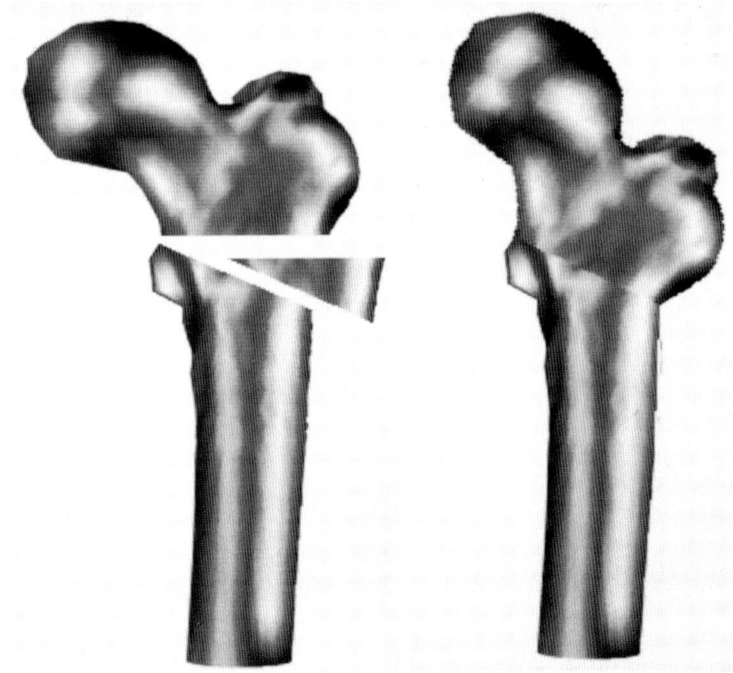

19a b

Fig. 18. Anterior-posterior computer view of the resultant optimal-fit stem inserted into the tranlucent femur

Fig. 19a, b. Simulated 3D views of a left femur demonstrating a proximal wedge osteotomy (**a**) and the resultant realignment of the femur following osteotomy (**b**)

and rocking, respectively) are to be retained in the process of whittling the canal-filling ideal stem down to an insertable geometry (Poss et al. 1987).

The second module designs the stem, starting with a precise endosteal match, or canal-filling model. This initial stem is vertically translated proximally in small increments. At each position, motion in the other five degrees of freedom is simulated and an overlap of stem with the canal surface is determined. A series of overlap scores is obtained by a formula multiplying overlap scores and priority scores; a position of minimalized score can be calculated by using a modified Newton's optimization algorithm. The stem is placed in this optimal position, and the portions of stem which overlap bone in this position are shaved off the hypothetical model so that the stem once more fits within the endosteal surface. The stem is again vertically translated to the next position, and the scoring and reshaping process repeated. Once the entire stem has been vertically translated in increments through the proximal femoral neck cut, the resultant shape should be the optimal compromise between the complete canal filling and the demands of insertion through the neck osteotomy. (Poss et al. 1987).

The third, postprocessing module verifies and edits the stem design. A graphics modeling package can now be used to generate actual 3D models of the stem, and of the stem implanted in bone. Finite element analysis is used on the mechanical environment of stem and bone. A computerized milling machine produces the femoral stem from the design program.

By filling plastic stem models, implanting them in cadaver bone, and repeating the initial transaxial CT endosteal cortical contour and analysis procedure, the stem-canal fit can be assessed. Adequate fit is defined as less than 1-mm gap between stem and endosteal surface. A standard off-the shelf symmetric (coronal plane) hip stem has up to 4% overall fit, with up to 7% fit at the high priority regions. In contrast, the 3D computer models of the optimal-fit stem predicted a total contact (or fit) of 68% with priority contact of 80%. The actual milled and reanalyzed specimens proved to have up to 38% overall contract (fit) and up to 41% at high priority regions (Poss et al. 1987).

While it is currently impractical to use this program for each hip implant, the implications are many. This system of analysis and design has been applied to series of femurs to produce an average 3D canal model. This simulated average canal was then used to design an off-the-shelf optimal-fit stem system, computer scaled into a range of six sizes, which is currently undergoing clinical trials (Poss et al. 1987). The custom-design approach can also be used for patients with unique problems of unique anatomy: the patient needing a revision, whose loss of bone stock precludes use of a standard stem; the patient with infection, gunshot wound, or other osteolytic process; or the patient with anomalous anatomy, either congenital or acquired. Since it is anticipated that the custom-fit stem will have improved biomechanics and presumably a longer functional life, it also may be appropriate to use this approach in the younger, healthier patient whose life expectancy and activity levels exceed that of the typical hip arthroplasty recipient (Rhodes et al. 1987; Woolson et al. 1986).

Three-dimensional CT technology has other potential applications. Bone stock loss can be mapped and analyzed for better understanding of the pathology involved, and for better design accommodating the biomechanical demands of suboptimal bone stock situations. Load simulation and analysis is analogous to using 3D computer simulations to study the aerodynamics of a new plane or car design. An external force system may be applied to the models, to study the response to axial load, torque, load transfer, and stress risers, and to determine the potential for motion once implanted. Since 3D models of both the bone and the hardware can be milled off of processed transaxial CT data, rehearsal surgery can be performed to train less experienced physicians in new techniques or in using new tools, and to test various design features of new tools or new implants.

4.6 Radiation Therapy Simulation and Planning

Destruction of cancerous cells without injury to normal tissue is the goal of chemotherapy and/or radiation therapy (Fig. 20). Unfortunately, achieving this goal may be difficult when ionizing radiation is used. A more realistic goal is the delivery of maximum dose to the tumor bed while limiting the dose to normal tissue. The development of CT and MRI has proven to be critical in radiation therapy planning. Better definition of tumor position and extent have led to more accurate therapy ports, as is documented in the literature. Studies have shown that 30%–40% of initial treatment plans are modified based simply on the use of CT.

Yet the standard CT therapy plan is a 2D representation while the tumor is truly 3D. This can be solved by using a true 3D planning system. The ideal system could incorporate data obtained from multiple imaging techniques including CT, MRI and positron emission tomography (PET). By combining anatomic and physiologic data a precise localization of the tumor could be obtained. Ideally, this process should be done interactively in real time. Initial work on this process has been done at the University of Michigan in Ann Arbor under the

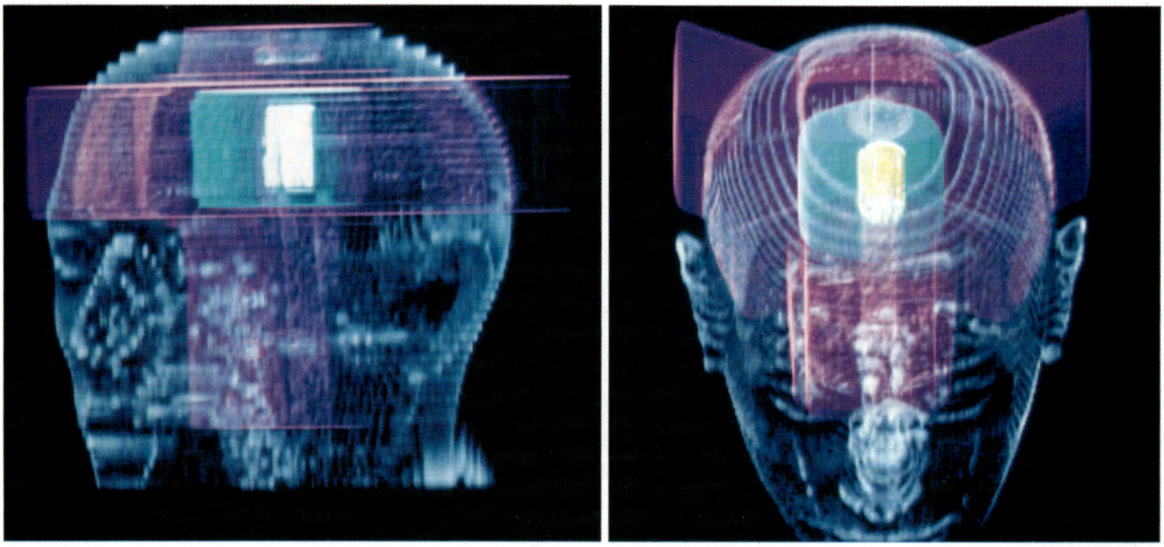

a b

Fig. 20 a, b. 3D radiation therapy planning image. This simulated 3D radiation therapy dose absortion profile was generated at the University of Southern California from CT head scans with superimposed beam reference data in place. (Image courtesy of Dr. Frederick W. George III) direction of Dr. Allen S. Lichter, Chairman of Radiation Oncology, and his colleagues (LICHTER 1987) (Fig. 19).

4.7 Other Clinical Applications of Three-dimensional Imaging

Three-dimensional medical imaging has been developing at a rapid pace, and will continue to do so (Fig. 21). The most visible development will be a rapid increase in the clinical use of 3D imaging. Although most 3D medical imaging is presently being done with CT data, it will be applied to many other modalities. The computing equipment for 3D imaging has been steadily increasing in performance in respect to price. This trend will result in faster and cheaper methods for solving current problems. It will allow tasks which are too grand for present-day computers to be solved in the future. All of these predictions point to a rapid increase in the amount of 3D medical imaging being done.

Oncology is a very natural application of 3D imaging (YANG et al. 1986; ETTINGER et al. 1985). It will allow for accurate visualization of tumor evolution. A combination of visualization and accurate volumetrics would be invaluable. Radiation therapy planning can and should be done in three dimensions. Eventually, beam placement and dose calculation will be combined in an interactive process that will result in very effective treatment (Fig. 20).

Interactive surgical simulation has and will be a hot topic in 3D medicine. The concept of simulating surgical methods upon the patient using a computer has obvious applications. However, much work needs to be done before this idea becomes a practical reality. Interactive simulation calls for 3D view generation at speeds approaching real time. This requirement calls for more computing power

Fig. 21. Orthotool reconstructions demonstrating complex right acetabular fracture. Notice how reformatting from coronal and sagittal clearly shows the full extent of injury and the deficiency in the weight-bearing surface. The full sequence of 3D images gives additional information on the extent of injury

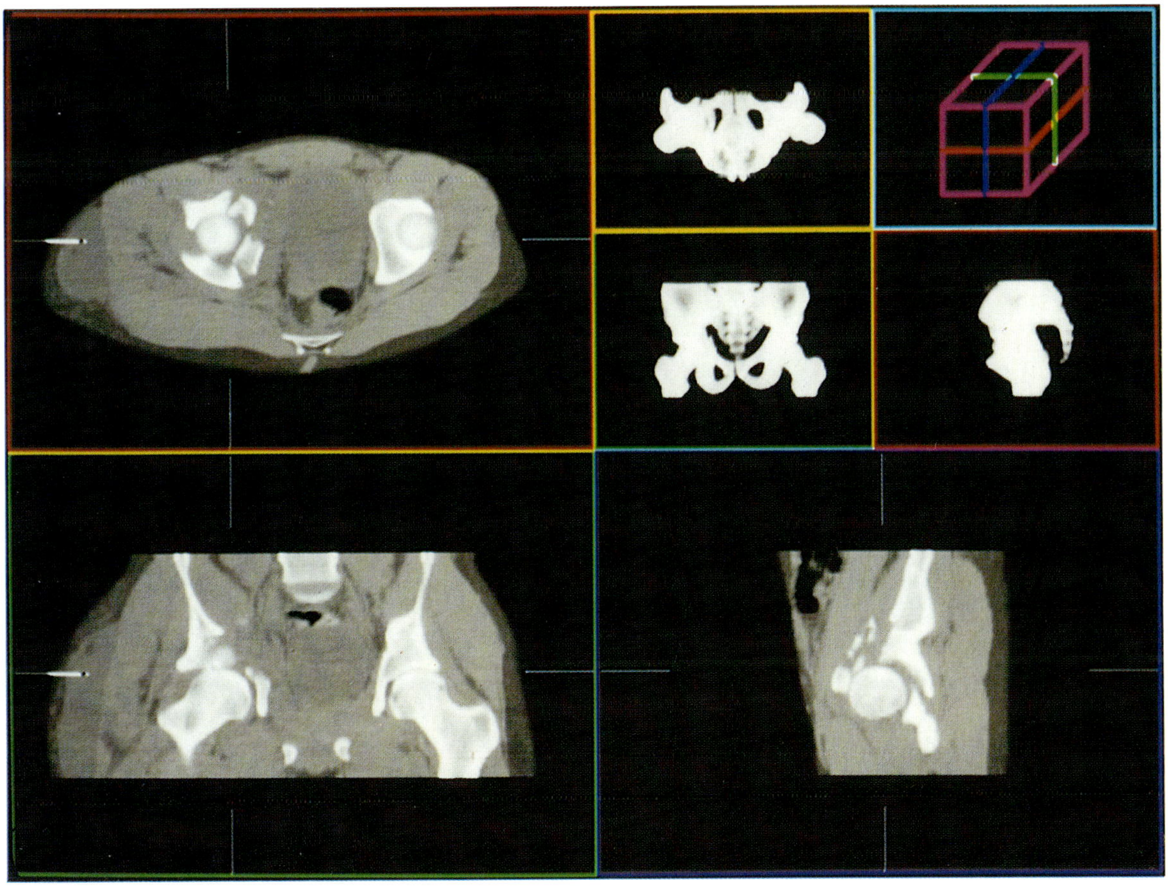

than is readily available now. If the rapid advancements in computer hardware architecture continue, this power will exist in less than 5 years. Methods for specifiying actions in 3D-space upon a volume also need to be refined. Present-day volume editors are, at their best, quite cumbersome and tedious to use.

Light microscopy generates data volumes which would benefit greatly from 3D visualization. The visualization of small structures in three dimensions will have application to detection and prevention of disease. Cellular biology will certainly benefit from 3D visualization of microstructures. Although little work has been done in this area, there is nothing intrinsically difficult about visualizing microvolumes. Visualization of microvolumes will become a very important and active part of 3D medical imaging.

The educational use of 3D medical imaging will become an important field on its own. Teaching images based on this technology will have clarity that is only matched by actual dissection. An educational video tape depicting anatomic relationships in three dimensions will have obvious impact on medical education. The ability to manipulate the image will undoubtedly prove useful in tracing surgical residue or in rehearsing difficult procedures. We have recently developed a new interactive imaging program called Orthotool which can be used for educational instruction. This tool takes a standard CT volume (Figs. 21, 22) and allows the physician or technologist to roam through the transaxial, coronal, and sagittal images in real time via simple mouse motion on the computer. The images can be viewed with different windows, can be zoomed to a 1:1 size, or distances and angles measured. An arbitrary oblique plane can be chosen and all images rotated in that plane. 3D views are also provided for easy orientation.

Magnetic resonance imaging has been gaining increasing acceptance in the medical community (HIGGINS et al. 1983) (Fig. 23). The data produced by the MR scanner are similar to those produced by CT scans. There are, however, a number of negative characteristics that are found in MR scans, and not

Fig. 22. Orthotool reconstruction of patient with lung cancer and right hip pain. Notice on all three views the presence of a blastic lesion in the right femur near the level of the greater trochanter. This was a metastasis. Plain film in this patient was negative and bone scan equivocal. The Orthotool provides an interactive mode for evaluating transaxial, coronal, and sagittal images with orienting 3D views also supplied

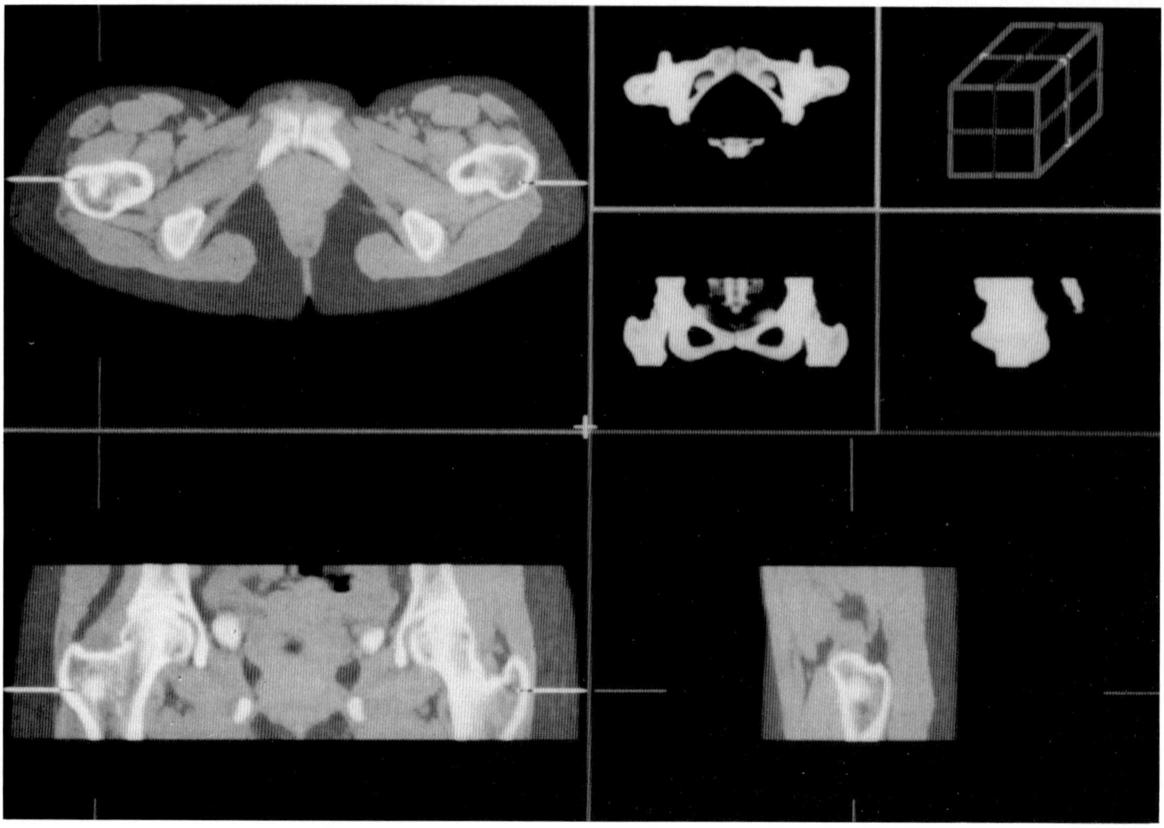

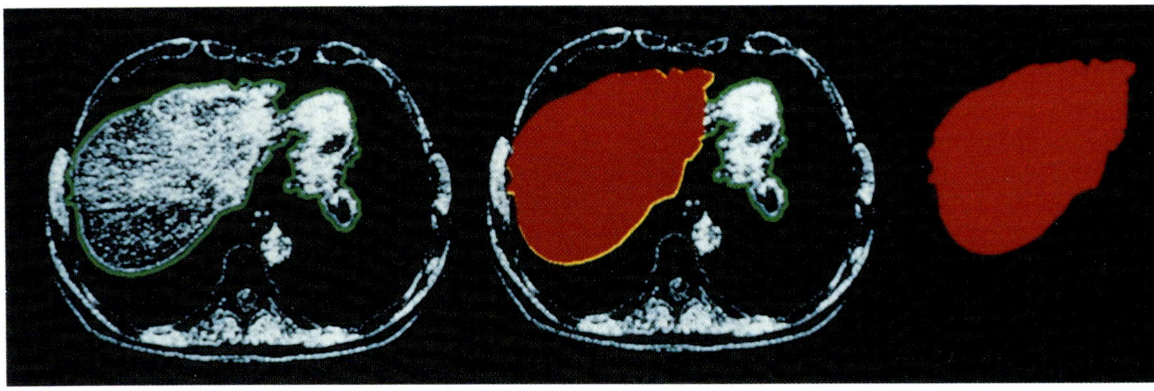

Fig. 23. Sequence of images demonstrating computer detection of boundaries of liver with demarcation of liver. This can be used for therapy planning or for tumor volumetrics

in CT scans. Obtaining slices that form a contiguous volume is more difficult with an MRI scanner. Each MRI scan is spatially nonlinear (warped) to some degree. The reading obtained from a given tissue scanned with a certain technique tends to vary considerably. The generation of 3D visualizations becomes highly dependent on scan technique. This can be turned into an advantage which MRI has over CT. Proper scan technique can increase differentiation of various tissues, allowing for better volume visualization. By correlating two or more scans that use different scan techniques (emphasizing different features) one can produce visualizations with exactly the desired information clearly indicated. In the future, 3D/MR imaging will grow to equal if not surpass 3D imaging with CT.

Nuclear medicine studies produce data which are generally of quite coarse spatial resolution. 3D visualizations of these data will not be the pleasing anatomic models that are produced with CT data. However, this does not indicate any lack in usefulness of such visualizations. 3D imaging of nuclear medicine data alone will suffer from difficulty in finding a reference point in the real anatomy. Correlation of nuclear medical data with MRI or CT will be very effective. See chap. 3 for additional information. Correlating sets of scan data of a given volume obtained from different modalities is difficult only because of registration. Many methods of registration have been suggested and tried. Automated registration with no human intervention is not yet available. Correction for spatial nonlinearities in the two data sets could conceivably be a problem. For many applications, the warping of the volume will be small enough that it can be ignored. A correction method for volume warping would still be useful. Once these problems are solved, the use of correlated modalities will be very common.

4.8 Tumor Volumetrics

Tumor volumetrics are essential to accurately follow the impact of oncotherapy. We have developed a technique, using the Sun/Pixar combination, to determine organ and tumor volumes intelligently, despite the use of noisy CT or MRI data (Fig. 23).

A number of factors may obscure the boundary between an organ and adjacent tissue. Let us consider a case which is of great clinical interest and which has many of the difficult features inherent in selecting out organs; that is the liver which has a hepatoma (liver cancer). In the case of the liver being imaged with a CT scanner, there may be no CT window that can be set which lets one differentiate between the liver and adjacent abdominal wall tissue. In this situation the computer must use information about the likely shape and location of the organ. If one is lucky, there may be only a small band of contact. This typically appears to be a finger-like protrusion. For the liver to develop such shapes is exceedingly unlikely, and so they can be omitted. Thus, after doing an edge detection based on CT values in an appropriate window and centered in the liver, any finger-like protrusion is replaced with a curve based on points adjacent to the protrusion. The curves used to do such a fit can be anything from a simple polygonal section to rational function, Bezier, spline, bi-cubic, etc. On the other hand, one may be unlucky, especially in cases involving advanced malignancies; then an entire edge of the enlarged liver may be indistinguishable from the abdominal wall. In such cases, one must make the computer do what one does by eye; that is, fit a reasonable curve which starts at the distinguishable parts of the edge and progresses through the difficult region. All these high likelihood regions are combined and made into a matte (mask) which is used to select out the liver from the data.

Scanners sample space in a rectangular lattice. In a given cell in that lattice one may have only one material or one may have multiple materials. Only one number comes out of that region for a given set up of the scanner. We will call that the "scan number." It is the CT (Hounsfield) number on CT scanners. On MR scanners the "MR" number depends on the pulse sequence that is chosen. Nonetheless, for a given pulse sequence each material will have a consistent signal strength. Realistic colors can be assigned to all scan numbers in a given scan number window. Since different CT densities correspond to different sorts of tissue, the CT window of values corresponding to bone, for example, can be mapped into a range of partially transparent whites (high and equal RGB values with a moderate degree of opacity in the alpha channel). Similarly "muscle" CT values can be mapped into a range of nearly transparent reddish brown, etc. These color mapped data are then combined to give a variable transparency color view through the subject. The colormaps can be changed to emphasize features of interest such as bones or soft tissue.

A further refinement is possible by making a "soft window." These windows are described using four numbers. Starting at the lowest scan number, the low value is that which is the last value for cells containing 0% of the material; the next is the first value for cells containing 100% of the material. This can be viewed as an upgoing line (if linearly interpolated). Then there is a set of values for cells containing 100% of the material. This ends at some upper value. This is a straight line segment. Next there is range of values going from 100% of that material down to 0% of that material. This is a downgoing line segment (if linearly interpolated).

Now, in fact, a given cell in the lattice may actually consist of several materials, but with only one data set one cannot differentiate more than two materials. Still, it is a significantly better approximation to the true data to model the region as two materials rather than one. However, two values work perfectly if one is interested in a region which is an organ versus its neighbors (versus not organ). Use of soft windows will yield a more accurate volume because all edge effects (including internal edges) are treated more accurately. Knowing the scale size of the scanner, the number of cells (e.g., 512×512), and the interslice distance gives a volume per cell. The total volume is computed by multiplying this number times the total of the partially contributing voxels in every high likelihood region.

Having selected the liver using a soft window, a scan number window appropriate to tumor densities is chosen. This window has soft edges in that values above or below are only permitted a partial contribution. All voxels in the liver that are also in that window are labeled. This yields the tumor volume by computing the total of the partially contributing voxels in every high likelihood region for the whole liver volume.

At this point in time the computer cannot handle all cases of arbitrarily complicated pathology. As a compromise a fit is suggested which can be improved through mouse interaction to control the location of the curve. Additional information about volumetrics can be found in chap. 3.

4.9 Three-dimensional Database and Combining Images

Three-dimensional image recontraction offers a number of benefits in comparison with 2D recontraction, including improved visualization of complicated fractures, reduction of noise with consequent ability to produce clear images even when pins or prostheses are present, etc. However, at present images are not computed in real time; rather they are precomputed for a preselected range of angles and then exhibited in rapid sequence (animated). Instead we construct a 3D database for CT, MR, or other scanner data that can be examined in as nearly real time as possible, given our equipment, from a user selectable set of angles. There is one angle for each of the three planes xy, yz, and xz. There are currently two levels of quality available. One of these is a rapid scan mode with some loss of detail, the other is high quality mode. This allows one to home in on the optimal view of a particular feature quickly and then produce a high quality picture once the view is found.

First we perform any preprocessing of the data that may be desired. This can include removal of extraneous objects such as the scanner table, or the data may be rescaled or rotated into a particular configuration. But, almost always it involves interpolation of the data in the longitudinal direction so that the vertical scale will be appropriate to the horizontal scale. This data set is then stored to disk.

These data, once loaded into the 24-Mbyte frame buffer of the Pixar, can be viewed from any perspective by projecting the data onto a plane which is oriented at the three user-selectable angles associated with the three mutually perpendicular planes which can be passed through the 3D database. The projection is performed using ray tracing techniques. Given a set of angles, one computes the set of point in the frame buffer corresponding to a ray The raw data which consist of scan number data (scaler data) are converted from an integer into RGB color plus opacity via a color lookup table. These four integers are generated so as to optimize the visual information. For example, in CT, those densities corresponding to bone are made into nearly opaque white; those corresponding to muscle are made into transparent red-brown, etc. The pixels along a ray are merged under their predecessors using the opacity information and a weighting factor. They are then stored to the scratchpad. The process is repeated for a line and then for the whole plane. When a line has been generated, it is sent out to the display unit. The difference in quality and speed of the two modes depends upon the fact that in the low quality mode some data points are skipped.

One major advantage of this system is that by simply changing the colormap both CT and MR data can be presented in a single unified manner. This permits intercomparison of scans from these different imaging modalities and from the same modality at different times. To optimize intercomparison we will add the ability to rescale along any axis. This is desirable because there can be both horizontal and vertical scaling differences between imaging techniques. Indeed, one may wish to utilize a reference grid and a deformation map, which must be three dimensional, at some future date. Needless to say, this can also be very useful for highlighting differences between serial scans taken on the same machine. Alternatively, the colormaps can be selected so that the two images can be superimposed and a new imaging modality "combined imaging" such as MR+CT becomes avilable. This can be especially exciting when the information from the two scanners is very different, for example, if one is a nuclear medicine scanner and the other is an "anatomic" scanner such as MR or CT. Thus if a patient had a hip abscess, it could be highlighted using a nuclear medicine scan and localized using a CT scan. The two images could then be superimposed so that a surgeon could plan his approach. Similarly, by creating a composite image of CT and MR scans one can combine the optimal bone definition of high resolution CT with the excellent soft tissue discrimination of MRI. More on multiple modality image registration can be found in chap. 3.

4.10 Pattern Recognition and Artificial Intelligence

So far we have mainly discussed techniques that are either currently done or very near completion. In this section we will discuss some things that are a little further down the road. This will undoubtedly entail significant changes in the hardware and software.

Ideally, it would be nice to have a system that knew enough about human anatomy and its representation via scanners that one could request an organ by name and the computer would locate it entirely on its own, isolate the organ, and present it to the viewer from an arbitrary, selectable perspective in real time. Furthermore, enough knowledge of standard pathologies should be available that the computer would suggest to the system user a prioritized list of the feature that it has found. One would hope that such a system would be flexible enough that the user would not be just a radiologist in a major hospital but any properly trained physician. Indeed the differential diagnoses might well be more useful to the nonradiologist, the surgeon or internist late at night, or even to a single physician at an isolated outpost.

To accomplish such a goal will require an extensive "expert system" coupled to pattern recognition features from the "robot vision" aspect of the computer sciences and fed by the expertise of radiologists. The computation problem of real-time presentation will probably be solved using highly parallel systems. Searching through large knowledge-based systems may also take a similar approach.

4.11 Conclusion

This chapter has provided at best a cursory glance at one of the most exciting areas in radiology; the application of cutting edge computer graphics to provide advanced solutions to practical medical imaging problems. Although many of these applications are used by only a handful of institutions at present we feel that the diffusion of this technology will occur over a short period of time due to its wide clinical acceptance and its positive effect on patient management. The speed of this diffusion will require the coordinated efforts of radiologists, computer scientists, and representatives of key subspecialties like orthopedic surgery and radiation therapy. In a combined effort, the only apparent visible limitation to its future development is our own imagination and ability.

References

Burks DL Jr, Mears DC, Kennedy WH, Cooperstein LA, Herbert DL (1985) Three dimensional computed tomography of acetabular fractures. Radiology 155: 183-186

Chandler HP, Reineck FT, Wixon RL, McCarthy JC (1981) Total hip replacement in patients younger than thirty years old. J Bone Joint Surg 63A: 1426-1434

Ettinger DS, Leichner PK, Siegelman SS, Fishman EK, Klein JL, Order SE (1985) Computed tomography assisted volumetric analysis of primary liver tumors as a measure of response to therapy. Am J Clin Oncol 8: 413-418

Fishman EK, Magid D, Mandelbaum BR et al. (1986) Multiplanar (MPR) imaging of the hip. RadioGraphics 6: 7-54

Fishman EK, Drebin RA, Magid D et al. (1987) Volumetric rendering techniques: application for 3-dimensional imaging of the hip. Radiology 163: 737-738

Fishman EK, Magid D, Ney DR, Drebin RA, Kuhlman JE (1988a) 3-Dimensional imaging and display of musculoskeletal anatomy. J Comput Assist Tomogr 12: 465-467

Fishman EK, Drebin RA, Hruban RH, Ney DR. Magid D (1988b) Technical note. Three-dimensional recontruction of the human body. AJR 150: 149-1420

Herman GT, Vose WF, Gomori JM, Gefter WB (1985) Stereoscopic computed three-dimensional surface displays, RadioGraphics 6: 825-852

Higgins CB, Goldberg H, Hricak H et al. (1983) Nuclear magnetic resonance imaging of vasculature of abdominal viscera: normal and pathologic features. AJR 140: 1217-1225

Lichter AS (1987) Radiation therapy treatment planning. CT, MR imaging and three dimensional planning. Radiology 165(P): 118-119

Magid D, Fishman EK, Mandelbaum BR, Brooker AF Jr, Siegelman SS (1986a) Computed tomography with multiplanar recontructions in the assessment and management of acetabular fractures. J Comput Assist Tomogr 10: 778-783

Magid D, Fishman EK, Brooker AF Jr, Scott WW Jr, Riley LH (1986b) A systematic approach to the hip: computed tomography with multiplanar recontruction. Contemp Ortho 13(6): 15-23

Nerubay J, Rubenstein Z, Katznelson A (1981) Technique of building a hemipelvic prosthesis using computer tomography. Prog Clin Biol Res 99: 147-152

Pellicci PM, Wilson PD, Sledge CB, Salvati EA, Renawat CS, Poss R (1982) Revision total hip arthroplasty. Clin Orthop 170: 3-41

Poss R, Robertson DD, Walker PS, Reilly DT, Ewald FC, Thomas WH, Sledge CB (1987) Anatomic stem design for press-fit and cemented application. In: Fitzgerald RH Jr (ed) Non-cemented total hip arthroplasty: the bone interface. Churchill Livingstone, New York

Rhodes ML, Azzawi Y, Chu E, Glenn W, Rothman S (1985) Anatomic model and prostheses manufacturing using CT data. Proc Conference and Exposition of the NCGA 110-124

Robertson DD, Huang HK (1986) Quantitative bone measurements using x-ray computed tomography with second order correction. Med Phys 13: 474-479

Scott WW Jr, Fishman EK, Magid D (1986a) Optimal imaging of acetabular fractures. Radiology (in press)

Scott WW Jr, Magid D, Fishman EK, Riley LH, Brooker AF Jr, Johnson CA, (1988b) Three dimensional imaging of acetabular trauma. J Orthop Trauma (in press)

Woolson ST, Dev P, Fellingham LL, Vassiliadis A (1986) Three dimensional imaging of the bone from computerized tomography. Clin Orthop 202: 239-248

Yang NC, Leichner PK, Fishman EK et al. (1986) CT volumetrics of primary liver cancer. J Comput Assist Tomogr 10: 621-628

5 NMR Imaging: An Appraisal of the Present and the Future

STEPHEN J. BLACKBAND

CONTENTS

5.1 Brief History and Introduction 69
5.2 Basic Principles 70
5.3 Imaging Techniques 71
5.4 NMR Imaging Hardware 72
5.4.1 General 72
5.4.2 Magnet 73
5.4.3 Gradients 74
5.4.4 Computer 75
5.4.5 rf Coils 75
5.4.6 The Spectrometer 76
5.5 The Information NMR Can Provide 76
5.6 High Speed Imaging 77
5.7 Flow Imaging and Angiography 78
5.8 Multinuclear Imaging 79
5.9 Chemical Shift Imaging 80
5.10 Spatially Localized Spectroscopy 82
5.11 NMR Microscopy 83
5.12 Solid Imaging 85
5.13 Biological Effects Associated with NMR Imaging 85
5.14 Clinical Applications of NMR Imaging 86
5.15 NMR Imaging of Nonmedical Systems 86
5.16 Electron Spin Resonance Imaging: Its Implications on NMR Imaging 88
5.17 New Developments with Potential Impact 88
5.18 Conclusions 89
References 90

5.1 Brief History and Introduction

Since its conception by LAUTERBUR in 1973 and independently by MANSFIELD and GRANNELL (1975), nuclear magnetic resonance (NMR) imaging has grown rapidly to become a viable clinical imaging modality that is now the method of choice for many applications (KRESSEL 1985; STARK and BRADLEY 1988). NMR imaging (often referred to as magnetic resonance imaging, MRI) times have decreased dramatically from hours to milliseconds and resolutions have improved in certain cases from centimeters to microns. A dramatic range of information is available from the technique that sets it apart from all other imaging modalities in terms of its flexibility, and we are still on the growing curve in terms of NMR imaging techniques and applications. The drive behind this virtual explosion of techniques has been the noninvasive nature of NMR imaging and its implications with respect to the diagnostic study of the human body. Most NMR imaging concerns the observation and spatial mapping of the hydrogen nucleus (^{1}H) in water, since water is the most abundant material in the human body and consequently ^{1}H gives the most signal with respect to other resonant nuclei.

Many good reviews of NMR imaging theory, techniques, and clinical applications now exist (MANSFIELD and MORRIS 1982; MORRIS 1986; STARK and BRADLEY 1988; BISESE 1988; DANIELS et al. 1987). The purpose of this chapter within the context of this book is to try to describe concisely the present state of the art of NMR imaging and to indicate where significant advances may be made in the next decade. With respect to these objectives, it will be impossible to give anything but a sparse account of the vast array of literature that now exists with regard to NMR imaging. Rather, the author hopes to indicate, albeit briefly, the vast scope and range of potential of NMR imaging applications in an effort to direct non-NMR imaging personnel towards ways of using this technique effectively within their own particular field. It is hoped that after reading this book, the reader will appreciate the complementary nature of all the imaging modalities described and will then be able to decide which methods may be suitable for his/her own particular requirements. It is felt that this cross-fertilization of imaging modalities can do naught but enhance the versatility of each individual modality and thus help to achieve the ultimate aims of medicine, namely better patient screening, diagnosis, treatment, and care.

Nuclear magnetic resonance imaging is also finding many applications outside the medical field, and an attempt is made to indicate some of these. It is felt that experience in nonbiological applications of NMR will produce feedback into the biological

STEPHEN J. BLACKBAND, Ph. D., Dept. of Radiology and Radiological Science, The Johns Hopkins University, School of Medicine, 600 North Wolfe Street, Baltimore, MD 21205, USA applications, and vice versa. Although this chapter predominantly concerns NMR imaging, it will make considerable reference to NMR spectroscopy and should be read in conjunction with the chapter on NMR spectroscopy within this book. Many recent advances in both fields involve a combination of the two. This is not surprising since they are based on the same phenomenon. Indeed there is no real distinction between the two, rather a gradual transition from one to the other.

5.2 Basic Principles

The phenomenon of nuclear magnetic resonance has been well documented and is addressed briefly in Chap. 6. Complete accounts of the phenomenon have been given in several works (Abragam 1961; Slichter 1978; Farrar and Becker 1971; Ernst et al. 1987). Essentially nuclei with an odd number of spins, when placed in a magnetic field, become dipoles and orientate in that field. Unperturbed they will all align in the same direction along that magnetic field, resulting in the system having a net magnetic moment in the field. By the application of a second magnetic field at resonance with the spins they can be perturbed from this equilibrium and effectively tipped over from the axis of the main field. For nuclei, this resonance occurs at radiofrequencies (rf). When perturbed, the spins precess around the main field vector. Whilst doing this they will induce a current in a receiver, usually referred to as the rf coil, that is placed around the sample. The rf pulse required to do this must be of a frequency equal to the resonant frequency (ω) of the nuclei in that particular field strength (B) and is given by $\omega = \gamma \cdot B$, where γ is the gyromagnetic ratio of the nuclei of interest. If the rf pulse tips the spin vector through 90° it is called a 90° rf pulse. A 180° pulse will tip the spins through 180° and so on. The angle through which the spins are displaced is often referred to as the tip angle. Since the amount of induced signal is a maximum when the spin vector is perpendicular to the main field, a 90° rf pulse will produce the largest signal. The induced signal from the precessing spins is oscillatory in nature and is referred to as the free induction decay (FID).

In the absence of any decay phenomena, this FID would be produced continuously. However, the spins lose energy through relaxation processes that can loosely be regarded as a sort of "NMR friction." The first is a loss of energy due to spin-spin interaction, i.e., an exchange of energy between the spins that causes them to precess at slightly different frequencies. The spins precess at different rates and fan out in the plane orthogonal to the main field. This causes the FID to decay in an exponential manner. The time constant of this decay is called T_2, the spin-spin relaxation time. After approximately five T_2 periods, the spins fan out until equal numbers of spin vectors point in all directions. The resulting current induced from all the spins thus cancels to zero. This decay process is incoherent and consequently the signal can only be regenerated by further excitation pulses. Thus to regenerate the full signal the system must be allowed to fully relax. In real systems, the FID actually decays away in a time shorter than T_2, usually given the notation T_2^* (and called "T_2 star"). This added relaxation is due principally to magnet inhomogeneities and imperfections. However, this decay process is coherent and the signal loss due to this process can be regenerated. If a 180° pulse is applied after the decay of the FID the precessional direction of the fanning spins is reversed. The spins thus reorder or rephase, causing a signal regrowth that forms a spin echo at a time TE (the echo time) after the initial excitation pulse. This signal is a regrowth and a redecay of the signal equivalent to that which would be produced if two FIDs were placed back to back. It is this spin echo, when spatially encoded, that is most frequently used for generating NMR images. A series of spin echoes may be generated by the further application of 180° pulses, and the magnitude of the echoes is modulated by the T_2 decay envelope. Thus after several T_2 time periods, no further spin echoes are generated.

The second decay mechanism occurs when spins interact with the lattice of the resonant material. This causes the spin vectors to realign parallel to the main field once again in an exponential manner. This exponential decay is characterized by a constant T_1 and is called the spin-lattice relaxation time. After several T_1s, most of the spins will have returned to alignment with the main field and the system must be reexcited to regain the NMR signal. The time between the initial and reexcitation pulse is often referred to as the repetition time, TR. Typical relaxation times for liquids (NMR imaging presently concerns mainly liquids) are approximately 10–200 ms for T_2 and 100–1500 ms for T_1. Since there can be no induced current when the spins are aligned along the main field, T_2 must always be less than or equal to T_1.

These interactions form the fundamental processes studied in NMR spectroscopy. The induced current is directly proportional to the number of resonant spins in the sample and consequently images of the spin density may be formed. Images can be acquired with differing timings, and pulse sequences that weight the image signal intensities according to the T_1 and T_2 relaxation times can be generated. These can then be used as contrast mechanisms in NMR imaging since different tissues generally have differing relaxation times. Further, the FID may be composed of many different resonances that may be excited simultaneously by a broadband rf pulse. The different resonances correspond to different nuclear species within the sample and it is these resonances that are examined in spectroscopy. They show considerable application and promise in the study of biological systems (RADDA 1986; Chap. 6).

As described above, the NMR signal observed comes from the whole sample, which is ideal if the sample is homogeneous. However, if the sample is heterogeneous, as in the case of the human body, the signal becomes difficult if not impossible to interpret. A way must be found of encoding the FID as a function of space, i.e., of producing spatial maps or images of the sample in terms of the NMR signal. Potentially it should then be possible to obtain images of the spin-density, the chemical content, and the T_1 and T_2 relaxation times of the sample. The most significant factor that makes NMR imaging possible is the introduction of magnetic field gradients. If a small magnetic field gradient is applied across a sample containing spins that initially resonate in the main field at the same frequency, then spins in different parts of the magnetic field gradient will be in slightly different fields and consequently will resonate at slightly different frequencies. Each frequency is thus directly proportional to the spins spatial coordinates. The FID from such a system can then be converted into a single one-dimensional projection of the spins by performing a Fourier transform. Imaging sequences can then be implemented that encode the FID in such a way that subsequently it may be processed into a two- or three-dimensional spatial map. Some of these sequences are described briefly in the next section.

Another basic tool used in imaging sequences is a method of restricting the signal from a sample to a single slice. This is desirable for performing simple two-dimensional imaging. This may be achieved via an oscillating gradient (HINSHAW 1974) but is most often and more accurately effected through the use of a selective excitation pulse (GARROWAY et al. 1974). The exciting rf pulse can be amplitude modulated, or "tailored," in time so that it only excites a small range of frequencies. When this pulse is applied in the presence of a gradient that generates a range of frequencies that are proportional to spatial coordinates, then only a small region or slice through the object is excited. The thickness of the slice is then controlled by the time duration of the rf pulse and the magnitude of the slice selection gradient. The longer the rf pulse, or the stronger the slice selection gradient, the thinner the slice is. A two-dimensional image may then be formed by suitably encoding the signal from this slice.

So far all the spatial discrimination has been achieved by frequency encoding of the spin system. However, we may also encode the phase of the precessing spins for spatial discrimination (KUMAR et al. 1975). As the excited spins precess around the main magnetic field they dephase under T_2 processes to produce the FID. A pulsed gradient applied during this period will cause the spins to dephase at a different rate proportional to the magnitude of that gradient and its duration. If this phase encoding gradient is stepped through a range of values in equal increments the resulting set of FIDs are spatially encoded in that gradient direction. This may be again decoded by Fourier transform techniques.

5.3 Imaging Techniques

Only the simplest and most frequently used techniques are described here. Since the concept arose of making spatial maps from the NMR signal of a system, methodologies have developed rapidly from single point methods, which acquire data for each voxel in the image separately and sequentially, through line scan methods, which acquire data from a line of voxels simultaneously, to planar methods, which acquire data from the whole plane (BRUNNER and ERNST 1979). The planar methods can be extended to three-dimensional acquisition techniques, variants of which are now being used for chemical shift imaging. However, for most clinical imaging studies, full three-dimensional data acquisitions can be too time consuming, and the imaging techniques used most often are planar methods implemented in a multislice mode. The TR repetition period leaves sufficient time to repeat the basic acquisition sequence several times at different slice offsets. Thus several slices can be obtained in the time taken to acquire a single slice.

The most common planar imaging method in current use is the two-dimensional Fourier trans-

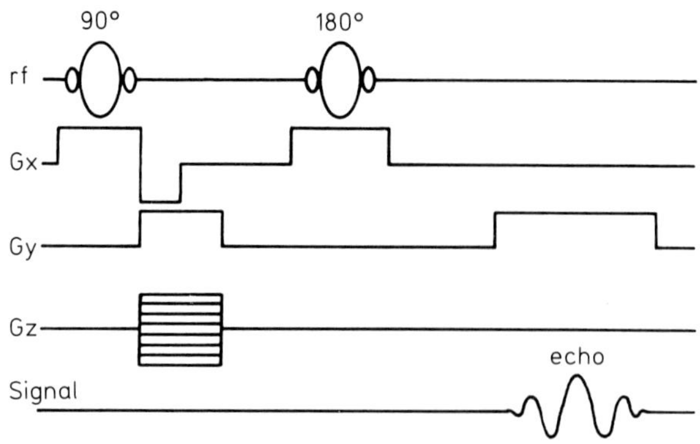

Fig. 1. A timing diagram for conventional 2-DFT imaging. *Gx*, slice gradient; *Gy*, read gradient; *Gz*, phase encoding gradient. The rf selective pulse is a one lobe sinc pulse

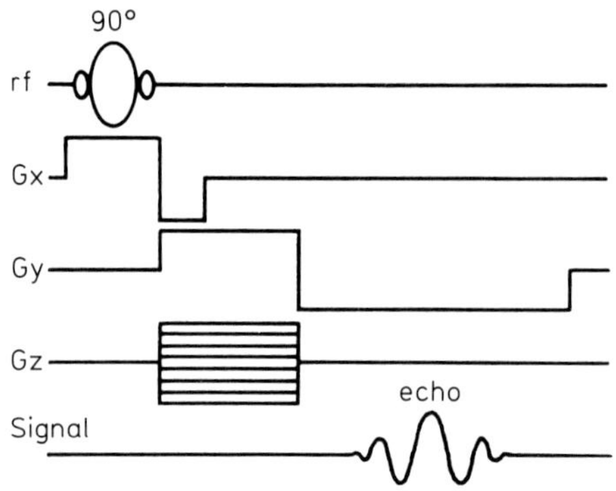

Fig. 2. A timing diagram for gradient echo imaging, labeled as in Fig. 1

form (2-DFT) spin echo imaging sequence (EDELSTEIN et al. 1980) depicted in Fig. 1. This utilizes a 90°, 180° rf pulse sequence which forms a spin echo at a time TE after the 180° pulse. Either the 90°, the 180°, or both rf pulses can be tailored and applied in the presence of a gradient to enable slice selection. The two-dimensional spatial encoding is achieved by a frequency encoding (or "read") gradient applied during the echo and by a phase encoding gradient applied between the 90° and the 180° rf pulses. A set of echoes is acquired with N different equally incremented phase gradient magnitudes and decoded via a 2-DFT into an $N \times M$ image, where M is the number of points sampled during the read gradient. The phase encoding and read gradients are perpendicular to each other and correspond to the x-y axis of the resultant image. Consequently by suitable choice of the physical gradients used, an image may be acquired of any plane of the object, i.e., transverse, coronal, sagittal, or oblique. Acquisition times using this basic technique range typically from 1 to 30 min depending upon the TR used (as determined by the contrast required) and the desired resolution. Since motion artifacts can cause considerable distortions in NMR images (STARK and BRADLEY 1988), especially in the chest and abdomen, where respiratory and cardiac motion are most prevalent, this imaging technique (and others) must usually be gated (SCHULTZ et al. 1984). This consists of timing each of the first 90° excitation pulses to occur at the same time point in the cardiac and/or respiratory cycle. Typically ECG leads (cardiac) and some form of pressure sensor (respiratory) are employed.

Another method, referred to as projection reconstruction imaging (LAUTERBUR 1973), uses a similar sequence. This time, however, the read gradient is a vector sum of the orthogonal imaging plane gradients, i.e., a gradient that can be placed at any angle across the imaging plane. This vector gradient is incremented around the axis of the object to produce a set of projections of the object that can be reconstructed by a mathematical algorithm into an image. Consequently the image is generated from purely frequency encoded data; no phase encoding is required. This technique is analogous to the method used for image reconstruction of X-ray CAT scans.

A method which has been used more often recently is gradient echo imaging (VAN DER MUELEN et al. 1985) as shown in Fig. 2. This time the echo is formed by reversing the read gradient, and the phase encoding is applied as before. This has the advantage that it only uses one rf pulse (180° pulses are more difficult to apply accurately than 90° pulses) and in general TE can usually be made smaller than it can in spin echo methods.

Many other techniques are used for imaging. There are many ways of refining these basic sequences, and many ways of adapting them to encode different information, some of which will be addressed briefly in this chapter. However, so many of these methods now exist that once again the reader is referred to the literature.

5.4 NMR Imaging Hardware

5.4.1 General

The principal components of an NMR imaging machine are illustrated in Fig. 3. Details of each of these components may be found in MANSFIELD and MORRIS (1982), and only a brief overview will be given.

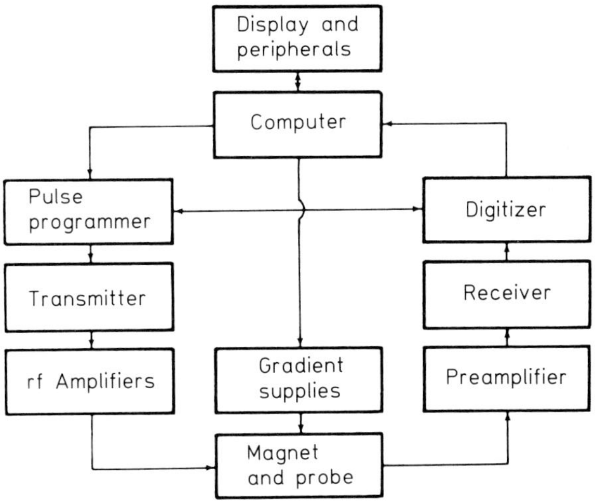

Fig. 3. The principal components of an NMR imaging machine

During the infancy of NMR imaging, the tendency was to build instruments designed specifically for NMR imaging within the constraints imposed by the available technology and the need for cost-effective clinical machines. NMR systems are very expensive, and from a commercial point of view it is important to keep costs low so that they become a realistic modality for hospital use. However, the discipline has developed so rapidly that by the time a given machine has been developed for the commercial market it is virtually obsolete! Although the pace in this regard now shows signs of slowing, there is still considerable room for improvement. It is becoming apparent that the NMR imaging machine is required to have the capabilities and flexibilities of a high resolution NMR spectrometer, a condition principally imposed by the merger of imaging and spectroscopy. Consequently the ideal imaging machine consists of a high resolution spectrometer which can be adapted to have a full range of imaging capabilities. This represents a considerable technical challenge that the NMR companies are now starting to address. The particular requirements are related especially to the bore size and field strength of the magnet which forms the heart of the system. Indeed two of the major companies are already responding to these requirements. Bruker are now selling imaging accessories that can be made to fit most of their high resolution spectrometers. Also, General Electric are marketing what are essentially spectroscopy consoles for their whole body systems, and other companies are developing similar approaches to design.

The necessity of making the NMR imaging machine a fully operational NMR spectroscopy machine will depend upon NMR spectroscopy fulfilling its potential as a clinical modality. Although the signs of this are encouraging, it may not prove viable for various reasons such as cost, difficulty, unspecificity, etc. In this case it may be more cost-effective to produce purely imaging machines. Ultimately a compromise is anticipated. A market will be established for both cheap, reliable imaging machines for small hospitals and satellite institutions, and for more comprehensive and expensive combined imaging and spectroscopy machines for the larger hospitals and specialized institutions.

5.4.2 Magnet

The magnet itself can be either permanent (i.e., made of permanently magnetized metal), resistive (i.e., coils of current-carrying wire at room temperature), or superconducting (i.e., coils of supercooled wire which exhibit no resistive loss). Although it was initially felt that superconducting systems would be too expensive for clinical use, stronger and more homogeneous fields can be achieved with these magnet designs and they are now the most predominant. Whole body superconducting magnets (1-m bore) are currently available with field strengths up to 2 Tesla (T), although the Federal Drug Administration (FDA) only gives clearance to date (1988) for fields up to 1.5 T for clinical studies. Several whole body 4-T magnets have been built recently and are being evaluated. It is not yet clear if such an increase in field strength will benefit human studies and these are issues of hot debate at the present time. These issues resurface each time a higher field instrument is built and it will be interesting to see what develops. It is also of interest to note that less than 8 years ago, it was anticipated that imaging above 10 MHz would be impractical (Mansfield and Morris 1982, Sect. 6.2) (the 1.5-T clinical magnets presently in use have a resonance frequency of 60 MHz for ^{1}H). However, these conclusions were based on data obtained from simple models (Bottomley and Andrew 1978) and it is now clear that a more realistic model is required for making such estimates (Bottomley et al. 1985). A range of magnets are available with smaller bore sizes, but higher field strengths. These are suitable for limited studies of the human limb, animals, and pathological specimens. For example, one can obtain 40-cm/4.7-T, 15-cm/7-T, 8.9-cm/9.4-T, and recently 5.2 cm/14.1-T superconducting magnets. The 8.9-cm and 5.2-cm diameter bore magnets are designed primarily for high resolution spectroscopy of liquids or solids, though recently the advent of NMR microscopy has made them attractive instruments for imaging of biological and nonbiological specimens. The intermediate bore machines, as well as being suitable for animal studies, provide valuable preliminary information about the feasibility of imaging on larger bore instruments at those fields for when it becomes technically possible to build such a magnet. There is no doubt that the successful imaging studies performed recently on 40-cm/4.7-T instruments influenced the decision to build the 100-cm/4-T magnets that are now being evaluated. Speculation and intense debate presently center on the possibility of imaging at even higher fields. The ultimate goal is to obtain improvement in the available signal (which increases with field strength) and spectral resolution. This is important with respect to the usefulness of chemical shift imaging and multinuclear studies. Indeed, serious investigations into the feasibility of building a 10-T whole body instrument have been undertaken, although as yet the author knows of no commitment to proceed with such an ambitious undertaking. The problems with such a machine include the effects of such a high field on biological systems, the amount and effect of the rf power required, the degree of rf attenuation, and the strategies required to build tunable rf coils of such diameters at such high frequencies, assuming that ^{1}H imaging is still required. It may be that such a machine will only be suitable for lower resonant frequency nuclei (such as phosphorus or sodium) or partial body imaging (surface coils), but this remains to be seen.

The smaller instruments designed for high resolution spectroscopy can be adapted for imaging, and the potential of such instruments is only just being realized. The smaller size of the rf coil required and the rf power needed on these smaller instruments mean that the rf penetration effects and rf coil design problems apparent on the larger instruments do not exist. These instruments will be useful for high resolution spectroscopy and microscopy on a wide range of small biological systems, and indeed can be used to study the potentially adverse effects of high fields on biological systems. Such instruments also have great potential for nonbiological studies.

Little attention has been given here to the other types of magnet mentioned above. These may be of use when relatively cheap systems are required, or when locating problems become too difficult with high field magnets. However, with respect to these problems, strategies for shielding large superconducting magnets are now being developed, and some are already available. The large fringe field of these magnets may by reduced radically by either an active or passive screening system. The active screen is in essence a second magnet winding around the main magnet in such a configuration that its field cancels the external field from the windings of the main magnet. The passive screen consists of large amounts of iron around the magnet that concentrate the field lines from the main windings, again reducing the range of these fringe fields. Although it is not certain which will prove to be the better strategy, the author feels confident that the installation restrictions of these instruments will be minimized and that the superconducting magnet will remain the principal instrument for imaging and high resolution studies.

Since NMR imaging is still a relatively new imaging modality and is still being assessed in terms of its clinical utility, whole body magnets are still the principal instruments of use. However, it may eventually prove that the construction of specialized magnets for specific anatomies may both generate better image quality of that specific anatomy and be cost-effective. Presently the same whole body magnet is used to image all parts of the human body, and the demand for NMR studies has increased so rapidly that most hospitals have been forced to acquire two or more whole body magnets. In the near future, when the clinical demand of NMR imaging is more stable, we may well see hospitals equipped with a range of magnets designed for specific anatomical studies. This may consist of, for example, magnets specifically for the body, the head, and the limbs.

5.4.3 Gradients

The gradient coils provide the means of obtaining spatial discrimination. Consequently it is desirable to produce the highest possible gradient strengths along with good gradient linearity. Of course, the frequency encoding produced by the gradient must correspond linearly with the spatial coordinates of the object so that images are not distorted. Several designs have been proposed and most are summarized by Mansfield and Morris (1982). The most frequently used geometry consists of a Golay (Golay 1971) and Helmholtz combination (Bottomley 1981). This is suitable for most basic imaging techniques used today. However, the recent improvements in imaging methodologies have placed more stringent demands on the gradients. For good spectroscopy studies using any gradients for localization, the gradients must be turned off completely before data acquisition to ensure there are no spectral distortions. With conventional gradients this usually requires a waiting period of several milliseconds before acquisition. This causes potential signal to be lost and causes distortions. Also, the echo planar techniques and their variants (see Sect. 5.6) require gradients which can be switched extremely quickly, in the order of tens of microseconds or less. This capability would also benefit less demanding imaging techniques. The main problem is that the gradients couple with the magnet. This mutual inductance reduces the rate at which the gradient field can change. Although it is feasible with powerful gradient supply control to switch gradients rapidly on resistive magnets, the problem becomes more difficult on superconducting magnets. The main magnet windings are made superconducting by immersing them in liquid helium, which in turn is surrounded by liquid nitrogen (to minimize helium boil off) in a large metallic container called a dewar. This dewar presents a large body with which the gradients can couple and hence greatly increases the mutual inductance.

The desire to minimize these coupling problems has led to the recent development of techniques to actively screen the gradients from the magnet and its dewar so that the field beyond the gradient windings is essentially zero (MANSFIELD and CHAPMAN 1986, 1987). Essentially a second set of gradient windings around the primary gradient windings are designed to produce a magnetic field distribution that cancels the magnetic field generated on the outside of the primary gradient windings. No field thus extends from the gradient windings to the magnet and its dewar and the coupling is then minimized. This development will improve the performance of all imaging machines and it will be interesting to see the impact this has on NMR imaging as a whole.

5.4.4 Computer

The computers associated with imaging systems are rapidly increasing in power. Not only are larger volumes of data being obtained, especially now that spectroscopy is becoming more practical, but these large volumes are being acquired more quickly and need more rapid processing. At present large microcomputers such as Vax and, more recently, Sun computers are being used, and no doubt more are on the way. The advent of the array processor shortened processing times considerably and more involved parallel processing should further improve matters. More complex data processing algorithms are being utilized and considerable computing power is required to implement these in acceptable times. This is especially crucial in clinical settings, where the results of an examination may be required as soon as possible. The arrangement preferred at present is to have one central computer to operate the spectrometer and to perform immediate processing. The data are then handed on to one or more "data stations" where they can be processed further without wasting expensive NMR machine time. This seems to be a suitable strategy that is unlikely to be superseded in the near future. This strategy also applies for research machines where once again machine time is at a premium. Needless to say the limiting factor is the initial financial outlay required to purchase the data stations.

5.4.5 rf Coils

There are now many designs for the rf coil (receiver and transmitter), which depend intimately on the sample geometry, ease of use, signal-to-noise ratio (S/N), and operating frequency. Popular low field coil designs are the saddle coil (GINSBERG and MELCHNER 1970), the solenoid (HOULT and RICHARDS 1976), and the Helmholtz coil (MANSFIELD and MORRIS 1982). Optimization of the S/N in experiments with such a relatively low sensitivity as the NMR phenomenon is of paramount importance. Of course, it is not beneficial to increase the signal in an experiment if this also results in a greater increase in the noise. In this case, the resultant S/N is lower and it is thus more difficult in a data set to distinguish the signal above the background noise. The solenoid gives the optimal S/N of the coil geometries named previously, but is difficult to tune to high frequencies. Furthermore access is often restricted since its central axis must be perpendicular to the main field. This limits its use with superconducting magnets for clinical studies where the main field is parallel to the bore of the magnet.

High field imaging of large objects introduces a relatively new problem. The resonant frequency of a coil is given by

$$f^2 = 1/(4\pi^2 LC) \tag{1}$$

where L and C are the inductance and capacitance of the circuit respectively. The inductance is essentially fixed by the length of the conductor in the coil, and thus to increase the frequency the capacitance must be reduced. However, at high frequencies this tuning capacitance becomes impractically small and may be overwhelmed by the stray capacitances inherent in the circuit. To sidestep this problem, coils have been designed that effectively reduce the apparent inductance of the coil by distributing the capacitance around it and breaking the inductance up into smaller segments, each of lower inductance. This must be incorporated with a coil design that maintains the homogeneity of the coil's rf excitation. Presently the bird cage (HAYES et al. 1985) and slotted tube resonator (LEROY-WILLIG et al. 1985) are popular designs that work well on whole body 2-T and 33-cm/4.7-T magnets. It remains to be seen just how effective this strategy will be at higher fields on larger bore magnets. Of course, these considerations are less crucial if only lower frequency nuclei are examined.

The S/N available in an NMR experiment is given approximately by MANSFIELD and MORRIS (1982) as

$$(S/N)^2 \simeq A \cdot (T_2/T_1) \cdot t \cdot r^{-2} \cdot f^{7/2} \cdot (x \cdot y \cdot z)^2 \qquad (2)$$

where r is the coil diameter, f is the resonant frequency, and x, y, and z are the voxel dimensions. (A data element in a two-dimensional image is called a pixel. The slice width from the image is the third dimension of each pixel which is then referred to as a voxel.)

It can thus be seen that the S/N is maximized by minimizing the coil diameter. The minimum size of a coil that completely surrounds the object to be imaged (i.e., a volume coil) is limited by the size of that object. If better S/N is required, this can be obtained at the expense of the field of view by the use of a surface coil. This usually takes the form of a simple loop of wire with the approximate shape and dimensions of the region of interest. Many designs are now available for imaging different parts of the anatomy. Problems may arise with the use of a surface coil, especially in localized spectroscopy studies, because, unlike the volume coil, it does not excite the region of interest homogeneously. The tip angle experienced by the spins in the sample decreases with the distance of the spins from the coil. This may be seen commonly in surface coil NMR images as a fall off in the image intensity with distance from the coil. To eliminate this inhomogeneous excitation problem, a common arrangement used for imaging and spectroscopy is to excite the whole object with a volume coil and then receive with a surface coil. In this way a homogeneous excitation is obtained over the region the surface coil receives signal from. Care must be taken, however, to ensure that the coils do not interact if they are not at right angles to each other (BENDALL et al. 1986).

5.4.6 The Spectrometer

The rest of the technology required for an NMR imager/spectrometer is already in existence and has been developed for the high resolution spectroscopy machines over the past 40 years. Fast data sampling, accurate pulse phase control, noise minimized preamplifiers, powerful rf transmitters, rf transmission cables, etc. are all available. Again it becomes a simple question of economics rather than of feasibility; high technology is expensive. As the techniques that are implemented on the whole body machines become more demanding, the quality of such instrumentation will, of necessity, improve. This trend is already evident in the real progress now being made towards the clinical use of multinuclear spectroscopy. With few exceptions, and with the provision that the promise of multinuclear spectroscopy is at least partially fulfilled, we can expect the capabilities of the whole body machines to rapidly approach those of the high resolution spectrometers.

5.5 The Information NMR Can Provide

As already indicated, NMR can be used to obtain information about spin densities and relaxation times, which may or may not be spatially discriminated. Clinically, differences in the relaxation times of tissues are most often used as contrast mechanisms. In certain cases it is possible to quantitate the relaxation times which may provide further, more specific information for tissue characterization. However, NMR is capable of providing us with more information than this, some of which is expanded upon in the rest of this chapter. This includes information on flow, chemical shift, nuclei other than ^{1}H, J-coupling, and chemical exchange rates. NMR has the potential to provide us with other sources of information, which are not discussed here because at the present time their applications appear to be limited. However, in the future such information may find a use in conjunction with other imaging techniques. An example is temperature mapping by monitoring T_1 relaxation times (PARKER et al. 1983; DICKINSON et al. 1986).

5.6 High Speed Imaging

There are several reasons to minimize the imaging time required for a conventional NMR scan. Obviously, very fast experiments are required to obtain unblurred images of the fast moving portions of an object, in particular the beating heart. This also reduces problems associated with the slower motions in the body, such as breathing or irregular patient movement. Faster acquisition times can potentially increase patient throughput, minimizing patient exposure and potentially decreasing the cost per patient of an NMR examination.

Several techniques are available for fast imaging. Some are more efficient than others, but essentially the price paid for speed is a decrease in the S/N ratio. When this becomes unacceptably low it is translated into a decrease in the spatial resolution which is required to retrieve the lost S/N. Faster images may be obtained by making the initial excitation pulse in conventional spin echo or gradient echo imaging techniques less than a full 90° excitation pulse so that only a portion of the available magnetization is read out for each echo that is acquired (HAASE et al. 1986). Consequently spatially encoded sequential echoes can be acquired without waiting for relatively long TRs for the magnetization to relax and return to equilibrium after excitation. Usually images can be obtained with such methods in seconds (EDELMAN et al. 1986) as opposed to minutes. More often than not, gradient echo images can be acquired a little faster than conventional spin echo images since it is usually possible to make TE shorter. A low tip angle may be used in combination with the gradient echo technique.

Echo planar imaging (MANSFIELD and PYKETT 1978) and its variants are by far the fastest of the imaging techniques available today, and they offer exciting prospects with regard to the future development of NMR. The basic pulse sequence is illustrated in Fig. 4. Essentially all the echoes required are recalled very quickly by a switched gradient which is applied simultaneously with an orthogonal broadening gradient which encodes the second spatial dimension. After suitable reordering, the data are decoded by conventional Fourier transform methods. This is very much an oversimplification and the reader is referred to the literature (MANSFIELD and MORRIS 1982). A complete image can thus be acquired in a single shot, resulting in imaging times as short as 64 ms or less. This is sufficient to freeze the heart motion in the human body, and indeed this represents one of the primary clinical

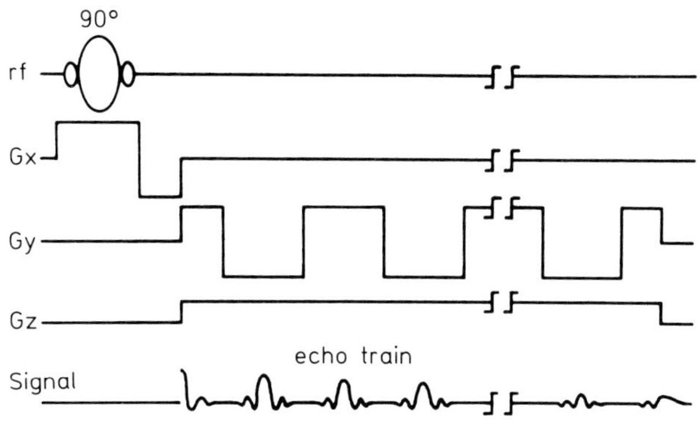

Fig. 4. A timing for echo planar imaging, labeled as in Fig. 1

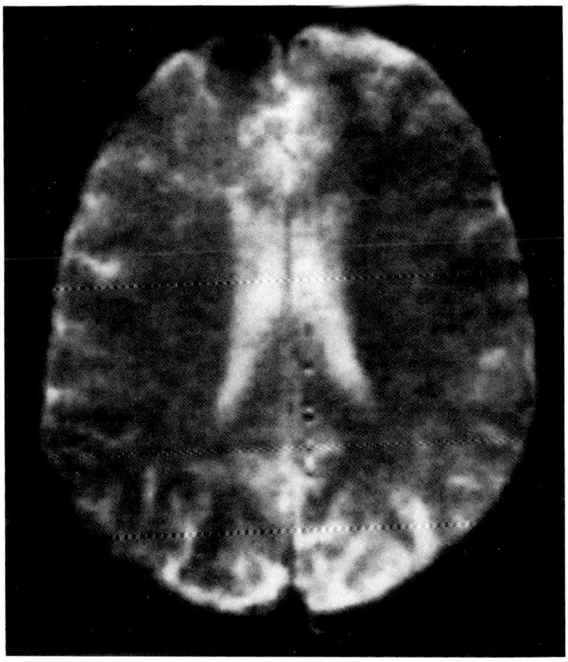

Fig. 5. A transverse image of a human head generated by a modified echo planar sequence. The slice thickness is 1 cm and the in-plane spatial resolution a little less than 2 mm. The image was acquired in 128 ms. (ORDIDGE et al. 1988)

applications of these techniques. Such images can also be displayed in real time to produce movie loops of the motion. Figure 5 shows an example of the image quality that can be obtained using the echo planar technique.

Echo planar imaging is technically very demanding. Large magnetic field gradients are required which must be able to switch rapidly (in tens of microseconds as opposed to approximately 1 ms in conventional techniques) and the acquisition bandwidth must be large in order to sample all the echoes sufficiently rapidly. Nevertheless, these technical difficulties can be overcome as described in the literature (Chapman et al. 1987; Ordidge et al. 1988), and advances in this respect are represented by the progression from the early image matrices of 16 × 16 pixels to ones of 128 × 128 pixels. Gradient screening techniques as described in Sect. 5.4.3 have contributed to these developments and we can expect still greater improvements in the future. Quite what the clinical utility of echo planar images will be has yet to be firmly established. Despite its real time capabilities the resolution of the technique is poor compared with images obtained by conventional methods using gating to freeze the motion. Such images can be acquired in several minutes and are of excellent quality and resolution. This will be important for studies of heart wall motion and changes of heart wall thickness. However, such images are composed from an average taken over many heart cycles and important real time information may be lost. Even if the clinical utility of simple echo planar ^{1}H imaging is limited at the moment, the implications of the technique and its associated technology will be far-reaching, and better gradients will be able to improve the capabilities and flexibility of any imaging technique. The first commercial machine with real time imaging capability became available in 1987 (Pykett and Rzedzian 1987), and it will be interesting to see what impact this has on the NMR imaging field as a whole. In principle, an instrument with the ability to perform echo planar techniques could also be capable of performing virtually any other imaging technique and potentially an extremely versatile machine could be developed.

5.7 Flow Imaging and Angiography

The development of NMR flow imaging and angiography has exciting potential, particularly with respect to their clinical applications. The sensitivity of NMR imaging to flow effects became apparent in some of the very first images obtained of biological systems; blood vessels showed up as dark holes in the image due to the motion of the excited spins in the blood moving out of the slice of interest before the signal was observed. Several mechanisms cause either a decrease or an increase in the signal intensity of flowing spins in images relative to stationary spins (Stark and Bradley 1988, Chap. 7). Care must be taken to allow for these effects when interpreting clinical images.

The flexibility of the NMR imaging experiment is such that the effects of flow can be controlled and discriminated against. Flowing material within a system may be selectively imaged and the flow rate quantified. At present, there are two principal classes of techniques for measuring flow. First, there are "time of flight" experiments. In their most basic form, these techniques involve exciting a slice of spins in one part of a sample and measuring the signal loss due to spins flowing away from that slice. Conversely, the signal increase in nearby slices is measured as the excited spins flow into them (Wehrli et al. 1984). The second class of techniques exploits a phase difference that can be generated between stationary and moving spins within a gradient. One recent and particularly successful method developed by Dumoulin and Hart (1986) is an example of the second class of techniques. In this method, a bipolar gradient pulse is inserted into a conventional imaging sequence. Stationary spins are dephased and then rephased by the bipolar gradient. However, moving spins will be in a different position in the magnet and hence in a different gradient strength. Consequently they do not fully rephase. This results in a net phase difference between the stationary and the flowing spins. The magnitude of the phase shift is controlled by the strength and duration of the bipolar gradient pulse. Two images are acquired with the phase encoding applied both in a positive and a negative sense by reversing the signs of the bipolar gradient pulse. A subtraction of the data sets then eliminates all signal except that from the flowing spins. Figure 6 shows an example of this technique. Because of the tortuous nature of the blood vessels in biological systems, the slice selection gradient is often made weak or zero so that the slice is relatively thick. In this way a projection of the vascular network is obtained. The images thus resemble conventional angiograms and the technique is referred to as magnetic resonance angiography. One of its major advantages over conventional angiographic techniques is that contrast agents are not required.

The amount of dephasing due to flow is directly proportional to the velocity of the flow. Consequently it is possible to quantitate the flow velocity (Moran 1982). This may have important clinical significance and requires further study. These flow imaging techniques are also expected to have significant application in the study of nonbiological systems.

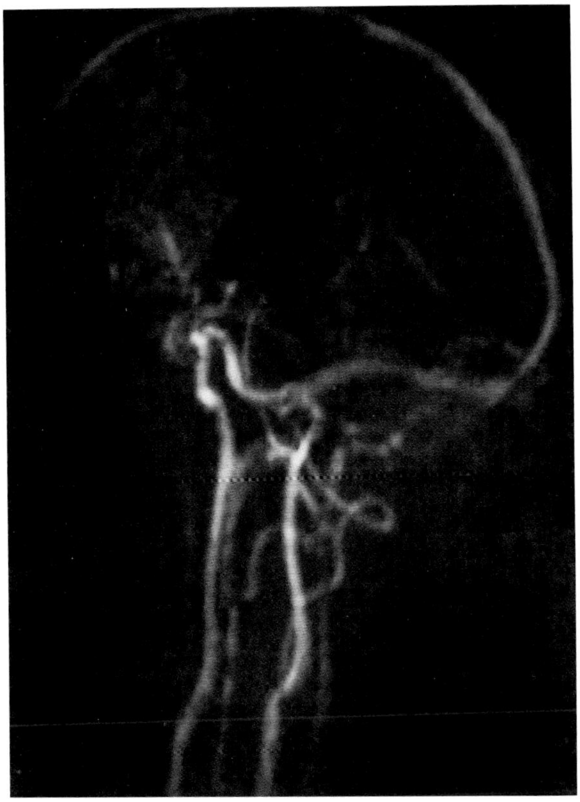

Fig. 6. A projection angiogram of a human head. The blood vessels are clearly isolated fron the signal arising from stationary tissue. The *lower half* of the image shows the blood vessels within the neck. (DUMOULIN and HART 1986)

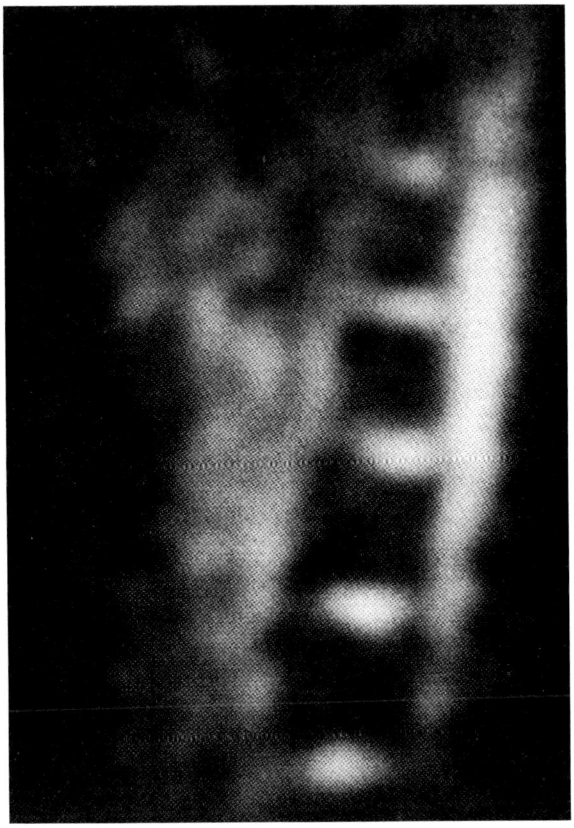

Fig. 7. A sodium image of the human spine. The disks are clearly defined. The image obtained at 1.5 T in 50 min and has a resolution of $2 \times 2 \times 2$ mm^3. (RA et al. 1988)

5.8 Multinuclear Imaging

Nuclear magnetic resonance imaging has predominantly involved the ^{1}H resonance because of the relatively high sensitivity of NMR for this nucleus and because of its relative abundance in biological systems. However, many other nuclei may be imaged under certain conditions. Unfortunately most other resonant nuclei give many times less signal in biological systems due principally to their much lower abundance and also to their lower sensitivity due to their lower gyromagnetic ratio. Typically they are present in only millimolar concentrations. For example, the ^{31}P resonances from ATP in vivo give approximately one million times less signal than the ^{1}H resonance that arises principally from water. Consequently they are not suitable for the production of high quality anatomical images. Some nuclear species give a little more signal than this. Recent developments have made sodium imaging a diagnostic reality and fairly high quality images have been produced using this nucleus (MAUDSLEY and HILAL 1984; RA et al. 1988). Figure 7 shows an example of the image quality that has recently been achieved. Because sodium has a relatively short T_1 it is possible to use a correspondingly shorter TR repetition period and average larger numbers of signals in a given time. Recently, such images have been shown to be useful for tumor localization (STARK and BRADLEY 1988, Chap. 31).

It is possible to distinguish between inter- and intracellular sodium (RA et al. 1986). This may well have far-reaching implications for biological research, although its diagnostic utility is not yet clear.

Imaging of phantoms, and in some cases of small biological systems and humans, has been demonstrated using fluorine (NUNNALLY et al. 1985; JOSEPH et al. 1985; CLARK et al. 1984), carbon (KORMOS et al. 1987), phosphorus (MAUDSLEY et al. 1983, 1984), lithium (RENSHAW et al. 1985), and deuterium (MULLER and SEELIG 1987). In all cases the S/N will almost always be much less than that available from ^{1}H imaging in biological systems and consequently the images will not be as useful for anatomical discrimination. However, they do show the distribution of the different nuclei, albeit coarsely, throughout the system providing useful chemical information. The best interpretation of such images is most likely to be achieved by overlaying them on ^{1}H images of the same region. However, such methodologies will only give information on the abundance of nuclear types. It may be more fruitful to obtain nuclear environmental information as a function of space, i.e., to perform chemical shift imaging or spatially localized spectroscopy as described in the following sections.

Nevertheless, since S/N, or effectively nuclear abundance, is the limiting factor with respect to multinuclear imaging, these techniques are most effective at higher fields where the S/N can be maximized, or on systems where the nuclear abundance can be significantly increased, i.e., by infusing labeled compounds. They may be particularly suitable for the study of nonbiological materials, where a particular nuclear abundance can be controlled more easily and probably made higher. Initial biological applications will be restricted to the study of small animal systems. If only one resonant species is present, then standard imaging methodologies are appropriate. If more than one resonance is present then chemical shift imaging, localized methods, or selective excitation or suppression techniques are required.

5.9 Chemical Shift Imaging

Although its clinical value is yet to be established, NMR spectroscopy (sometimes called magnetic resonance spectroscopy) promises to have considerable biological application (Chap. 6; RADDA 1986). The ability to distinguish between, and possibly quantitate, chemical shift species within a biological, or for that matter a nonbiological system, is indeed an exciting prospect. The first forays into this dimension have been made over the last several years. Again, the principal restriction will be the S/N achievable for nuclei at low concentrations.

Unless some method of spatially localizing the signal is employed, NMR spectroscopy itself will not be useful on an inhomogeneous system. To this end, localized techniques may be implemented and are discussed in the following section. Probably the most elegant and efficient way of obtaining such information is to perform chemical shift imaging. In these methods one, two or three dimensions in space are acquired along with one dimension of chemical shift (i.e., a spectral dimension, see Chap. 6). This is most easily achieved by extension of the 2-DFT imaging technique with the introduction of one or two more orthogonal phase encoding gradients to encode spatial information, the resulting FID being collected in the absence of a read gradient so as to encode spectral information (BROWN et al. 1982; MAUDSLEY et al. 1983). The data may be decoded with conventional Fourier transforms. Such methods can lead to long single acquisition imaging times, since the one shot imaging time is multipied by the number of steps required for the second and third phase encoding gradients. However, for many nuclear species it is likely that a considerable degree of averaging will be required because of the low S/N ratio. Since each phase encoded acquisition corresponds in effect to a signal average (signal is acquired from the whole slice in each step), the one shot imaging time may be less than or equal to the time required to obtain sufficient S/N with respect to averaging. Consequently the long single acquisition time required by this technique may not be a limitation. The multidimensional nature of chemical shift images allows several display modes. Most commonly, the spectra from single voxel elements can be examined, or alternatively an image may be reconstructed that corresponds to a particular chemical shift within the spectrum. Spatial maps of particular metabolites can then be generated. The low spatial resolution of the metabolite images usually requires the acquisition of a high resolution ^{1}H image from the same region so that the distributions of the metabolites can be correlated with the anatomical structures. Figures 8 shows a three-dimensional chemical shift image data set and one mode of display of such data.

To date, the phosphorus nucleus has been the most extensively studied with regard to spectroscopy on in vivo systems. Consequently it has been the principal nucleus examined to date in human studies. Recent work by BOTTOMLEY et al. (1988) (see Fig. 8) illustrates the present state of the art of phosphorus chemical shift imaging on a human head. The S/N is the limiting factor and consequently the resolution achieved was 27 cm^3 in 17 min (a voxel of sides $3 \times 3 \times 3$ cm^3). The spectra are quite noisy and although they may be improved a little in the near future, an improvement in the resolution of up to 8 cm^3 (a voxel of sides $2 \times 2 \times 2$ cm^3) is not expected (this would require an im-

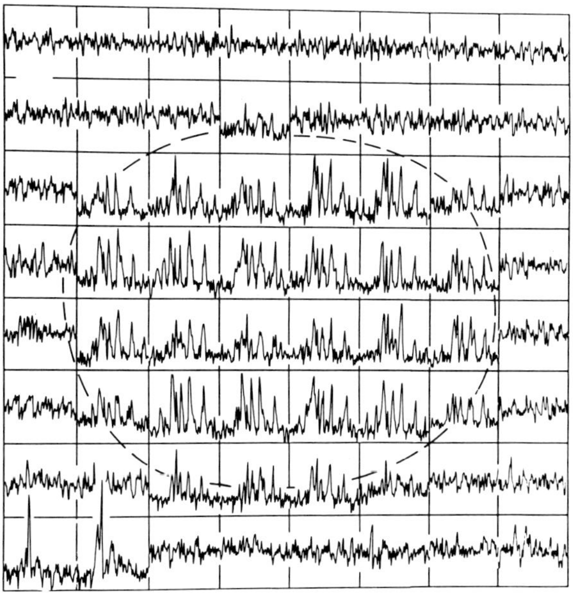

Fig. 8. A 3-DFT chemical shift ^{31}P image of a human head. Each image voxel is $3 \times 3 \times 3$ cm^3 and the spectrum from each voxel is displayed within it. The *dashed ellipse* shows the position of the head. The data took 17 min to acquire. (BOTTOMLEY et al. 1988)

provement in the S/N ratio by a factor of approximately 11). Phosphorus offers considerable promise for evaluating the energetic state of tissues since the most significant nuclei contributing to phosphorus spectra are incorporated in the molecules of ATP and phosphocreatine. By monitoring the chemical shift of the phosphocreatine peak, regional pH information may be inferred and pH maps may be generated (HALL and TAKAGALA 1985). The question therefore is whether or not spectra from such relatively large voxels will be useful in the clinical setting. Certainly, they are unlikely to be utilized as a screening modality for tumors, for example. However, they may be useful for the monitoring of the response to treatment. A clinical data base is required before this can be evaluated. The collection of such data is underway at the time of writing and it is likely to be a few years before it is completed.

Although the utility of clinical phosphorus chemical shift imaging may prove to be limited, such data are already very useful in the study of small animal systems and consequently are expected to play a major role in animal research studies. The examination of other nuclei, such as carbon or fluorine, may prove to have greater clinical utility.

Echo planar techniques may be used for chemical shift imaging (MANSFIELD 1984), and indeed a full two-dimensional spatial image with a chemical shift dimension can be obtained in a single experiment (GUILFOYLE and MANSFIELD 1985). Nevertheless, this method is limited by the number of echoes that can be formed within the T_2 decay period and consequently the spatial and spectral resolution will be poor. However, it is possible to combine echo planar methods with conventional methods to produce hybrid techniques. Although such methods are slower than the pure echo planar methods, they are faster than the pure spin echo techniques and may provide useful resolution (DOYLE and MANSFIELD 1987). It is expected that in principle the echo planar portion of the hybrid method may be used to obtain a coarse image quickly and the conventional portion may be used to improve the spectral resolution. As with all the chemical shift imaging methods, however, the limiting factor will again be the S/N available, and so the echo planar based techniques will only be of advantage in situations where the S/N is relatively high.

A special situation is encountered in vivo if high resolution ^{1}H spectroscopy is required. The human body is composed of approximately 66% water, which corresponds to an effective concentration of approximately 36 M. However, ^{1}H nuclei are also components in many interesting metabolities, e.g., lactate, which are only present in the body in millimolar concentrations. The water signal is thus approximately 10000 times greater than that from such metabolites. It is extremely difficult and to date technically impractical to build receiver hardware that can accomodate such a large dynamic range. The interesting metabolic information is thus swamped by the water signal. The large water signal must thus be suppressed (or not initially excited). Many techniques for specific applications with varying degrees of flexibility, success, and ease of implementation are available (HORE 1983 and references therein). In general, the larger the system to be imaged is, the less efficient the techniques; it becomes more difficult to control the rf pulses accurately as the coil volume increases. Successful water suppression has thus to date only been achieved adequately on small animal systems. Progress is expected in this area in humans over the next few years. Further, some parts of the body also have relatively large amounts of lipids that cause a problem similar to that presented by water. In these cases, both the water and the lipid ^{1}H signal must be suppressed.

5.10 Spatially Localized Spectroscopy

To exploit the potential of NMR spectroscopy on inhomogeneous systems, a method must be employed to spatially discriminate the spectroscopic response. This may be achieved by full chemical shift imaging as described above, or by restricting the NMR response of the system to some specified region. This is achieved by rf (BENDALL and GORDON 1983), magnetic field gradient (AUE et al. 1984; LUYTEN et al. 1986; ORDIDGE et al. 1986; FRAHM et al. 1987), or a combination of rf and magnetic field gradient techniques (BOTTOMLEY et al. 1984a, 1985). The rf techniques utilize a surface coil to localize a region corresponding to the excitation profile of the rf coil. Further localization within the excitation profile can be achieved by the application of a carefully designed rf pulse sequence. The main limitations of such methods are that the use of a surface coil restricts studies to the surface of the sample, and that the size, shape, and position of the localized region are difficult to determine and control.

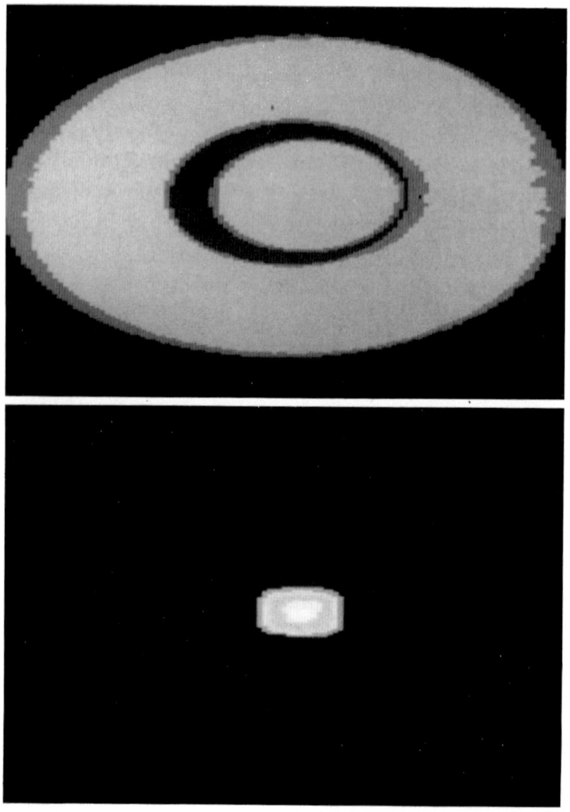

a

b

Fig. 9. a An image of a coaxial phantom containing dimethylacetamide in the outer tube and triethylamine in the inner tube. b An image of a region centered on the inner tube using selective excitation techniques (BLACKBAND et al. 1988)

This situation may be improved by combining the rf excitation with a selective excitation slice selection through the profile, thus restricting the NMR response to a disk. This technique, called DRESS (BOTTOMLEY et al. 1984b), is relatively simple to implement and gives good S/N because of the use of the surface coil. It has given some of the best results to date. However, it is still difficult to examine deep structures in this manner, and the volume and precise shape of the disk are not easily controlled. Further improvement is possible with a purely magnetic field gradient localization method. Several of these now exist and all are variants on the same theme. Although an oversimplification, essentially all the methods apply three orthogonal slice selective pulse trains in such a way that only the signal from the intersection of the three planes is observed. Since these are magnetic field gradient techniques, the size, shape, and position of the selected volume may be accurately and electronically controlled. Accurate volume determination is the first step towards the possible quantitization of the resulting spectra by some method, possibly by referencing the spectra to a standard that may be internal or external to the sample. Figure 9 shows images of a phantom illustrating the localization of a specific region from the sample. Figure 10 shows subsequently that spatially localized spectra can be obtained from these volumes. For clinical examples see chapt. 6.

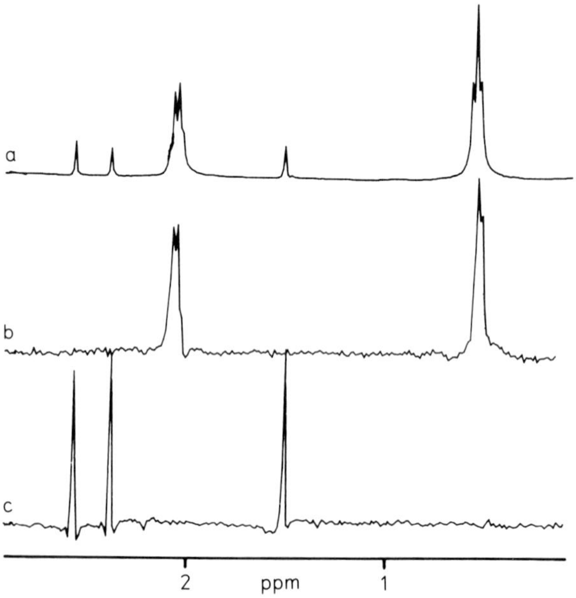

Fig. 10a–c. Spectra of the phantom of Fig. 9: a of the whole phantom; b of a volume centered on the inner tube; and c of a volume centered on the outer tube. The isolation of the spectra from the inner and outer tubes is clear. (BLACKBAND et al. 1988)

The choice between localized spectroscopy and chemical shift imaging remains controversial at the time of writing. Each acquisition for each phase increment of a chemical shift imaging technique averages the NMR signal. Consequently a spatially localized technique that is averaged the same number of times as the total number of phase increments for a one shot chemical shift image will have ideally the same S/N. This is providing that the localized volume is the same size as each of the chemical shift image voxels (GRANOT 1986). There are significant differences between the two methodologies. With the chemical shift image all the voxels across the subject are acquired whereas the localized techniques collect only one voxel in the same time. Further, any localized technique will suffer to some degree from contamination with residual signal outside of the required volume. However, the localized technique will be time saving when there is more S/N available than requires the number of averages to produce a full chemical shift image at least by 2-DFT techniques. This advantage may be circumvented if hybrid or pure echo planar based chemical shift imaging techniques become practical. Localized techniques also offer the ability to shim on the localized region of interest and thus to obtain a better homogeneity (and consequently a better resolved spectrum) than is possible when shimming on the whole sample (shimming is a process of optimizing the main magnetic field homogeneity by using weak magnetic field gradients called shim gradients). It seems likely, therefore, that the preferred technique will probably depend on the system to be studied. Thus both spatially localized spectroscopy and chemical shift imaging techniques will play roles in the future of NMR imaging.

5.11 NMR Microscopy

From Eq. (2) it can be seen that there are essentially three significant ways of increasing the S/N in an NMR experiment: by increasing the acquisition time, increasing the operating field strength, or decreasing the diameter of the receiver coil. Assuming that the acquisition time is to be limited (i.e., an hour or less), then small receiver coils must be used, preferably at high field strengths, in order to increase the S/N. This applies particularly when biological samples are involved. This limits one to the study of very small objects, or at least to the examination of very small regions of larger objects. With a corresponding increase in gradient strength (which is technically feasible since the gradient coils can also have a small diameter) this increased S/N can be translated into improved resolutions which approach microscopic dimensions. Such an instrument thus constitutes an NMR microscope and resolutions of up to $10 \times 12 \times 250$ μm have been reprorted (AGUAYO et al. 1986). Several groups are now working on microscopic imaging techniques (AGUAYO et al. 1987; JOHNSON et al. 1986; MANSFIELD and GRANNEL 1975; HALL and SUKUMAR 1982; LAUTERBUR 1974, 1984; MEYER and BROWN 1988; ECCLES and CALLAGHAN 1986). Generally, the larger the field of view that is required, the lower the resolution that can be achieved. This new domain of NMR imaging is only recently being explored and holds considerable promise in the near future for the microscopic examination of small biological systems and pathological specimens. Figure 11 shows the range of resolutions which can be achieved with respect to the field of view (i.e., the diameter of the receiver coil) to date. The in-plane resolution improvement from 210 μm in Fig. 11a to 10 μm in Fig. 11d is due principally to the reduction of the diameter of the receiver coil, which consequently improves the S/N.

The sequences used for microscopic imaging should be optimized to maximize the available S/N, but this is also true for most conventional imaging. It is as desirable to decrease the imaging time as it is to increase the resolution. However, different acquisition methods will be necessary when resolutions below approximately 5 μm are required. This is because at these high resolutions the effect of self-diffusion of the spins becomes significant and leads to an added loss of signal (STEJSKAL and TANNER 1965). In the interval between excitation of the system and observation of the induced signal, the spins will on average diffuse within the sample by an amount approaching or greater than the voxel dimensions. A spin which is excited in one voxel and which moves into an adjacent voxel before the observation window will not rephase properly and thus there is a loss of signal. Sequences for NMR microscopy must thus be designed to eliminate or minimize these effects at high resolutions.

Nuclear magnetic resonance microscopy also has considerable implications with respect to future nonbiological applications of NMR imaging, some of which are described later in this chapter. Microscopic resolutions are required to examine questions related to diffusion, porosity, and structure in materials. Several options are available with nonbiological samples in order to improve the S/N (and hence the resolution) that are generally not appli-

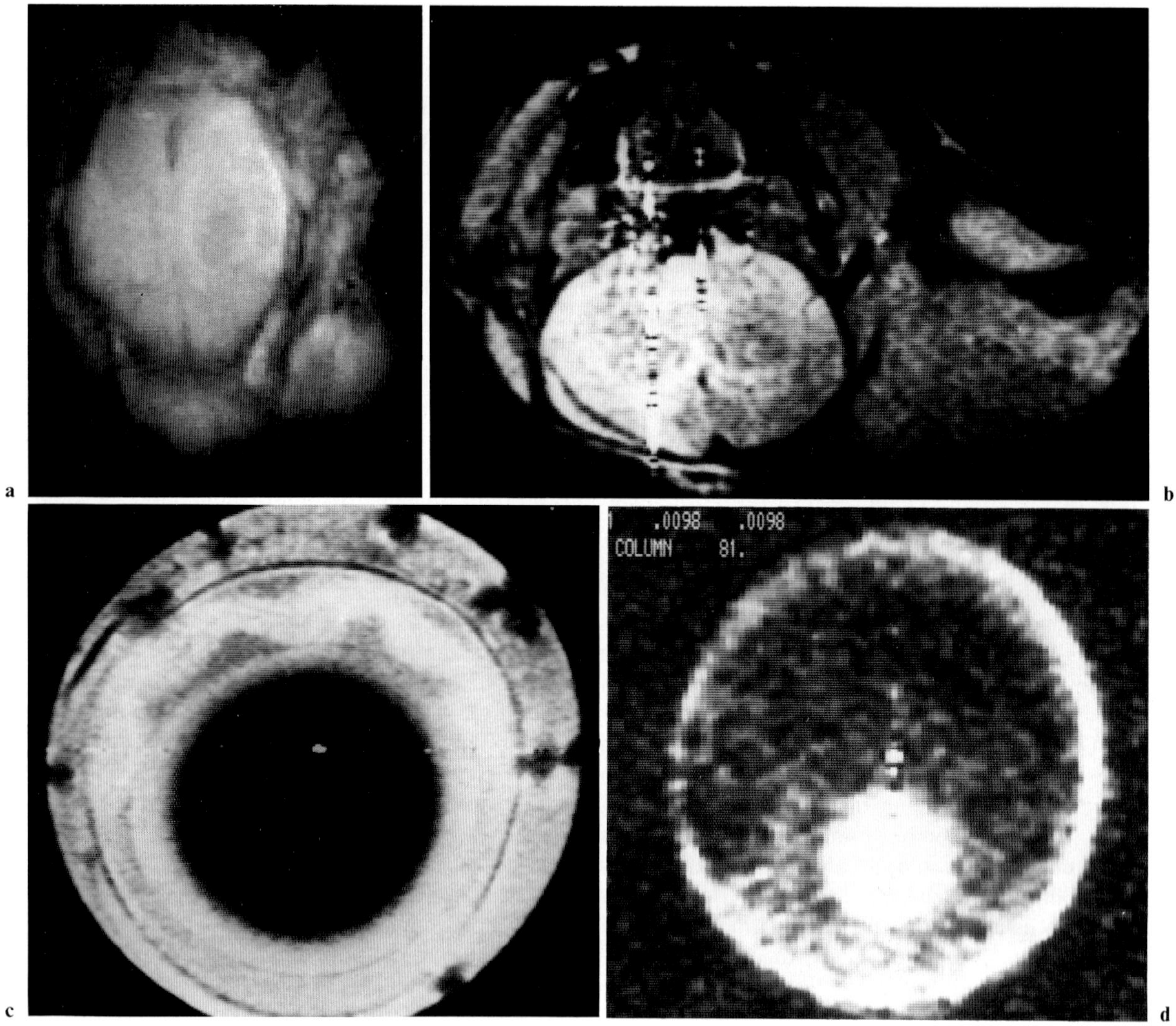

Fig. 11. a A transverse ^1H image of a rabbit brain containing a VX tumor (the darker round structure in the middle of the right hemisphere). The image resolution is $210 \times 210 \times 2000$ μm and it was obtained at 4.7 T. **b** An image through the head of a mouse obtained at 8.5 T. The large mass on the right-hand side of the head is a subcutaneously implanted RIF-1 tumor. The resolution is $88 \times 88 \times 1000$ μm: **c** An image of a mouse eye inside a 4.1 mm diameter capillary tube. the dark mass in the center of the eye is the lens nucleus. The resolution is $16 \times 27 \times 250$ μm. **d** An image of a frog ova inside a 1 mm diameter capillary tube. The white mass in the center of the image is the cell nucleus. The resolution is $10 \times 13 \times 250$ μm. **b:** Aguayo et al. (1987); **c, d:** Aguayo et al. (1986). See references for more details

cable when biological samples are examined. In particular, materials with lower self-diffusion coefficients may be examined; in many cases it may be possible to cool the NMR receiver and/or the sample, which can improve the sensitivity (Styles et al. 1984; Hall et al.1988), and generally such samples can be imaged for much longer time periods without the problems of sample maintenance commonly associated with biological samples (anesthesia, motion respiration, etc.)

Generally it is expected that the resolutions will gradually improve with technique and probe development. Applications will predominantly include the study of small biological organisms (e.g., dividing frog ova) from a research point of view. It remains to be seen if the examination of pathological samples can have a significant impact in the clinic. The noninvasive microscopic study of nonbiological materials is expected to have a more significant impact in industry and indeed may become a major tool for materials reserarch.

5.12 Solid Imaging

The nuclear spins in a system can be considered to be small magnetic dipoles. These dipoles, like tiny bar magnets, interact with each other; this is called the dipole-dipole interaction. In liquids (and gases), the random tumbling motion of the molecules causes this interaction to average to zero and consequently it is not significant in liquid spectroscopy and imaging. However, in solids the molecules are held in a rigid lattice and their motion is restricted. In this case the dipole-dipole interaction does not average to zero and it becomes a significant factor in the relaxation processes. Effectively the spins, when excited by an rf pulse, can dissipate their energy much more quickly between each other and the spin-spin relaxation time (T_2) becomes very short. In concert with this effect, the spins interact much less frequently with the lattice due to their restricted motion and cannot dissipate their energy to it as efficiently. Consequently the spin-lattice relaxation time (T_1) becomes very long. Both of these effects are detrimental with respect to NMR imaging. The long T_1 relaxation times translate into long TR times, and the short T_2 relaxation times demand very short TEs (tens of microseconds). With such short TEs, it is very difficult to spatially encode the FIDs or spin echoes when switched magnetic field gradients are involved. Short T_2 signals also require very fast sampling rates. Also, it can be shown that impractically large gradients are required (MANSFIELD and MORRIS 1982, Sect. 6.1.5).

Although it may be possible to overcome these problems in the future, the widespread imaging of solids is not yet feasible. However, the situation is not completely lost and some success has been achieved in imaging solids in a few specific samples. All the methods implemented to date use some method of averaging the dipole interaction to zero and consequently the NMR response looks liquid in nature (ABRAGAM 1961). In some special materials where the spin system of interest is sparsely distributed within the solid, the dipole-dipole interaction is minimal because of the relatively large distance between the spins (SZEVERENYI and MACIEL 1984). Some favorable solids exhibit rapid exchange between chemical species of the resonant nuclei of interest which again averages out the dipole interaction (CHINGAS et al. 1985). Multiple quantum methods offer some degree of success (GARROWAY et al. 1984). The most successful technique to date that has the broadest applicability utilizes a special sequence of rf pulses that are designed to average the dipole interaction to zero (CHINGAS et al. 1986). Figure 12 shows an example of such an image. However, these techniques are not at all simple, and they require very good rf pulse amplitude and phase control, and considerable rf power. Consequently they work most effectively on small samples. Their effectiveness also depends on the type of solid, i.e., the "more solid" or harder it is the less effective these techniques are. Although they work well on rubbers they are not effective on, for example, most metals.

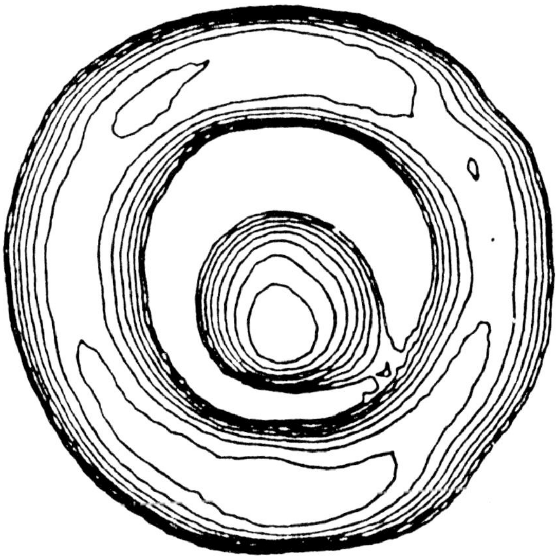

Fig. 12. A multipulse ^{1}H solid NMR image of a coaxial phantom of which the outer ring is made of rubber and the inner ring of adamantane. (CHINGAS et al. 1986)

Although the imaging, for example, of the solid component of human bones in vivo (as opposed to the liquid content of bone marrow) is not yet feasible, there does appear to be potential for solid imaging in the near future, at least on small samples. This should have an enormous impact on the applicabitity of NMR imaging in the material sciences.

5.13 Biological Effects Associated with NMR Imaging

To date, no detrimental biomagnetic effects from NMR imaging have been demonstrated, at least in human studies. Several effects have been documented, but all have been either anecdotal or badly reported and have not been reproduced by other workers. Many of these have been reviewed by MANSFIELD and MORRIS (1982). The basic consensus of their review is that there are as yet no substantiated detrimental effects of static magnetic fields at least up to approximately 1 T, of linear fields of 100 $\mathrm{Gcm^{-1}}$, of rf field effects providing that the rf power output is limited to the present government guidelines, or of time dependent fields up to at least 10 $\mathrm{Gcm^{-1}}$, which is well below the strengths used for clinical imaging. It is apparent from their review and from a survey of the current literature that there is a distinct paucity of information with respect to these problems. Now that whole body 4-T magnets have become feasible, and consequently even more powerful ones are being developed, it is crucial that some very careful and complete studies be undertaken to address these matters.

Certainly, high field imaging instruments of sufficiently large bore are available for animal studies of biomagnetic effects. Unfortunately the situation is extremely complex and it is difficult to retain control over all the variables in a given experiment. Also, at the "intermediate effect" field strengths the effects are likely to be very subtle and difficult to measure, especially when the experimentalist is not at all sure exactly what it is he or she should be looking for! Nevertheless, attempts must be made, and it is anticipated that the best results will be obtained by systematically looking for measurable effects at the highest available fields on biological systems, and then working backwards from that viewpoint.

Certainly, at high enough magnetic field strengths damaging or detrimental effects will be observed. Clinical imaging will probably not progress to such high fields for another decade or so because of technical limitations. When it does, however, the physician will need relevant information so that he can weigh patient exposure time against the risk/benefit ratio, as he does today with the diagnostic modalities that utilize damaging ionizing radiation. These problems will first need to be addressed in animal studies and will be of particular significance in microscopy, where the highest fields are currently being used. Indeed the effects of high fields may actually be exploited in this area. For example, the NMR response of a biological system that is disrupted from its normal function by very high magnetic fields may provide information that sheds light on the very nature of the sample, in particular on its metabolic and physiological processes.

One of the very real dangers associated with NMR imaging is that the high magnetic field attracts loose metallic objects, and can turn them into potentially harmful projectiles. It may also interact with metallic implants and, in particular, affect the performance of magnetically sensitive pacemakers. These problems can be avoided with careful screening and vigilance and the use of only nonmagnetic materials for implantation. Successful imaging has been demonstrated on patients with metallic implants. Only minor distortions occur due to the presence of the metal.

5.14 Clinical Applications of NMR Imaging

Virtually all human anatomy has now been examined by NMR imaging and many disease states have been studied. Figure 13 shows a selection of images of normal human anatomy that illustrate the kind of image quality that can be presently obtained on a commercial instrument. NMR imaging is now the diagnostic method of choice for many clinical applications, its most major impact to date being in the study and diagnosis of brain abnormalities. Discussion of these applications is outside of the scope of this chapter and the reader is referred to a small selection of the expanding array of literature on the subject (Stark and Bradley 1988; Bisese 1988: Daniels et al. 1987). The relative importance of NMR imaging as a clinical modality is expected to increase as the technique is developed. In particular the introduction of higher main magnetic field strengths, the more widespread clinical use of flow imaging methods, echo planar techniques, and associated technology, and the rapid integration of NMR imaging and NMR spectroscopy should dramatically increase the scope of NMR as a whole in clinical medicine.

5.15 NMR Imaging of Nonmedical Systems

The principal driving force behind the rapid development of NMR imaging has been its potential for the noninvasive investigation of the human body. Consequently rapid developments were made in building magnets large enough to accommodate the human body and in obtaining NMR images of diagnostic quality. However, the applications of NMR imaging extend far beyond these horizons and are now being explored more intensively. NMR imaging has already produced useful information on liquid ingress into building materials and polymers (Gummerson et al. 1979; Blackband and Mansfield 1986; Rothwell et al. 1984) and on the

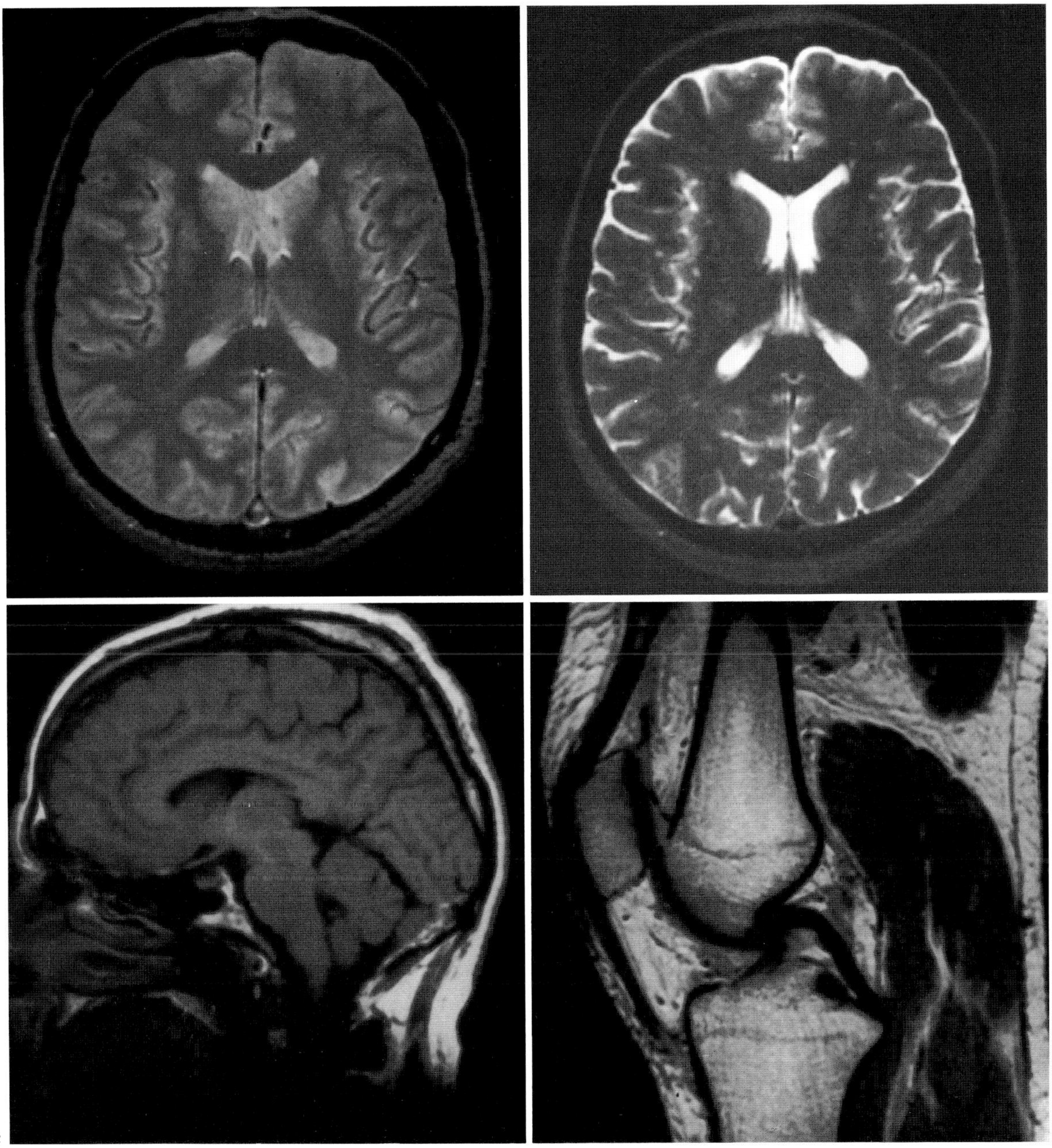

oil and water content of bore cores (BLACKBAND et al. 1986; HALL et al. 1986; HALL and RAJANAYAGAM 1987), and may find application in the examination of foodstuffs and explosives (MANSFIELD and MORRIS 1982). It also has potential for the study of plant materials, and has been used to examine the oil content of oil bearing seeds (LAUTERBUR 1974) and to monitor plant growth and examine plant root systems intact in their soil.

Until recently a principal limitation with regard to these applicatons has been the relatively poor spectral and spatial resolution attainable. Although

Fig. 13a–d Typical ^{1}H NMR images of human anatomy demonstrating the quality that can be obtained on a day-to-day basis in the clinic. They were obtained with standard clinical protocols in a General Electic 1.5-T instrument. **a** and **b** show transverse images of a human brain obtained with different imaging timings that change the T_1 and T_2 weightings in the images. A striking contrast difference is evident which is obviously clinically valuable. **c** shows a saggital image of a human head and **d** shows an image through a human knee. See references in text for examples and clinical descriptions.

one-dimensional resolutions of 240 μm have been used to study liquid ingress into polymers, it is apparent that better resolutions are required before the information obtained with NMR imaging techniques has a practical relevance for the study of such systems. Resolutions of 10 μm or less, made possible by the recent advances in NMR microscopy, open up new and far-reaching possibilities for such studies. With high field spectroscopy and microscopy machines, high resolution spectroscopy by localized or chemical shift imaging techniques offers new potential for nonmedical NMR imaging. In particular, many of the problems associated with biological systems will not be encountered in many nonbiological systems. Motion, limited temperature ranges, and exposure times will not be a problem in many cases. Indeed, sample shape design, as well as experimental design, can be manipulated to provide optimum conditions within the requirements and limitations imposed by a particular experiment or experimental apparatus. There are certain to be a myriad of other applications for NMR imaging just waiting to be uncovered and even more will be found if techniques for solid imaging become practical.

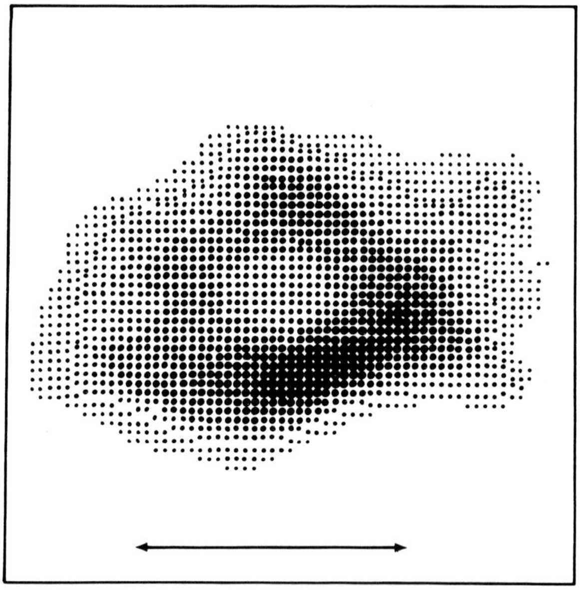

Fig. 14. A two-dimensional projection reconstruction ESR image of a live murine tumor. The data were acquired in 8 min. Although only four projections were acquired, the in-plane resolution is sub-millimeter and structure within the tumor is evident. (Berliner et al. 1987)

5.16 Electron Spin Resonance Imaging; Its Implications on NMR Imaging

Nuclear magnetic resonance imaging involves the exploitation of the resonant interaction between nuclei and a radiofrequency magnetic field. At higher frequencies, specifically at microwave frequencies, the magnetic field interacts with free electrons. This is the domain of electron spin resonance (ESR) spectroscopy (Wertz and Bolton 1972). Recently it has been demonstrated how this interaction can also be exploited to produce images (Eaton and Eaton 1984; Berliner and Fujii 1985; Demsar et al. 1988). Although fundamentally the same, this technique produces significantly different problems to those associated with NMR imaging. In particular, microwave frequencies can be harmful to biological systems, causing extensive heating. Thus the dose must be kept low. Also, only unpaired or free electrons such as those associated with free radicals give detectable signals and usually these radicals have to be introduced into or generated within biological systems. However, the ESR resonance induces in a receiver approximately one thousand times more signal than does the NMR resonance. Although ESR imaging has been performed on intact biological specimens (Berliner adn Fujii 1985; Berliner et al. 1987) as shown in Fig. 14, it is very unlikely that it could work on a human whole body basis. However, it does hold considerable promise for the study of small systems, and could become a complementary technique to NMR imaging on high resolution spectrometers, especially in the material sciences. An exciting prospect is possible utilization of the double resonance effects (Lurie et al. 1988). In some special systems the nuclear and electronic energy levels can be coupled. These techniques cause enhancement of the nuclear or electron resonance respectively by stimulating at the electron or nuclear frequency respectively. Thus with respect to NMR imaging it should be possible to obtain significant increases in the NMR sensitivity. This may be particularly useful for microscopy studies.

5.17 New Developments with Potential Impact

Nuclear magnetic resonance imaging is still a relatively new modality and considerable development of techniques and applications can be expected over the next decade. In harmony with this will be the integration of new technology with NMR imaging (and other imaging modalities), which will further improve its capabilities. Many of the improvements will involve better performance of the various standard components of NMR imaging systems such as receivers, rf amplifiers, and power supplies.

In particular we will see improved data aquisition, processing, and display capabilities associated with computer technology developments. Fast and interactive three-dimensional data processing capabilities will facilitate the more efficient use of three-dimensional data sets. A possible scenario is that of a surgeon using a light pen instead of a scalpel to perform imaginary surgery on a three-dimensional patient data set, thus planning his approach before actual surgery. This should help to minimize invasion in exploratory surgery and represents a sort of "flight simulator" for surgeons. The sequel to this would be some sort of computer guided surgery. The feasibility of displaying NMR data as a hologram has been demonstrated and offers promise as a possible method for displaying data of more than two dimensions in a concise and readable manner (TURNER 1985). Three or more dimensional data can be difficult to display in a useful format on video display screens and most often slices are extracted from the data for examination. NMR data are particularly amenable for hologram display; the NMR time data acquired is the Fourier transform of the actual image and consequently may be reconstructed by optical components, i.e., a lens, and filtered with apodizers, thus obviating the need for a conventional computer. However, some method of data storage for more complex processing will be required and it seems unlikely that this will replace the computer. Rather it may represent a real time image reconstruction and display facility for preliminary data examination and for NMR study set-up procedures. Should optical computers become a viable prospect in the future, then a display modality such as the hologram will be particularly appropriate.

Developments in several areas more specific to NMR are also expected to have an impact. Further improvements in magnet technology should maintain the progress towards higher field magnets and larger bore magnets at a given high field, which may in turn improve the available S/N and the spectroscopic performance of the instruments. It has been shown to be technically possible to improve the S/N in an NMR experiment by cooling the receiver to eliminate thermally generated noise (STYLES et al. 1984; HALL et al. 1988). Although feasible, this is not carried out in most applications, mainly because of the added complexities it introduces into the probe design. In particular, for significant improvements the coils must be cryocooled to the temperature of liquid helium or nitrogen and consequently a dewar system has to be maintained around the coils. This reduces the flexibility of the receiver and the usable magnet bore and can make access difficult. Further, in many biological systems, especially at high field strengths, the dominant noise source is not the coil itself but the sample. Biological systems generally contain moving electrolytes that induce random currents in the receiver coil that contribute to the noise. This coil cooling approach may thus have the most significant application in nonbiological studies where the dominant noise source is the coil.

A promising prospect is the introduction of the new high temperature superconducting materials (BEDNORZ and MULLER 1986; VOSS 1988; POOL 1988). If these materials can be fabricated into a wire that is superconducting at room temperature the implications are, of course, tremdendous in many areas of technology. With respect to NMR, they may be used to make receiver coils for all NMR machines (imaging and spectroscopy) without imposing any of the limitations of cryocooled coils. Eventually it may even be possible to use the material to construct the main magnet. Although there are many technological problems to overcome before this may be feasible, and most certainly it will not happen in the next decade, the prospect is highly attractive since it obviates the need for cryogens, will make the actual magnet lighter and physically smaller, and should facilitate the generation of stronger magnetic fields.

5.18 Conclusions

It is hoped that this brief chapter has indicated the wide scope of NMR imaging and its rapid and continuing development. It is already a prominent diagnostic modality and is expected to become one of the, if not the, most useful tomographic technique. In particular, the scope and utility of NMR imaging will increase dramatically if the promise of combined imaging and spectroscopy is fulfilled. Much useful noninvasive in vivo chemical information should become available. The echo planar techniques and their technological spin-offs are increasing the imaging quality and versatility of imaging machines and it is expected that these high speed imaging techniques should shortly become more widely available for clinical use. The issue associated with high field imaging is yet to be resolved, and it is expected that optimum field choices will depend specifically on the particular system to be studied. Certainly the trend to higher field magnets is a healthy one with respect to spectroscopy, microscopy, and nonbiological imaging studies, and it remains to be seen when possible detrimental effects of high field imaging and its associated consequences will become limiting factors with respect to in vivo studies.

The high cost of NMR imaging machines has so far restricted the nonbiological applications of the techniques. However, the recent introduction of comparatively cheap add-on imaging units to conventional spectrometers which are widely available is expected to expand these applications. Such instruments are also providing valuable information on the integration of imaging and spectroscopic techniques that is a useful precursor to such undertakings on larger bore instruments.

More widespread development and evaluation of relatively new areas of high speed imaging, flow imaging, and microscopy are expected to enhance the versatility of NMR imaging in the biological and material sciences. This versatility will further improve, at least on small samples, should solid imaging techniques become more practical.

Several new technologies will enhance the capabilities of NMR imaging. In particular new and more powerful computing facilities will improve the power of not only NMR itself, but also the correlation of NMR with other radiological modalities. The prospect of room temperature superconductors is extremely exciting, although one must not let the tremendous possibilities override the reality of the technological difficulties that must be overcome. However, governments are expected to provide considerable resources for the development of these materials because of their widespread implications in all areas of science and technology. All in all, the future of NMR imaging is increasingly exciting.

Acknowledgment. Many thanks to Dr. C. Hutchinson for her careful proofreading of this manuscript and helpful editorial comments.

References

Abragam A (1961) The principles of nuclear magnetism. Clarendon, Oxford

Aguayo JB, Blackband SJ, Schoeniger J, Mattingly M, Hintermann M (1986) Nuclear magnetic resonance imaging of a single cell. Nature 322: 190–191

Aguayo JB, Blackband SJ, Wehrle JP, Glickson JD, Mattingly MA (1987) NMR microscopic studies of eyes and tumors with histological correlation. Ann NY Acad Sc 508: 399–413

Anderson WA (1961) Electrical current shims for correction magnetic fields. Rev Sci Instrum 32: 241

Aue WP, Muller S, Cross TA, Seeling JJ (1984) Volume-selective excitation. A novel approach to topical NMR. J Magn Reson 56: 350

Bednorz JG, Muller KA (1986) Possible high T_c superconductivity in the Ba-LA-Cu-O system. Z Phys B 64: 189–193

Bendall MR, Gordon RE (1983) Depth and refocusing pulses designed fo multipulse NMR with surface coils. J Magn Reson 53: 365–385

Bendall MR, Connelly A, McKendry JM (1986) Elimination of coupling between cylindrical transmit coils and surface-receive coils for in vivo NMR. Magn Reson Med 3: 157–163

Berliner LJ, Fujii H (1985) Magnetic resonance imaging of biological specimens by paramagnetic resonance of nitroxide spin labels. Science 227: 517

Berliner LJ, Fujii H, Wan X, Lukiewicz SJ (1987) Feasibility study of imaging a living murine tumor by electron paramagnetic resonance. Magn Reson Med 4: 380–384

Bisese JH (1988) MRI: a teaching file approach. McGraw-Hill, New York

Blackband SJ, Mansfield P (1986) Diffusion in liquid-solid systems by NMR imaging. J Phys C 19: 149–152

Blackband SJ, Mansfield P, Barnes JR, Clague ADH, Rice SA (1986) Discrimination of crude oil and water in sand and in bore cores with NMR imaging. SPE Formulation Evaluation: February

Blackband SJ, McGrovern KA, McLennan IJ (1988) Spatially localized two-dimensional spectroscopy. SLO-COSY and SLO-NOESY. J Magn Reson 79: 184–189

Bottomley PA (1981) A versatile magnetic-field gradient control system for NMR imaging. J Phys (E) 14: 1081–1087

Bottomley PA (1985) Noninvasive studies of high energy phosphate metabolism in human heart by depth-resolved ^{31}P NMR spectroscopy. Science 229: 769–772

Bottomley PA, Andrew ER (1978) RF magnetic field penetration, phase shift and power dissipation in biological tissue: implications for NMR imaging. Phys Med Biol 23: 630

Bottomley PA, Edelstein WA, Hart HR et al. (1984a) In vivo ^{1}H imaging fo the head at 1.5T. Magn Reson Med 1: 113

Bottomley PA, Foster TB, Darrow RD (1984b) Depth-resolved surface coil spectroscopy (DRESS) for in vivo ^{1}H, ^{31}P, and ^{13}C NMR. J Magn Reson 59: 338–342

Bottomley PA, Redington RW, Edelstein WA, Schenck JF (1985) Estimating radiofrequency power deposition in body NMR imaging. Magn Reson Med 2: 336–349

Bottomley PA, Charles HC, Roemer PB, Flaming D, Engeseth H, Edelstein WA, Mueller OM (1988) Human in vivo phosphate metabolite imaging with ^{31}P NMR. Magn Reson Med 7: 319–336

Brown TR, Kincaid BM, Ugurbil K (1982) NMR chemical shift imaging in three dimensions. Proc Natl Acad Sci USA 79: 3523

Brunner P, Ernst RR (1979) Sensitivity and performance time in NMR imaging. J Magn Reson 33: 83–106

Chapman B, Turner R, Ordidge RJ et al. (1987) Real-time movie imaging from a single cardiac cycle by NMR. Magn Reson Med 5: 246–254

Chingas GC, Milliken J, Resing HA, Tsang T (1985) Graphite-AsF5 intercalation kinetics and diffusion by NMR imaging. Synth Met 12: 1–2, 131

Chingas GC, MillerJB, Garroway AN (1986) NMR images of solids. J Magn Reson 66: 530–535

Clark LC, Ackerman JL, Thomas SR, Millard RW (1984) High-contrast tissue and blood oxygen imaging based on fluorocarbon ^{19}F NMR relaxation times. Magn Reson Med 1: 135

Daniels DL, Haughton VM, Naidich TP (1987) Cranial and spinal magnetic resonance imaging. Raven, New York

De Luca F, Maraviglia B (1986) Magic-angle NMR imaging in solids. J Magn Reson 67: 169–172

Demsar F, Walczak T, Morse PD, Bacic G, Zolnai Zsolt Swartz HM (1988) Detection of diffusion and distribution of oxygen be fast-scan EPR imaging. J Magn Reson 76: 224–231

Dickinson RJ, Hall AS, Hind AJ, Young IR (1986) Measurement of changes in tissue temperature using magnetic resonance imaging. J Comput Assist Tomogr 10: 468–472

Dixon WT (1984) Simple proton spectroscopy. Radiology 153: 189

Doyle M, Mansfield P (1987) Chemical-shift imaging: a hybrid approach. Magn Reson Med 5: 255–261

Dumoulin CL, Hart HR (1986) Magnetic resonance angiography. Radiology 161: 717–720

Eaton SS, Eaton GR (1984) EPR imaging. J Magn Reson 59: 474

Eccles CD, Callaghan PT (1986) High-resolution imaging. The NMR mircoscope. J Magn Reson 68: 393–398

Edelman PR, Hahn PF, Buxton R, Wittenberg J, Ferrucci JT, Saini S, Brady TJ (1986) Rapid NMR imaging with suspenden respiration: clinical application in the liver. Radiology 161: 125

Edelstein WA, Hutchinson JMS, Johnson G, Redpath TW (1980) Spin warp NMR imaging and application to whole-body imaging. Phys Med Biol 25: 751–756

Ernst RR, Bodenhausen G, Wokaun A (1987) Principles of nuclear magnetic resonance in one and two dimensions. Clarendon, Oxford

Ferrar TC, Becker ED (1971) Pulse and Fourier transform NMR. Academic, New York

Frahm J, Merboldt KD, Hanicke W (1987) Localized proton spectroscopy using stimulated echoes. J Magn Reson 72: 502

Garroway AN, Grannell PK, Mansfield P (1974) Image formation in NMR by a selective irradiative process. J Phys C 7: L427–L462

Garroway AN, Baum J, Munowitz MG, Pines A (1984) NMR imaging in solids by multiple-quantum resonance. J Magn Reson 60: 337

Ginsberg DM, Melchner MI (1970) Optimum geometry of saddle shaped coils for generating a uniform magnetic field. Rev Sci Instrum 41: 122

Golay MJE (1971) US Patent Number 3569523 and 3622869

Granot J (1986) Selected volume spectroscopy (SVS) and chemical shift imaging. A comparison. J Magn Reson 66: 197–200

Guilfoyle DN, Mansfield P (1985) Chemical shift imaging. Magn Reson Med 2: 479–489

Gummerson RJ, Hall C, Hoff WD, Hawkes R, Holland GN, Moore WS (1979) Unsaturated water flow within porous materials observed by NMR imaging. Nature 281: 56

Gupta RK (1977) A new look at the method of variable nutation angle for the measurement of spin-lattice relaxation times using Fourier transform NMR. J Magn Reson 25: 231

Haase A, Frahm J, Matthaei D, Hanicke W, Merboldt KD (1986) FLASH imaging. Rapid NMR imaging using low flip-angle pulses. J Magn Reson 67: 258

Hall LD, Sukumar S (1982) Chemical microscopy using a high-resolution NMR spectrometer. A combination of tomography/spectroscopy using either ^{1}H or ^{13}C. J Magn Reson 50: 161

Hall LD, Talagala SL (1985) Mapping of pH and temperature distribution using chemical-shift-resolved tomography. J Magn Reson 65: 501–505

Hall LD, Rajanayagam V (1987) Thin-slice, chemical-shift imaging of oil and water in sandstone rock at 80 MHz. J Magn 74: 139–146

Hall LD, Rajanayagam V, Hall C (1986) Chemical-shift imaging of water and *n*-dodecane in sedimentary rocks. J Magn Reson 68: 185–188

Hall AS, Barnard B, McArthur P, Gilderdale DJ, Young IR, Bydder GM (1988) Investigation of a whole-body receiver coil operating at liquid nitrogen temperatures. Magn Reson Med 7: 230–235

Hayes CE, Edelstein WA, Schenck JF, Meuller OM, Eash MJ (1985) An efficient, highly homogeneous radiofrequency coil for whole-body NMR imaging at 1.5 t. J Magn Reson 63: 622

Hinshaw WS (1974) Spin mapping: the application of moving gradients to NMR. Phys Lett 48A: 87–88

Hinshaw WS, Bottomley PA, Holland GN (1977) Radiographic thin-section image of the human wrist by nuclear magnetic resonance. Nature 270: 722

Hore PJ (1983) Solvent suppression in Fourier transform nuclear magnetic resonance. J Magn Reson 55: 283–300

Hoult DI, Richards RE (1976) The signal-to-noise ratio of the nuclear magnetic resonance experiment. J Magn Reson 24: 71–85

Johnson GA, Thompson MB, Gewalt SL, Hayes CE (1986) Nuclear magnetic resonance imaging at microscopic resolution. J Magn Reson 68: 129

Joseph PM, Fishman JE, Mukherji, Sloviter HA (1985) In vivo ^{19}F NMR imaging of the cardiovascular system. J Comput Assist Tomogr 9: 1012–1019

Kormos DW, Yeung HN, Gauss RC (1987) NMR imaging of carbon-13. J Magn Reson 71: 159–162

Kressel HY (1985) Magnetic resonance annual. Raven, New York

Kumar A, Welti D, Ernst RR (1975) NMR fourier zeugmatography. J Magn Reson 18: 69-83

Lauterbur PC (1973) Image formations by induced local interactions: examples exploying nuclear magnetic resonance. Nature 242: 190–191

Lauterbur P (1974) Magnetic resonance zeugmatography. Pure Appl Chem 40: 149

Lauterbur P (1984) Spectroscopic imaging of microscopic objects. IEEE Trans Nucl Sci NA-31: 4

Leroy-Willig A, Darrasse L, Taquin J, Sauzade M (1985) The slotted cylinder: an efficient probe for NMR imaging. Magn Reson Med 2: 20–28

Lurie DJ, Bussel DM, Bell LH, Mallard JR (1988) Proton-electron double magnetic resonance imaging of free radical solutions. J Magn Reson 76: 366–370

Luyten PR, Marien AJH, Sijtsma B, den Hollander JA (1986) Solvent-suppressed spatially resolved spectroscopy. An approach to high-resolution NMR on a whole-body MR system. J Magn Reson 67: 148

Mansfield P (1984) Spatial mapping of the chemical shift in NMR. Magn Reson Med 1: 370–386

Mansfield P, Grannell P (1975) Diffraction and microscopy in solids and liquids by NMR. Phys Rev B 12: 3629

Mansfield P, Pykett IL (1978) Biological and medical imaging by NMR. J Magn Reson 29: 355
Mansfield P, Morris PG (1982) NMR imaging in biomedicine. Adv Mag Res, Suppl 2. Academic, New York
Mansfield P, Chapman B (1986) Active magnetic screening of coils for static and time dependent magnetic field generation in NMR imaging. J Phys E 19: 540
Mansfield P, Chapman B (1987) Multishield active magnetic screening of coil structures in NMR. J Magn Reson 72: 211–223
Maudsley AA, Hilal SK, Perman WH, Simon HE (1983) Spatially resolved high resolution spectroscopy by "four-dimensional" NMR. J Magn Reson 51: 147
Maudsley AA, Hilal SK (1984) Biological aspects of sodium-23 imaging. Br Med Bull 40: 165–167
Maudsley AA, Hilal SK, Simon HE, Wittekoek S (1984) In vivo MR sprectroscopic imaging with P-31. Radiology 153: 745
Meyer RA, Brown TR (1988) Diffusion measurements by microscopic NMR imaging. J Magn Reson 76: 393–399
Moran PR (1982) A flow velocity zeugmatographic interlace for NMR imaging in humans. Magn Reson Imaging 1: 197–203
Morris PG (1986) Nuclear magnetic resonance imaging in medicine and biology. Clarendon, Oxford
Muller S, Seelig J (1987) In vivo NMR imaging of deuterium. J Magn Reson 72: 456–466
Nunnally RL, Babock EE, Horner SD, Peshock RM (1985) Fluorine-19 NMR spectroscopy and imaging investigations of myocardial perfusion and cardiac function. Magn Reson Imaging 3: 399
Ordidge RJ, Connelly A, Lohman JAB (1986) Image-selected in vivo spectroscopy (ISIS). A new technique for spatially selective NMR spectroscopy. J Magn Reson 66: 283–294
Ordidge RJ, Coxon R, Howseman A, Chapman B, Turner R, Stehling M, Mansfield P (1988) Snapshot head imaging at O·5T using the echo planar technique. Magn Reson Med 8: 110–115
Park HW, Cho ZH (1986) High-resolution human in vivo spectroscopic imaging using echo-time encoding technique. Magn Reson Med 3: 448–453
Parker DL, Smith V, Sheldon P, Crooks LE, Russel L (1983) Temperature distribution measurements in two dimensional NMR imaging. Med Phys 10: 321–325
Pool R (1988) New superconductors come through. Science 240: 1613–1615
Pykett IL, Rzedzian PR (1987) Instant images of the body by magnetic resonance. Magn Reson Med 5: 563–571
Ra JB, Hilal SK, Cho ZH (1986) A method for in vivo MR imaging of the short T2 component of sodium-23. Magn Reson Med 3: 296–302
Ra JB, Hilal SK, Oh CH, Mun IK (1988) In vivo magnetic resonance imaging of sodium in the human body. Magn Reson Med 7: 11–22
Radda GK (1986) The use of NMR spectroscopy for the understanding of disease. Science 233: 640–645
Ratner AV, Hurd R, Muller HH et al. (1987) ^{19}F magnetic resonance imaging of the reticuloendothelial system. Magn Reson Med 5: 548–554
Renshaw PF, Haselgrove JC, Leigh JS, Chance B (1985) In vivo nuclear magnetic resonance imaging of lithium. Magn Reson Med 2: 512–516
Rothwell WP, Holecek DR, Kershaw JA (1984) NMR imaging; study of fluid absorption by polymer composites. JAJ Polym Sci Polym Lett 22: 241
Rzedzian R, Mansfield P, Doyle M et al. (1983) Real-time nuclear magnetic resonance clinical imaging in paediatrics. Lancet II: 1281–1282
Schneider HJ, Dullenkopf P (1977) Slotted tube resonator: a new NMR probe head at high observing frequencies, Rev Sci Instrum 48: 68–73
Schultz CL, Alfidi RJ, Nelson AD, Koppiwoda SY, Clampitt ME (1984) The effect of motion on two-dimensional Fourier transformation magnetic resonance images. Radiology 152: 117
Slichter CP (1978) Principles of magnetic resonance. Springer, New York
Stark DD, Bradley WG (1988) Magnetic resonance imaging. 1st edn. C.V. Mosby, St. Lois
Stejskal EO, Tanner JE 81965) Spin diffusion measurements: spin echoes in the presence of a time-depentent field gradient. J Chem Phys 42: 288
Styles P, Soffe NF, Scott CA, Cragg A, White DJ, White PCJ (1984) A high-resolution NMR probe in which the coil and preamplifier are cooled with liquid helium. J Magn Reson 60: 397–404
Szeverenyi NM, Maciel GE (1984) NMR spin imaging of magnetically dilute nuclei in the solid state. J Magn Reson 60: 460–466
Tanner IE (1965) Pulsed field gradients for NMR spin echo diffusion measurements. Rev Sci Instrum 36: 1086
Turner R (1985) Optical reconstruction of NMR images. Proc of the Fourth Meeting of the Soc Magn Reson Med, London, pp 1262–1263
van der Muelen P, Groen JP, Cuppen JJM (1985) Very fast MR imaging by field echoes and small angle excitation. Magn Reson Imaging 3: 297
Voss DF (1988) Superconductivity: The FAX factor. Science 240: 280–281
Wehrli FW, MacFall JR, Azel L (1984) Approaches to inplane and out-of-plane flow imaging. Noninvasive Med Imaging 2: 127–136
Wertz JE, Bolton JR (1972) Electron spin resonance; elementary theory and applications. McGraw-Hill, New York

6 NMR Spectroscopy and Its Application to the Study of Cancer

JANNA P. WEHRLE, CYNTHIA PAELLA MARTIN, and JERRY D. GLICKSON

CONTENTS

6.1	Introduction	93
6.2	Basic Principles of NMR Spectroscopy	93
6.2.1	The NMR Spectrum	94
6.2.2	NMR-Visible Nuclei in Biological Systems	95
6.2.3	Measurement of Reaction Rates by NMR	96
6.2.4	Techniques for NMR Spectroscopy In Vivo	97
6.3	NMR Studies of Murine Tumors	99
6.3.1	Untreated Tumor Growth	100
6.3.1.1	^{31}P NMR Spectra of RIF-1 Tumors	100
6.3.1.2	A Model for Growth-Associated Changes in the Energy Metabolism of Tumors	101
6.3.2	Treated Tumors	102
6.3.2.1	Chemotherapeutic Agents	102
6.3.2.2	X-Irradiation	106
6.3.2.3	Hyperthermia	107
6.3.2.4	Other Therapeutic Modalities	108
6.4	NMR Spectroscopic Studies of Humans	108
6.5	Status of Cancer Studies	109
6.6	A Look at the Future of NMR Spectroscopy	111
	References	113

6.1 Introduction

In this chapter the application of nuclear magnetic resonance (NMR) spectroscopy to the study of cancer will be discussed. As cancer continues to be a leading cause of death and primary focus of physicians, biomedical researchers, and health care adminstrators throughout the world, interest remains high in the utilization of diagnostic technologies that provide unique capabilities for the detection and management of this disease. In vivo NMR spectroscopy is one of the most promising of the new diagnostic methods. This technique holds considerable promise for diagnosis and staging of cancer, for prediction and detection of therapeutic response, for monitoring pharmacokinetics of antineoplastic agents, and for detection of toxicity of anticancer agents to vital normal tissues. In addition to these potential clinical capabilities, NMR spectroscopy has already demonstrated its utility in experimental investigations of the biochemical and physiological characteristics of cancer.

This chapter will include a brief overview of the principles of NMR spectroscopy to provide a basic understanding of the information obtained during an NMR experiment. The application of these techniques to the investigation of cancer growth and treatment will then be discussed using an experimental mouse tumor as a model. The potential clinical utility of this method will be considered in light of these experimental data and the initial clinical applications recently reported. Throughout this chapter future trends in NMR spectroscopy will be emphasized. Chapter 5 presents a discussion of NMR imaging (magnetic resonance imaging, or MRI), a newer NMR technique which already has had a significant impact on diagnostic radiology. Whereas NMR imaging primarily provides anatomical information, NMR spectroscopy monitors biochemical processes. Both methods are noninvasive and apparently free of hazard. The combined use of these modalities holds great promise in the diagnosis and treatment of cancer and other diseases and in providing information about basic physiological and biochemical processes in living tissues.

6.2 Basic Principles of NMR Spectroscopy

A thorough discussion of the basic principles of NMR spectroscopy can be found in texts by GADIAN (1982) and FARRAR and BECKER (1971). Here we present a brief, heuristic description of the method and emphasize its applications to cancer. NMR experimentation is based upon the intrinsic ability of certain atomic nuclei to spin about their axes and generate a magnetic field. This spin axis will rotate around the direction of a strong external magnetic field applied to the sample much as the axis of a

JANNA P. WEHRLE, Ph.D., CYNTHIA PAELLA MARTIN, M.S., Dept. of Radiology and Radiological Science, The Johns Hopkins University, School of Medicine, 600 North Wolfe Street, Baltimore, MD 21205, USA

JERRY D. GLICKSON, Ph.D., Depts. of Radiology and Radiological Science, and Biological Chemistry, The Johns Hopkins University, School of Medicine, 600 North Wolfe Street, Baltimore, MD 21205, USA spinning top rotates around the direction of the gravitational field. This motion is called precession. In the presence of the external magnetic field, the simplest nuclei orient themselves in one of two possible spin states, which arise from quantum mechanical considerations. These nuclei, with a spin quantum number of 1/2, include ^{1}H, ^{13}C, ^{19}F, and ^{31}P. Because one spin state is slightly preferred, a net magnetization of the sample under investigation occurs. In an NMR experiment, a radiofrequency (rf) coil is employed to induce a transition between these two spin states and detect the resulting changes in the bulk magnetization of the sample.

The rate at which nuclei precess in the presence of the applied field is called the Larmor frequency. Not only is the Larmor frequency proportional to the magnitude of the external field, but it also reflects the specific chemical environment of any given nucleus within a molecule. Detection of the presence of neighboring atoms ultimately makes possible the elucidation of chemical structure.

Nuclear magnetic resonance experiments were originally performed by what was called continuous wave NMR spectroscopy (CW-NMR). The experiment could be performed by continuously varying the frequency of the rf coil while the external field was kept constant (i.e., at constant Larmor frequency) or by varying the external field (i.e., at varying Larmor frequencies) while the rf was kept constant. Spin transitions occurred when the rf exactly matched the Larmor frequency of specific nuclei in the sample. This condition, called *resonance,* was detected by current induced in the detector coil as a consequence of changes in bulk magnetization of the sample. By sweeping the entire range of Larmor frequencies, each chemically distinct nucleus was sequentially excited, thus producing a series of deflections or *resonance peaks*. These peaks, when plotted as a function of rf, constituted the NMR *spectrum* of the sample. The NMR spectrum contains one peak for each chemically distinct nucleus; the intensity of each peak is proportional to the concentration of the corresponding nucleus. The resonance frequency and shape of each peak are sensitive indicators of the chemical nature of the nucleus. Still, the CW-NMR experiment is an inefficient method for obtaining the spectrum, requiring on the order of 500 s to sweep the entire spectral frequency range (for protons).

Modern spectrometers use a far more efficient procedure called *Fourier transform* or *FT-NMR* spectroscopy. The NMR spectrum in these experiments is obtained by applying a short pulse of rf power to induce spin transitions in all the nuclei within the sample. Once the pulse is discontinued, the sample magnetization returns to its equilibrium state by a process termed *relaxation,* which is several seconds in duration. Many experiments can be performed and averaged together to improve sensitivity (which increases as the square root of the number of experiments). The data obtained during this return to equilibrium, called the *free induction decay* (FID), are converted to an NMR spectrum via a mathematical computation called Fourier transformation.

During the FID, additional information is also acquired. The relaxation time of a particular spin varies significantly in biological tissues, and during an NMR study two different relaxation times are measured, the spin-lattice relaxation time (T_1) and the spin-spin relaxation time (T_2). T_1 measures the time required for the sample to dissipate its excess magnetic energy to the environment, while T_2 refers to the time required for the spins to lose phase coherence after a pulse. The water ^{1}H T_1 and T_2 values in many tumors are significantly longer than in nonmalignant tissues (DAMADIAN 1971). Measurement of T_1 and T_2 times is critical to the acquisition of high contrast NMR images of tumors and other tissues (see Chap. 5).

6.2.1 The NMR Spectrum

An NMR spectrum contains a discrete peak for each chemically distinct nucleus in the sample under investigation, the intensity of which is proportional to the number of equivalent nuclei in the sample. A spectrum can thus provide information not only about the nature but also about the concentration of NMR-detectable compounds. For example, in the ^{31}P spectrum of a mouse tumor shown

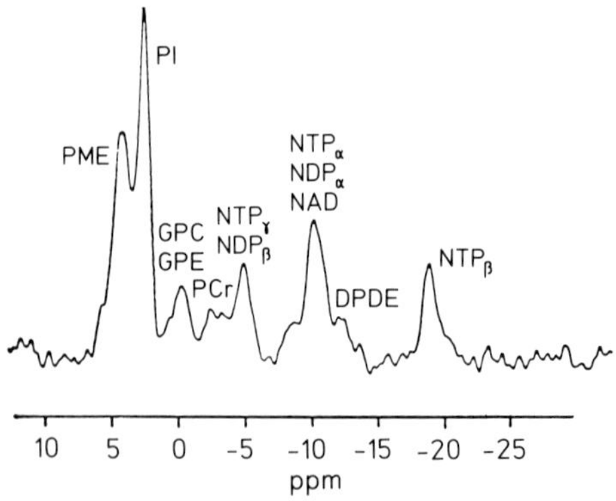

Fig. 1. ^{31}P NMR spectrum (80.96 MHz) of a 1.1-g RIF-1 tumor. Peaks of key metabolites are assigned. (GLICKSON et al. 1987)

in Fig. 1, separate peaks can be observed for each of the phosphorus atoms in ATP and for other phosphorus-containing compounds. Other nuclei produce similar spectra in which the number of lines correspond to the number and complexity of existing compounds. Compounds in solution produce sharp, narrow lines which are easy to resolve; living samples, on the other hand, yield broader resonances which can contain overlapping peaks from nuclei which have similar chemical properties (for instance, the α resonance of ATP and one of the phosphates of NAD in Fig. 1). Because both the intensity of peaks in the spectrum and the separation between them increases as external field strength increases, the newer, higher-field magnets are extremely useful for spectroscopy. Peaks or resonances in the spectrum are assigned to specific nuclei by applying a variety of NMR, biochemical, and chromatographic techniques (EVANOCHKO et al. 1984b).

6.2.2 NMR-Visible Nuclei in Biological Systems

Because of the relative simplicity of ^{31}P spectra and their ability to reveal key metabolites in cellular bioenergetics and phospholipid metabolism, ^{31}P has been the nucleus most often employed in in vivo studies of tumors and other biological tissues, as suggested by Fig. 1. The component resonances of the mouse tumor shown in this figure have been identified by analysis of the perchloric acid extracts of freeze-clamped tumors. These include phosphocreatine (PCr); inorganic phosphate (P_i); nucleoside triphosphates (NTPs), including ATP, UTP, GTP, and CTP; corresponding nucleoside diphosphates; phosphomonoesters (PMEs), including phosphorylethanolamine (PE), phosphorylcholine (PC), and trace quantities of AMP (not labeled in the figure); phosphodiesters (PDEs), the glycerol esters of PE and PC (GPE and GPC, respectively); and pyridine diphosphonucleotides (e.g., NAD^+), the resonance of which include contributions from reduced and oxidized forms of these compounds. In in vivo tissue the concentration of ADP is too low to observe by NMR techniques.

Nuclear magnetic resonance spectra of tumors generally exhibit resonances from P_i, PMEs, PDEs, and NTPs. Conflicting claims have surfaced about the presence or absence of PCr in tumors, with some investigators proposing that this metabolite originates from peripheral normal tissues. However, studies of numerous tumor cells in culture have demonstrated that tumor cells can produce NMR-detectable levels of PCr (EVANOCHKO et al. 1984b), while careful calibration of surface (NG et al. 1982a) and solenoidal coils (NG and GLICKSON 1985) confirms that PCr signals do originate from the tumor. Overall, PCr appears to be present in some, but not all, tumors.

The resonance frequency of the P_i peak is used to determine the pH of the tumor. In spectra of perfused tumor cells, detection of distinct resonances from intracellular and extracellular P_i has been possible, thereby allowing measurement of pH in these compartments. However, under in vivo conditions only average tissue pH is detected.

Changes in ratios of phosphate metabolites and pH have been observed in in vivo ^{31}P NMR spectra of tumors during untreated growth and following effective therapeutic interventions. The relative levels of high energy phosphates (PCr and NTPs) compared to low energy phosphates (P_i) serve as indices of the bioenergetic status of the tumor (see Sect. 6.3). Since PE and PC have been identified as phospholipid precursors in some tumors (DALY et al. 1987), and since GPE and GPC have been shown to be products of phospholipid catabolism, the ratio of PMEs to PDEs serves as a measure of the relative extent of phospholipid synthesis and degradation.

The most sensitive nucleus, ^{1}H, is ubiquitous in biological tissues. Detection of ^{1}H resonances of key metabolites is impeded by the diversity and abundance of overlapping resonances and by the intense resonances of water and lipids, which obscure the spectra of small molecular weight metabolites present in low concentrations in biological tissues. With appropriate pulse sequences, contributions from water and lipid resonances can be minimized and signals from key biomolecules such as amino acids, lactate, creatine, and glucose can be detected (ROTHMAN et al. 1984a, b). Refinement of these spectral editing techniques will play a key role in the clinical application of ^{1}H NMR spectroscopy. Application of these methods to tumors, which has proven more difficult than with nonmalignant tissues (HETHERINGTON et al. 1985; GADIAN et al. 1987), promises to provide information which complements information obtained from other nuclei.

Carbon plays a central role in metabolism, and ^{13}C NMR provides a noninvasive method for monitoring critical biochemical pathways in tumors and normal tissues. In some cases compounds are present in such high concentrations that they can be monitored by natural abundance (e.g., the extremely high levels of citrate in normal prostate; SILLERUD et al. 1988). More often, isotopically labeled reagents are required to overcome the intrinsic low sensitivity and low natural abundance of carbon 13. Relative rates of glycolysis and oxidative metabolism, synthesis and degradation of glycogen, and many other important biochemical processes can be monitored in vivo following infusion of ^{13}C-labeled glucose or other substrates.

^{19}F NMR spectroscopy offers two key advantages: (1) high sensitivity (83% that of ^{1}H NMR), and (2) the absence of background signals from naturally occurring compounds (since fluorine is absent from normal metabolites). Hence, only exogenous compounds containting fluorine are detected. These compounds include perfluorinated blood substitutes and the commonly used chemotherapeutic agent 5-fluorouracil (5FU). The accumulation, activation, and inactivation of 5FU both in tumors and the liver has been detected by ^{19}F NMR spectroscopy (STEVENS et al. 1984; WOLF et al. 1987). Monitoring molecular pharmacology in the patient promises to lead to the development of therapeutic protocols specifically designed for the individual patient under examination.

A major emphasis of R&D in NMR spectroscopy and imaging is placed on adapting current techniques to additional nuclei. Deuterium (^{2}H) NMR holds considerable promise for applications to cancer. KIM and ACKERMAN (1988) have recently measured blood flow and perfusion in tumors by monitoring the washout of HDO using in vivo ^{2}H NMR spectroscopy. The significance of blood flow and perfusion in the effectiveness of cancer treatment is addressed in Sect. 6.3.1.2. MCCOY et al. (1988) have monitored ^{2}H-labeled misonidazole in tumors by ^{2}H NMR spectroscopy. In addition, our laboratory (LI et al. unpublished) has measured the absolute concentrations of phosphorus metabolites in murine tumors by comparing their ^{31}P resonance intensity with the ^{2}H intensity of the natural abundance of trace deuterated water, which is a constant in tissues.

Nuclear magnetic resonance studies of the alkali metals sodium and potassium continue to be performed to a greater extent. Next to ^{1}H, ^{23}Na is the most sensitive naturally occurring nucleus. Under normal conditions the intracellular concentration of this metal is low and the extracellular concentration is high, a situation which forms the basis for distinguishing between tumor and edema by ^{23}Na imaging of tumors (GRIFFEY et al. 1988). Controversy exists over this technique since aberrant Na,K-ATPase activities have been reported for some tumors and breakdown of ATPase activity occurs during cell death. Hence, ^{23}Na may actually serve as a marker of cell death. Although ^{39}K is a nucleus with low sensitivity, it recently has been monitored with whole body instruments that can be adapted for clinical applications (WANG et al. 1988). While the spatial resolution of ^{39}K spectroscopy will likely remain poor, this nucleus should be of increasing biomedical interest, particularly as more sensitive, higher-field instruments are introduced.

6.2.3 Measurement of Reaction Rates by NMR

Because concentrations of many key metabolites such as ATP are controlled by homeostatic mechanisms, changes in steady-state levels of these metabolites may be limited even in response to pathological conditions. However, the effects of disease or environmental stress (e.g., changes in blood flow, substrate concentrations, oxygenation) are strongly reflected in flux changes that occur to compensate for these stresses. For this reason flux measurements by NMR, using magnetization-transfer and isotopic labeling, hold great promise for studies related to cancer and other disorders.

A unique capability of NMR spectroscopy is its ability to measure unidirectional reaction rates by magnetization-transfer experiments. These experiments are performed at chemical equilibrium, do not require introduction of any exogenous reagents, and only involve electronics (i.e., monitoring the changes in magnetization of one resonance when another is irradiated). Magnetization-transfer has been used to measure the rates of important biological reactions in vivo, including the ATP synthetase reaction rate, k_1:

$$P_i + ADP + H^+ \underset{k_{-2}}{\overset{k_1}{=}} ATP \qquad (1)$$

and the creatine kinase reaction rate, k_2:

$$PCr + ADP + H^+ \underset{k_{-2}}{\overset{k_2}{=}} ATP \qquad (2)$$

In principle measurement of the reverse reactions is also possible, but these measurements are complicated by the numerous reactions in the cell which are formally identical but involve different enzymes and are defined by different rate constants (e.g., in reaction 1). In addition, some reactants may be involved in multiple, simultaneous reactions (e.g., ATP in reactions 1–2).

Magnetization-transfer studies of tumors have thus far been limited to perfused cells (NEEMAN et al. 1987). This technique has also been employed in in vivo studies of the heart (KINGSLEY-HICKMANN et al. 1987) and other tissues (HSIEH and BALABAN 1987) and should prove useful for characterization of in vivo tumors.

Another NMR technique for measuring flux through specific biochemical pathways is monitoring the transfer of ^{13}C labels from isotopically labeled substrates. This procedure is analogous to the use of radioactive labels, but NMR allows the experiment to be performed in situ without the need for isolation procedures.

6.2.4 Techniques for NMR Spectroscopy In Vivo

Traditional NMR spectrometers employed vertical bore magnets which held samples in narrow tubes of 5–25 mm in diameter. The earliest studies of living samples performed on these instruments were restricted to samples with manageable geometries, such as yeast and ascites tumor cells, isolated perfused hearts, and tumors in the tails of animals. However, as soon as the potential of in vivo spectroscopy became clear, NMR probes were designed specifically for in vivo applications. More recently the development of large horizontal bore magnets has permitted large animals and humans to be examined under comfortable conditions. The two most important spectroscopic requirements are localization of the signal to the tissue under study and sensitivity adequate to produce data in a reasonable (short) amount of time.

Initial studies in small animals have used tumors that have been implanted in a subcutaneous (sc) manner. These tumors are already somewhat isolated from the body, and their growth and response to therapy can be followed noninvasively, if approximately, by volume measurement. Figures 2 and 3 illustrate two types of coil that are employed to measure in vivo NMR spectra of sc tumors in mice. A surface coil (Fig. 2), introduced by ACKERMAN et al. (1980), consists of one or more turns of copper wire connected to an appropriate resonance circuit. The "sensitive region," the area from which signal is detected by the coil, extends in a perpendicular direction away from the coil to a distance approximately equal to the radius of the coil. By appropriate placement of the coil and choice of coil dimensions, measurements can be restricted to tissue within the tumor, while contributions from external normal tissues can be excluded. Exclusion of signals from beyond the tumor is further improved by introducing a Faraday shield (NG et al. 1982a) between the body of the mouse and the coil. The Faraday shield consists of a sheet of grounded copper foil with a hole through which the tumor protrudes. Further localization within specific regions of the tumor can be achieved with sophisticated pulse techniques such as rotating frame zeugmatography (HOULT 1979) or DEPTH pulse sequences (NG et al. 1984). While these techniques eliminate the need for Faraday shields, the sensitive regions generated by these methods can have odd shapes.

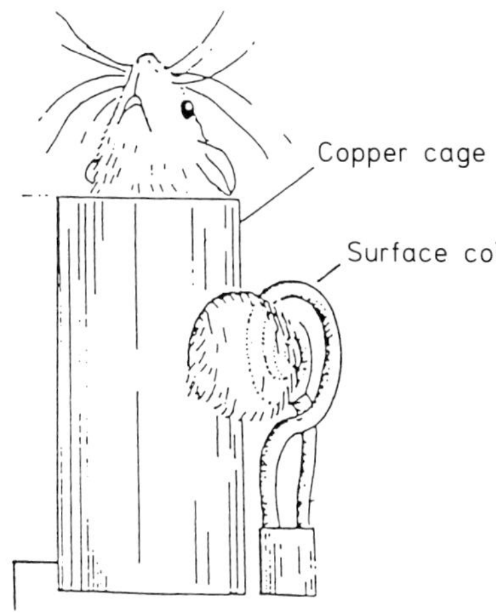

Fig. 2. Schematic diagram of a surface coil employed in the detection of a subcutaneously implanted murine tumor. Nonmalignant tissues are shielded with a Faraday shield consisting of a grounded copper cage. (EVANOCHKO et al. 1984a)

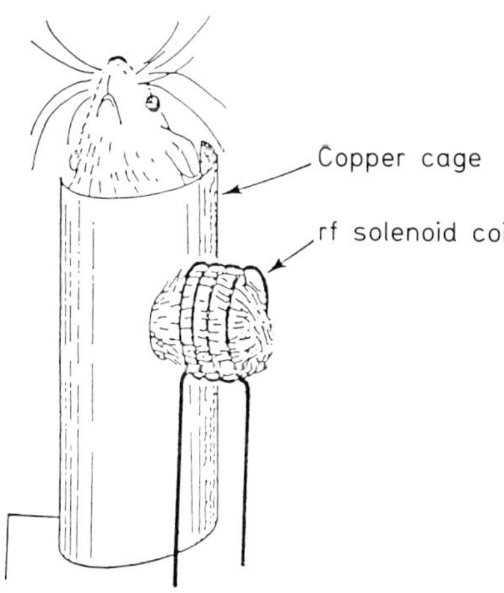

Fig. 3. Schematic diagram of a solenoidal coil employed in the detection of a subcutaneously impanted murine tumor. Nonmalignant tissues are shielded with a Faraday shield consisting of a grounded copper cage. (EVANOCHKO et al. 1984a)

Tumors are intrinsically heterogeneous, consisting of regions of cells that are well-perfused, poorly perfused, and necrotic. Because surface coils generate rf fields that are also heterogeneous, they do not sample the tumor uniformly. Sampling artifacts can occur when tumors which exhibit gross histological heterogeneity are examined with surface coils. This problem does not occur with tumors having more uniformly distributed microregions of histological heterogeneity.

One way of avoiding these artifacts is to employ a solenoidal coil, which can be wrapped around the sc tumor (Fig. 3). Solenoidal coils uniformly excite spins encompassed by the coils and offer the additional advantage of providing significantly greater sensitivity than surface coils of comparable dimensions. As with surface coils, Faraday shields or appropriate pulse sequences need to be employed to avoid excitation of spins extraneous to the tumor (NG and GLICKSON 1985). One drawback of current in vivo NMR probes, compared to traditional high resolution probes, is that spectroscopic conditions cannot be reproduced perfectly from one animal to another. For comparison of in vivo spectra, *ratios* of the different peaks in the spectrum are commonly used; these ratios, in turn, can be compared among spectra.

In vivo spectra of human tumors were first obtained using surface coils. New techniques have been developed in which NMR spectroscopic and imaging techniques have been combined to obtain spectra from well-defined, localized regions anywhere in the body. Although these techniques are generally not sensitive enough for small animal studies, they hold considerable promise for clinical application of NMR techniques in the detection and monitoring of cancers.

One technique for localization is image-guided, spatially localized spectroscopy. SEGEBARTH et al. (1987) employed this technique in a study of human brain tumors. In this study ^{31}P NMR spectra were obtained from a prolactinoma using a spatial localization technique called ISIS, as demonstrated in Fig. 4. A scout MR image was initially obtained to delineate the location of the tumor and a control region uninfiltrated by the tumor. The tumor is identified by distortions of normal anatomy and by characteristic modifications of water relaxation times (which are usually longer in the tumor). ^{31}P NMR spectroscopy is then performed on the region containing the tumor. In these studies the tumor spectrum, obtained from a sensitive region consisting of a cube 3.4 cm on a side, revealed an increase in the relative intensity of the PME resonance and a decrease in the relative intensity of PCr compared to the spectrum of a region of noninfiltrated brain (which was identical to the spectrum obtained from brain of normal volunteers).

Another localization technique, chemical shift imaging (CSI), will also play a vital role in future cancer studies. With this method an entire "slice" of tissue can be excited to generate a two-dimensional matrix of voxels per plane. Spectra from each of these voxels are then obtained simultaneously. BOT-

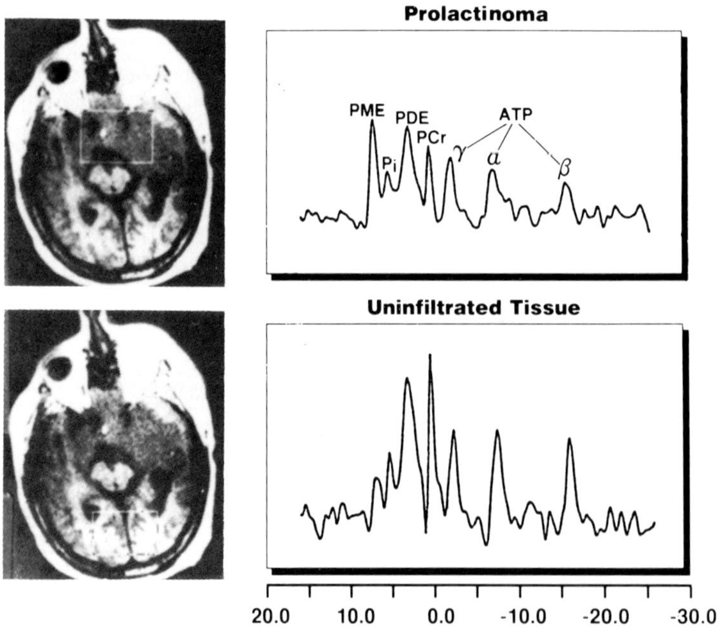

Fig. 4. Proton images and ^{31}P spectroscopy results obtained during examination of a patient with a prolactinoma. Phosphorus 31 spectra from two volumes of interest are presented at *right;* the spectra are scaled to take into account differences in volume size. The tumor spectrum *(upper)* shows an increase of PME and a decrease of PCr, while the uninfiltrated tissue spectrum *(lower)* resembles a normal ^{31}P brain spectrum. (SEGEBARTH et al. 1987)

TOMLEY et al. (1988) employed CSI to examine human brain tissue in 34 min with an 8×8 matrix of voxels consisting of cubes 3 cm on a side. Acquisition times for this kind of study have been decreased to approximately 17 min. Using interleaved techniques, which allow time-shared performance of CSI experiments on multiple slices, spectra of the entire human brain should be possible to obtain in approximately 45 min on commercially available 1.5-T instruments.

Both of these localization methods can be correlated with high resolution NMR images. While the CSI technique appears more efficient than the ISIS method, there may be considerable volume averaging artifacts if the tumor only partially fills one or more voxels. In contrast, the dimensions of the region of interest in the ISIS experiment can be selected to fall within the tumor or to minimize contributions from extraneous tissues. Both methods suffer from the intrinsic low sensitivity of ^{31}P NMR spectroscopy, which results in relatively large voxel dimensions. Although these dimensions will diminish as instruments operational at higher fields become available, they will still remain on the order of $2 \times 2 \times 2$ cm for fields up to approximately 4–5 T. Spatial resolution for spectroscopy on the order of 1 cm may be achievable with more sensitive nuclei (e.g., ^{1}H, ^{19}F, or perhaps ^{23}Na).

Surface coils are employed in the third class of methods used to obtain spatially localized spectra. These methods are most useful for studies of tissues located on or near the surface of the body. For these applications the surface coil offers higher sensitivity than is available with body or head coils. Both image-guided, spatially localized spectroscopy and CSI can be applied in conjunction with surface coils. Surface coil spectra can then be correlated with images obtained with other coils.

6.3 NMR Studies of Murine Tumors

Studies of animal models have played a critical role in the development of all diagnostic modalities, including in vivo applications of NMR. Much of the confusion generated by initial clinical studies employing NMR spectroscopy results from a failure to base clinical studies on a firm foundation of experimental animal data. Close integration of animal and clinical experiments promises not only to dispel much of this confusion but also to properly delineate the clinical capabilities and limitations of NMR spectroscopy.

Individual variability can create problems in biological experiments, particularly in studies of tumors. Although NMR spectroscopy offers the unique capability of individually monitoring each patient and tumor, interpretation of the spectra obtained requires strict attention to statistical considerations. With animal models the same tumor can be implanted in a syngeneic population of hosts, and statistical evaluation of the reproducibility of the spectral, biochemical, and histological characteristics of these tumors can be performed. To establish the ability of NMR to detect therapeutic response, determination of the characteristics of the tumor during untreated growth is essential. This determination, which cannot be made in the clinical setting, can be made with animal models.

Even though one of the greatest potential advantages of in vivo NMR spectroscopy is its ability to obtain information noninvasively, evaluation of the physiological meaning of NMR spectra still requires comparison of NMR data with data from numerous invasive techniques. These invasive analyses include evaluation of tissue histology; analyses of cell extracts; cytokinetic characterization; measurement of various physiological parameters such as blood flow, blood oxygenation, and extracellular pH; and measurement of traditional therapeutic endpoints such as clonogenic cell killing. For these studies well-described animal models are essential. Studies of cells in tissue culture are also required to distinguish direct biochemical effects from physiological or systemic effects.

A good model for the study of tumors by NMR spectroscopy must meet several criteria: it must resemble common human tumors; it must grow both in vivo and in culture; and it must respond to important therapeutic modalities. In addition, it must not metastasize, at least until late in growth, so that response to therapy is actually due to treatment of the primary tumor. The tumor should be nonimmunogenic in its host; if the tumor stimulates the host immune system, distinguishing between tumor regression induced by exogenous therapeutic agents and effects arising from the immune response is difficult.

The following sections will present NMR studies of experimental murine tumors during untreated growth and following treatment with several therapeutic modalities. Examples have been taken from our work with the radiation-induced fibrosarcoma (RIF-1) developed in the laboratory of Robert Kallman (TWENTYMAN et al. 1980). This tumor model was chosen because it largely satisfies the criteria outlined above. However, since tumor lines vary substantially in all aspects of their growth, no single tumor model will provide universal answers. Results from other laboratories studying different tumors have revealed similarities and differences in patterns of growth and response to therapy.

6.3.1 Untreated Tumor Growth

6.3.1.1 ^{31}P NMR Spectra of RIF-1 Tumors

Unlike normal adult tissues, which have a constant ^{31}P NMR spectrum unless disturbed, growing tumors have a constantly changing spectrum which tends toward lower and lower apparent energy status. Figure 5 presents ^{31}P NMR spectra of a representative RIF-1 tumor grown sc in the flank of a C3H/HeN mouse. Compared to the spectrum labeled day 0, which was obtained on the 12th day after tumor implantation, a substantial increase in the relative intensity of the P_i resonance and a concomitant decrease in the PCr peak (relative to the resonance of the β phosphorus of NTP) is evident. In addition, the pH of the tumor decreases from 7.5 to 6.9. Figure 6 summarizes data on 15 RIF-1 tumors monitored during 14 days of growth (LI et al. 1988). The P_i/NTP and P_i/PME ratios increase for 2 weeks after implantation and stabilize thereafter. The PCr/P_i ratio decreases to approximately 0.1.

These spectral changes are similar to those exhibited by a variety of tumors, including the sc murine mammary 16/C adenocarcinoma (EVANOCHKO et al. 1983, 1984a) and human tumors of the breast, lung, and colon implanted subcutaneously in immunodeficient mice (EVANOCHKO et al. 1982). In other tumors, such as sc MOPC 104E myeloma (NG et al. 1982b) and sc 9L glioblastoma (STEEN et al. 1988), NMR spectra indicate high levels of high energy phosphates in early stages of growth (as reflected in a higher initial PCr/NTP ratio) but very low levels in late stages of growth, when both PCr and NTP fall below the level of detection by ^{31}P NMR spectroscopy.

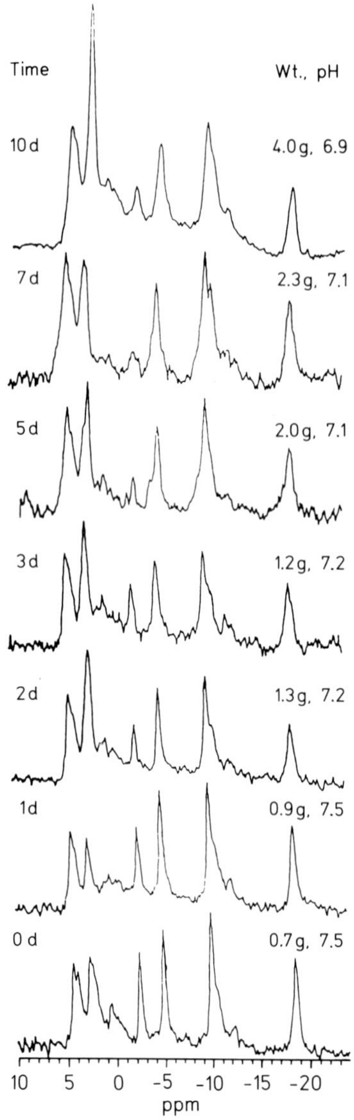

Fig. 5. Typical in vivo ^{31}P NMR spectra of a subcutaneous RIF-1 tumor during untreated growth, beginning on day 12 after implantation of 10^5 cells. Tumor weight (by volume approximation) and pH (by P_i chemical shift) are indicated

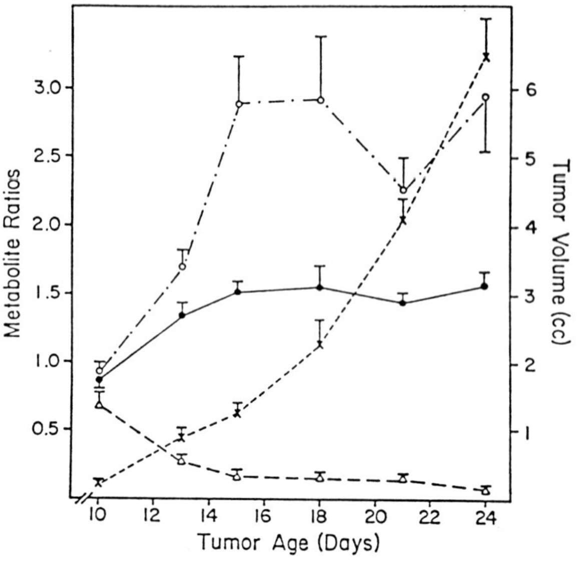

Fig. 6. Changes in tumor volume and phosphorus metabolite ratios of RIF-1 tumors during untreated growth. Data shown indicate mean (±SEM). ● P_i/PME, ○ P_i/NTP, △ PCr/P_i, × Volume. (LI et al. 1988)

6.3.1.2 A Model for Growth-Associated Changes in the Energy Metabolism of Tumors

The energy changes occurring during tumor growth and reflected in the ^{31}P NMR spectra are consistent with tumor growth unaccompanied by the vascularization required to maintain a constant level of perfusion in the tumor. In this situation the tumor tends to outgrow its blood supply. The extent to which this phenomenon occurs varies from tumor to tumor. The ability of ^{31}P NMR spectroscopy to detect this phenomenon may prove one of its most useful attributes because it would provide a basis for predicting tumor response to certain therapeutic modalities. For instance, perfusion directly influences delivery of drugs and response modifiers, while oxygen levels influence radiosensitivity. In addition, many types of therapy are affected by the proliferative state of the tumor, which is determined in part by the quality of tumor perfusion.

The NMR data for untreated solid tumors can be explained in terms of a model similar to that introduced by THOMLINSON and GRAY (1955) to explain variations in tumor radiosensitivity during various stages of growth. In this model the energetic and proliferative status of tumor cells was determined by their distance from tumor capillaries. The model, which focused on the state of oxygenation of subpopulations of tumor cells, considered only chronic, structural aspects of oxygenation. In a more complete model, perfusion must be seen as responsible not only for oxygen delivery but also for delivery of substrates such as glucose and for removal of toxic wastes. In addition, regions of tumors are now known to become transiently ischemic as capillaries collapse and then reopen, a phenomenon referred to as "acute" hypoxia (BROWN 1979).

Three subpopulations of tumor cells exist. The first subpopulation consists of well-perfused cells that are in close proximity to blood vessels. These cells not only have supplies of oxygen and substrates capable of sustaining a high level of metabolic activity and proliferation but also are able to efficiently eliminate toxic waste products such as lactic acid. Well-perfused tumor cells generally obtain energy by a combination of oxidative phosphorylation and aerobic glycolysis. The extent to which these metabolic pathways are employed will depend on the particular tumor and on environmental conditions. Poorly differentiated, rapidly proliferating tumors tend to exhibit mitochondrial deficiencies (PEDERSEN 1978) and rely more heavily on glycolytic pathways even at oxygen concentrations that sustain oxidative metabolism in normal tissues. The well-perfused tumor cells will have high levels of ATP, and in tumors which contain the creatine kinase energy storage system PCr will tend to be high. Due to efficient elimination of any lactate formed, the tumor pH will be neutral or slightly alkaline.

The second subpopulation consists of cells more remote from blood capillaries. These cells are poorly perfused and will tend to be hypoxic. The efficient oxidative pathway of ATP synthesis is increasingly replaced by the inefficient glycolytic pathway. Glucose delivery may also be reduced. PCr, if present, is lost first, followed by a reduction in ATP itself. Inorganic phosphate accumulates. Increased glycolysis increases lactic acid production, and reduced perfusion reduces washout. Proliferative capacity decreases as levels of ATP diminish.

Far from the capillaries, under conditions of very poor perfusion, tumor cells eventually die and decompose. These dead and necrotic tumor cells constitute the third major cellular compartment of the tumor. Little is known about the spectral characteristics of these cells. Cell death is generally accompanied by depletion of all high energy phosphates and accumulation of P_i and lactate, but these latter constituents will tend to diffuse away as the cells necrose (i.e., as their membranes decompose). The pH of hypoxic cells is expected to be acidic, but necrotic regions of tumors have been reported to be alkaline (VAUPEL et al. 1981).

At any stage of tumor growth the observed spectrum is the superposition of spectra of the well-perfused, the poorly perfused, and the dead and necrotic constituents. In early stages of growth, well-perfused cells predominate in well-vascularized tumors, while in later stages of growth poorly perfused cells predominate. The tumor exhibits a gradual transition to the metabolically inactive state. In still later stages, the metabolically less active and necrotic cells predominate. The relative proportions of these cells vary not only with the age of the tumor but also with expression of angiogenesis factors and other factors that determine the extent of tumor perfusion.

Variations in the levels of NMR-detectable PME and PDE compounds appear to be related to phospholipid metabolism. DALY et al. (1987) have demonstrated that PE and PC are precursors of phospholipids in the MDA-MB231 tumor and that the glycerol esters of these PMEs are products of lipid catabolism. Since increased levels of phospholipids are required in cell replication, this ratio may serve as an index of tumor growth. This explanation is consistent with elevated levels of PE observed in neuroblastomas (MARIS et al. 1985) and in neonatal dog brains (GYULAI et al. 1984).

Experimental confirmation of the relationship between tumor perfusion and the ^{31}P NMR spectrum of the RIF-1 tumor has been obtained by EVELHOCH et al. (1986). These investigators found that in sc RIF-1 tumors, tumor pH, PCr/NTP, and P_i/NTP were correlated with the size of the well-perfused fraction of the tumor as measured by washout of ^{15}O generated in the tumor. This situation was true even though no simple correlation of NMR parameters with tumor volume existed. Further studies are now needed to determine the properties of perfusion that determine tumor energy status, such as oxygen, glucose, pH, or other factors. Measurement of substrate delivery and metabolism is best achieved with ^{13}C NMR spectroscopy employing isotopically labeled substrates such as [1-^{13}C]glucose. Measurement of blood flow by NMR methods has been performed by measuring washout of injected D_2O (ACKERMAN et al. 1987; KIM and ACKERMAN 1988). Determination of the glucose and oxygen available to cells far from blood vessels is critical. CHEN et al. (1988) have proposed that the rate of reduction of nitroxide spin labels may serve as an index of cellular hypoxia. This group continues to develop nitroxide contrast agents for MRI mapping of tissue oxygenation.

Over the next few years research on solid tumors can be expected to focus on developing NMR and other noninvasive methods to measure blood flow, perfusion, and oxygenation. Research will also focus on examining the effect of these variables on the relative success or failure of various therapeutic regimens.

6.3.2 Treated Tumors

Treatment of experimental tumors with effective antineoplastic therapy results in prompt changes in the ^{31}P NMR spectrum. Two general patterns of response have been observed. In the first, changes in the NMR spectra of treated tumors, usually observable beginning 24 h after treatment, resemble a reversal of the changes observed during untreated growth. This response has been observed in many tumors responding to chemotherapy and in the RIF-1 responding to radiation. An entirely different response is observed following hyperthermia or photodynamic therapy. Spectral changes, which are visible within hours, resemble acute ischemia or metabolic injury, with a dramatic decline in high energy phosphates, a rise in P_i, and an acid shift in the pH. This response has also been observed following treatment of certain tumors with chemotherapy (NARUSE et al. 1985) or radiation (SIJENS et al. 1986; SKOG et al. 1986), and following treatment with a variety of cytokines and metabolic inhibitors (see below).

6.3.2.1 Chemotherapeutic Agents

An example of the first response pattern is the response of RIF-1 to cyclophosphamide, a commonly used alkylating agent. Figure 7 displays ^{31}P NMR spectra of a representative RIF-1 tumor treated with an intraperitoneal (i.p.) injection of cyclophosphamide 12 days after implanting 10^5 tumor cells in the flank of the mouse. The spectrum before treatment contains an intense P_i resonance and smaller NTP, PCr, PME, and PDE peaks. The pH of the tumor is 6.9 before treatment. Within 1 day of drug administration, the intensity of the P_i peak (relative to the resonance of the β phosphorus of NTP) decreases dramatically, with the minimum relative P_i intensity observed on day 3. Between days 1 and 7, the pH increases to a value of 7.5, while the mass of the tumor remains constant within experimental error. By day 10 tumor regrowth occurs and the pH returns to 6.9.

Figure 8 presents average values of spectral parameters 3 days posttreatment for groups of mice ($n = 10$–15) treated with various doses of cyclophosphamide (LI et al. 1988). The P_i/NTP and P_i/PME ratios decrease with dose and stabilize at a dose of approximately 150 mg/kg. The PCr/P_i ratio and the pH increase, with limiting levels reached at doses of approximately 200 and 150 mg/kg, respectively. Thus, at this early time point the magnitude of the NMR response is related to the effectiveness of treatment over part, but not all, of the dose-response range.

A positive correlation can be observed between tumor pH and the PCr/P_i ratio in age-matched tumors examined by NMR spectroscopy on day 15 after treatment with cyclophosphamide or saline on day 12 postimplantation (Fig. 9). This relationship is consistent with the prediction that aerobic tumors should exhibit relatively high PCr/P_i ratios and normal pH. The data from drug-treated and sham-treated animals cluster in two distinct groups.

Useful NMR spectra will reflect the time course and magnitude of cell killing by the drug. An assessment of the efficacy of cancer therapy can be made by measuring changes in the population of clonogenic cells in the tumor. These are the cells in

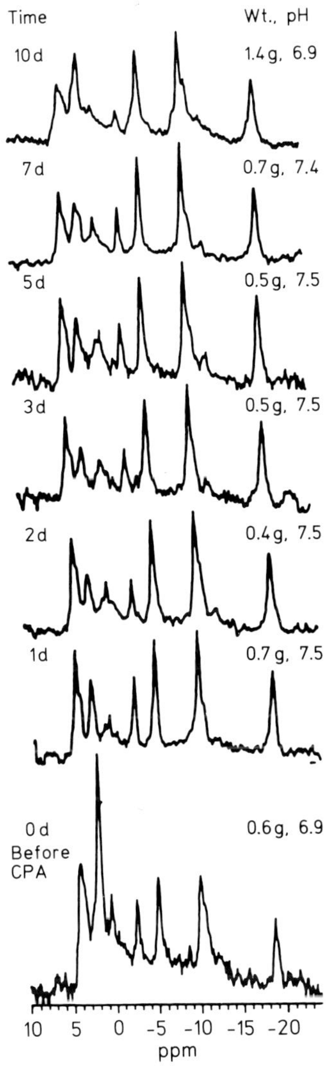

Fig. 7. ^{31}P NMR spectra of an RIF-1 tumor before and after i.p. treatment with 150 mg/kg cyclophosphamide *(CPA)*. Treatment was performed on day 12 after inoculation of 10^5 cells. Tumor weight (by volume approximation) and pH (by P_i chemical shift) are indicated

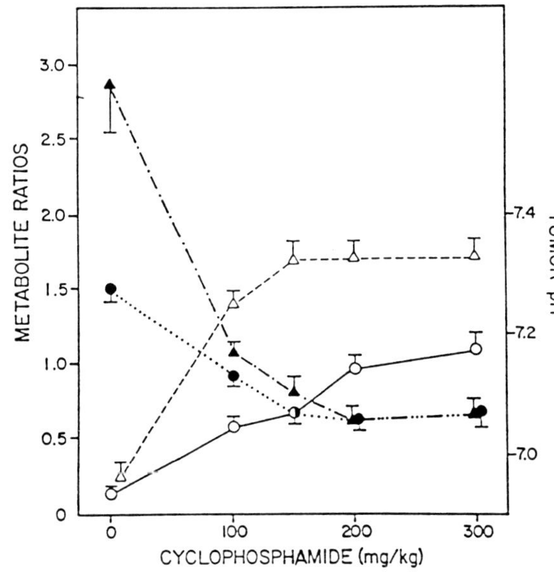

Fig. 8. Phosphate metabolite ratios and pH on 3rd day following treatment with cyclophosphamide (or sham). Data shown indicate mean (±SEM) of 10–15 animals. ● P_i/PME, ○ PCr/P_i, ▲ P_i/NTP, △ pH. (LI et al. 1988)

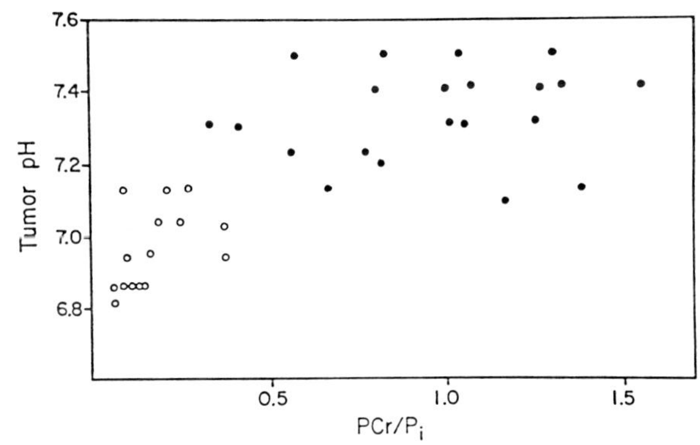

Fig. 9. Relationship between tumor pH and PCr/P_i ratio. Values for individual treated (200 mg/kg) or control tumors on 3rd day after treatment or sham treatment (○, control tumors; ●, treated tumors). (LI et al. 1988)

the tumor which retain the capacity for unlimited replication. Figure 10 shows that following treatment the population of these important cells falls, after which it begins to recover (WEHRLE et al. 1987). In Fig. 11 a dose-response curve of cyclophosphamide treatment of RIF-1 is presented (LI et al. 1988). The tumors were excised and assayed 24 h after treatment. Even at the lowest dose employed in these studies (100 mg/kg), the clonogenic cell fraction is reduced by at least one log order. The higher dose of 150 mg/kg corresponds to a two-log reduction in clonogenic capacity.

Another indication of therapeutic effectiveness is the delay in tumor growth as measured by size, although this measurement is an indirect assessment of tumor cell killing. Figure 12 displays growth curves for RIF-1 tumors for cyclophosphamide doses of 100, 200, and 300 mg/kg. With these doses, growth delays (the extra time it takes the tumor to reach four times its pretreatment volume) of 6, 13, and 21 days, respectively, were obtained.

Figure 13 presents ^{31}P NMR spectra of perfused RIF-1 tumor cells before and after treatment in vitro with 4-hydroperoxycyclophosphamide, an ac-

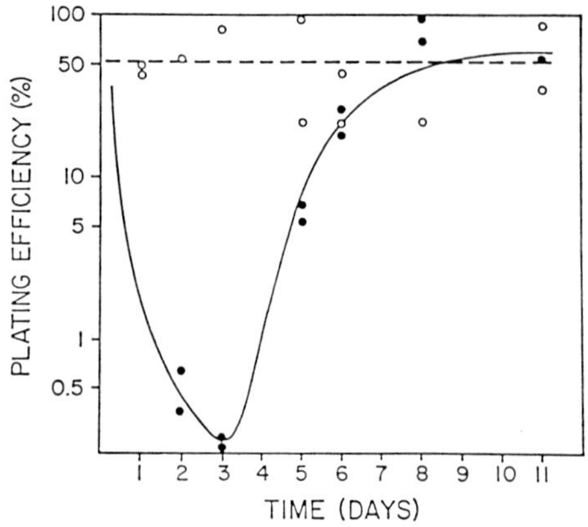

Fig. 10. Response of RIF-1 tumor to cyclophosphamide. Calculated clonogenic cell fraction on different days following i.p. treatment (150 mg/kg). (WEHRLE et al. 1987)

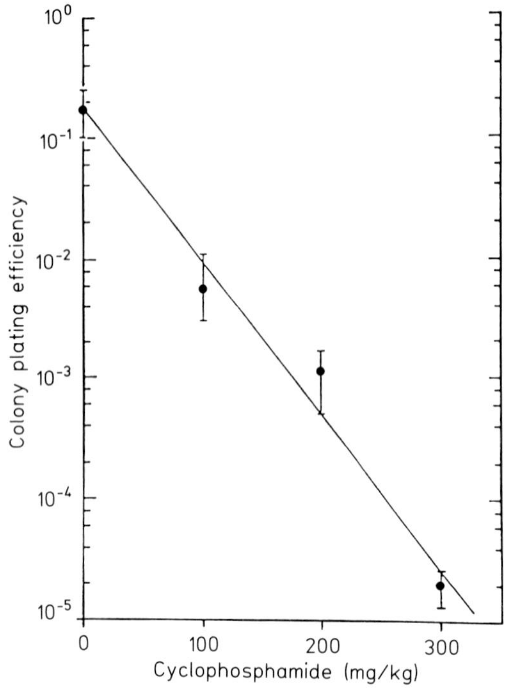

Fig. 11. In vitro colony forming efficiency following in vivo treatment with cyclophosphamide on day 12 after tumor implantation. Assays were performed 24 h after treatment or sham treatment. Data indicate mean (±SD) of four animals. (LI et al. 1988)

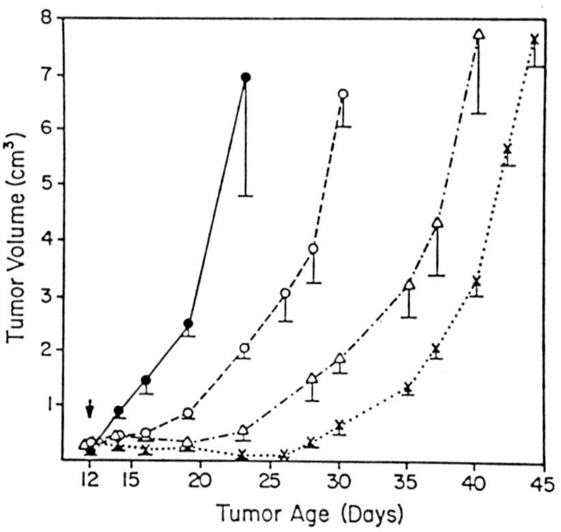

Fig. 12. Tumor growth delay induced by cyclophosphamide. All animals were treated on day 12 after tumor implantation with saline (●), 100 (○), 200 (△), or 300 (-X-) mg/kg cyclophosphamide. Data shown indicate mean (±SD) of six animals epr treatment group. (LI et al. 1988)

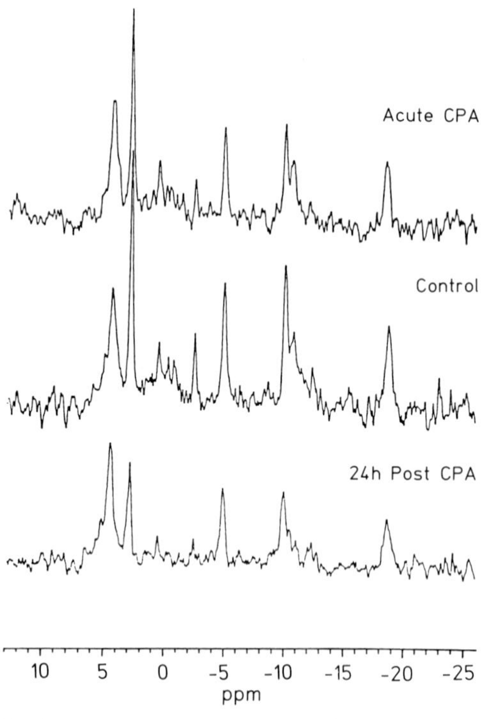

Fig. 13. Cyclophosphamide treatment of RIF-1 in culture on microcarrier beads. Control spectrum: untreated confluent monolayer perfused with P_i-free Eagle's minimal essential medium with 20 mM HEPES and 5% fetal bovine serum, saturated with 95% O_2/5% CO_2. Acute: same cells shown in control spectrum, 2 h after adding 4-hydroperoxycyclophosphamide (4-HC, 100 μM) to the perfusion medium. Twenty-four hours: cells were treated with 100 μM 4-HC for 60 min, washed, and returned to culture in drug-free medium on the day before NMR examination

tive metabolite of cyclophosphamide. The control spectrum resembles the spectrum of an in vivo tumor. The dramatic decrease in P_i observed in vivo was exhibited by the perfused cells 24 h after, but not immediately after, treatment. Similar spectral changes have also been observed in cultured human breast cancer cells treated with actinomycin D or Adriamycin under conditions of constant perfusion (H. DEGANI, personal communication). These changes suggest that in addition to the tissue effects described above, cellular effects of the antineoplastic agents increase the relative levels of high energy phosphates compared to low energy phosphates. This situation could occur if cell growth were inhibited without a corresponding decrease in ATP production, in which case a net increase in the levels of high energy phosphates would be observed.

In an estrogen-dependent mammary adenocarcinoma in vivo, RODRIGUES et al. (1985) found that ovariectomy performed to reduce tumor growth rate without direct cell killing resulted in an enhanced PCr/P_i ratio. Such decoupling of energy production from energy demand is more likely to occur in tumors than in normal tissues in which energy supply and demand are usually tightly coupled. These conclusions are clearly preliminary. Investigations are in progress to determine the mechanism of this phenomenon.

The time course of NMR changes may also reveal the time course of important cytokinetic changes which occur after treatment, thus aiding in the scheduling of doses of anticancer agents. SCHIFFER et al. (1985) examined the relationship of these parameters to drug-induced perturbations in NMR spectra in the RIF-1 tumor. Figure 14 demonstrates that cell proliferation reaches a minimum level by 2–3 days after cyclophosphamide treatment and returns to an elevated level by day 5. The minimum rate of DNA synthesis coincides with the day on which the NTP/P_i ratio reaches its maximum value (top of Fig. 15). As shown in Fig. 14, the time of the return to plateau levels of DNA synthesis is the optimal point for administration of a second dose of chemotherapeutic agent (SCHIFFER et al. 1985). As seen in Fig. 15, the maximal alkaline shift in the pH of the tumor nearly coincides with this day, suggesting that NMR may prove useful for optimizing the sequential timing of doses of anticancer agents. A number of cell types have been shown to undergo an alkaline shift in pH during mitosis (HESKETH et al. 1985). In the RIF-1 tumor this shift in pH could reflect transition of some of the tumor cells into a state of active cell division.

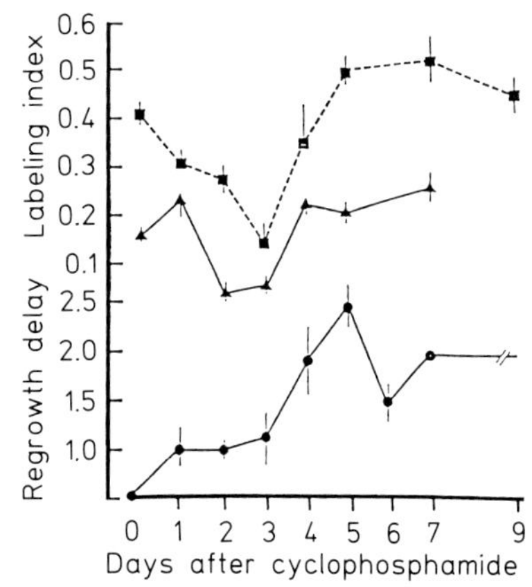

Fig. 14. Proliferative phenomena of the RIF-1 tumor. The [^{3}H]TdR labeling index (▲) and the PDP index (■) are shown during the experimental period of 9 days. Cyclophosphamide was administered on day 0. Represented on the *lower curve* (●) is regrowth delay, normalized to tumor doubling time, after 150 mg cyclophosphamide (day 0) and 100 mg cyclophosphamide (other days). (SCHIFFER et al. 1985)

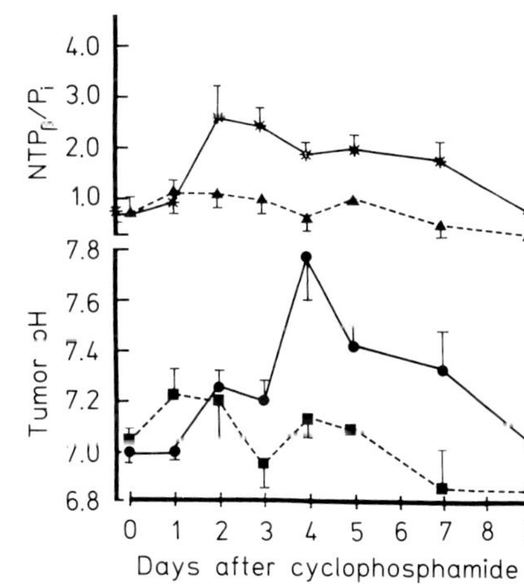

Fig. 15. Phosphorus 31 NMR studies of the RIF-1 tumor. The *upper graph* represents the ^{31}P NMR NTP/P_i ratio of treated (150 mg/kg cyclophosphamide) and control animals during the experimental period of 9 days. The *lower graph* represents the pH as measured by chemical shift of P_i. Same symbols as in Fig. 13. (SCHIFFER et al. 1985)

This response pattern, in which the spectral changes of uncontrolled growth are reversed during the growth delay period, has been observed with many tumors and drugs. These studies include RIF-1 tumors treated with 5 FU (LI et al. to be published), 9 L glioblastoma treated with 1,3-bis(2-chloroethyl)-1-nitrosourea (BCNU; STEEN et al. 1988), MOPC 104 E myeloma treated with cyclophosphamide or BCNU (NG et al. 1982b), mammary adenocarcinomas 16/C (EVANOCHKO et al. 1983) and 17/A (EVELHOCH et al. 1987) treated with Adriamycin, as well as a human breast tumor xenograft (MX-1) treated with Adriamycin (EVANOCHKO et al. 1982). Current and future investigation of tumor response to therapy will focus on the following paradox: subsequent to treatment producing more than 90% cell kill, tumor cells appear to be *more* metabolically active than they were prior to treatment. One possible explanation for this phenomenon is that ultimate therapeutic response reflects genetic damage, which may not be reflected in the metabolic state of the overall tumor cell population at the time of spectral measurements. The relative rates of cell death and dead cell clearance clearly influence the overall spectrum. Several changes in tumors in the days following chemotherapy would tend to improve the energy state, even of cells "doomed to die."

Increases in tumor blood flow have been measured in RIF-1 following treatment with cyclophosphamide (BRAUNSCHWEIGER 1988). In addition, as some cells die and are cleared from the tumor, the residual cells may experience less competition for available oxygen and nutrients and may thus exhibit an improved bioenergetic state. In another tumor line, histological study supports this explanation; in the 9L gliosarcoma treated with BCNU (STEEN et al. 1988), the number of necrotic cells decreased and the extracellular volume increased following treatment. This tumor exhibited spectral changes following treatment with BCNU similar to those described in this chapter for RIF-1 treated with cyclophosphamide.

Another use of NMR in chemotherapy is observation of the delivery of chemotherapeutic agents and the alterations in these agents as they are metabolized. To date this use has been restricted to ^{19}F NMR spectroscopy of fluorinated agents, which takes advantage of the high sensitivity of the ^{19}F nucleus. Studies with deuterated drugs (MCCOY et al. 1988) and ^{13}C-labeled drugs (GAMCSIK et al. unpublished) are at the preliminary stage.

Studies of the chemotherapeutic agent 5 FU by STEVENS et al. (1984) demonstrated the feasibility of directly monitoring the metabolism of 5 FU in situ via ^{19}F NMR spectroscopy. This group observed catabolism of the drug in the liver of mice and detected synthesis of 5-fluorodeoxyribonucleotides, including the active form of 5 FU (5-fluorodeoxyribonucleoside monophosphate, or FdUMP), in the tumor. FU-derived ribonucleotides may also be cytotoxic. Study of the effects of 5 FU on the RIF-1 tumor has revealed activation of 5 FU (Fig. 16) within 20 min of administration of the agent (LI et al. to be published). These nucleotides, labeled as

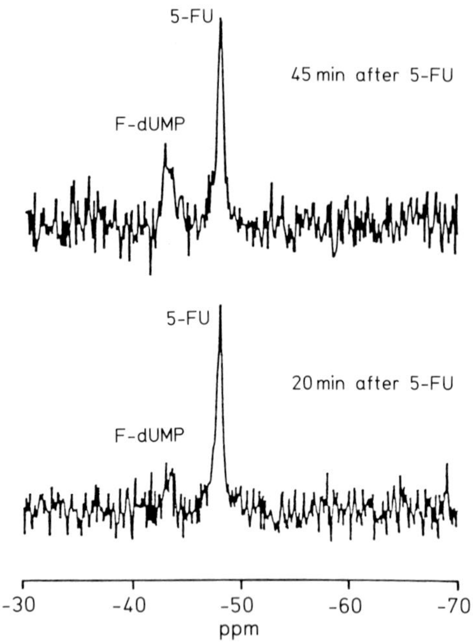

Fig. 16. In vivo ^{19}F NMR spectra (8.5 T) of an RIF-1 tumor following intracarotid infusion of 5FU (200 mg/kg). The spectra were obtained with a home-built, ^{19}F/^{31}P doubly tuned solenoidal coil. The lower spectrum was begun 20 min after infusion. The upper spectrum was begun 45 min after infusion. The peak labeled FdUMP also contains other fluoronucleotides. ^{31}P NMR spectra obtained during the intervening period indicated no alterations in tumor bioenergetic status

FdUMP in the figure, may also contain the corresponding nucleoside di- and triphosphates. Compared to cyclophosphamide treatment, 5 FU treatment produces a longer growth delay and more pronounced ^{31}P NMR spectral changes (Fig. 17). Prior administration of the vasodilator hydralazine to diminish blood flow in the tumor resulted in an increase in the P_i/βNTP ratio and a dramatic decrease in the production of ^{19}F NMR-detectable 5-fluoronucleotides. Decreased activation of the drug can be attributed to the reduced level of ATP, which is required for the synthesis of nucleotides. These observations suggest that 5 FU activation is directly related to tumor bioenergetics and that ^{19}F and ^{31}P NMR spectroscopy provide noninvasive methods for monitoring the extent of drug activation and the bioenergetic status of the tumor, respectively.

6.3.2.2 X-Irradiation

Treatment of an sc RIF-1 tumor with γ-radiation (Fig. 18) produces ^{31}P NMR spectral changes similar to those induced by treatment with cyclophos-

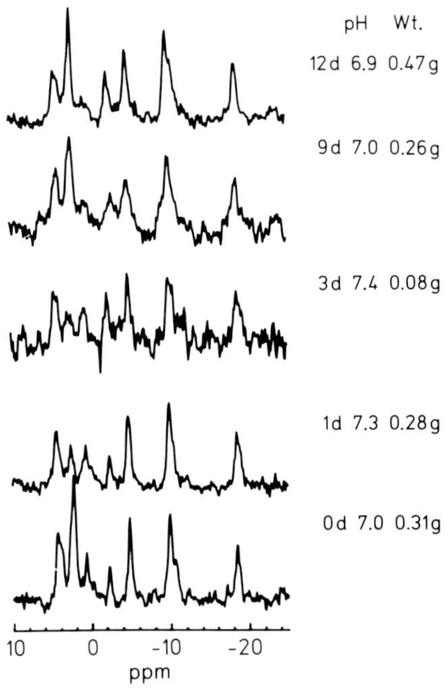

Fig. 17. In vivo ^{31}P NMR spectra of an RIF-1 tumor before and at intervals after i.p. treatment with 200 mg/kg 5FU. Tumor weight (by volume approximation) and pH (calculated from chemical shift of P_i) are indicated

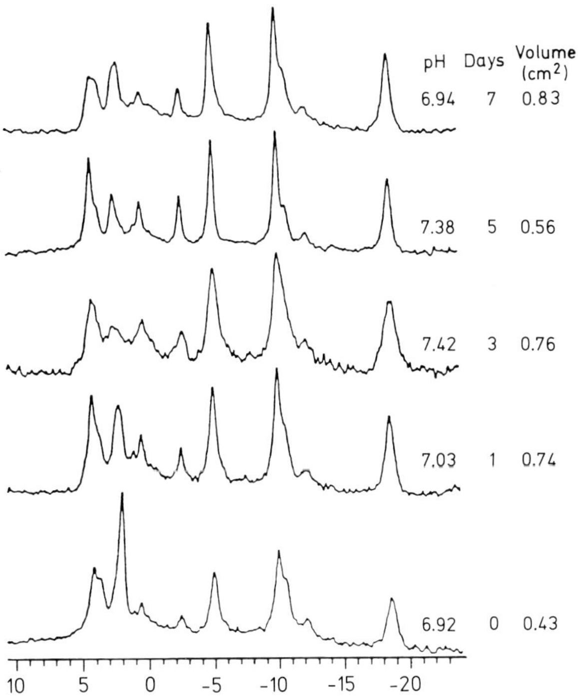

Fig. 18. Typical in vivo ^{31}P NMR spectra of a subcutaneous RIF-1 tumor before and after localized X-irradiation. The tumor was irradiated on day 14 after implantation of 10^5 cells (day 0). Tumor volume (size) and pH (by P_i chemical shift) are indicated

phamide or 5FU. Most prominent is the decrease in the intensity of the P_i resonance relative to the intensities of other phosphorus metabolites. In the days following treatment, the tumor appears to be better energized than it was prior to treatment, illustrating the paradox previously noted in discussion of cyclophosphamide treatment on the RIF-1 tumor. In these studies the magnitude and time course of the ^{31}P spectral changes were a function of the dose of radiation delivered (5, 15, or 25 Gy). The parameters most affected in the days following treatment were tumor pH and metabolite ratios $P_i/\beta NTP$ and PCr/P_i (RAJAN et al.). An increase in ATP/P_i following irradiation of RIF-1 has also been observed by GRIFFITHS et al. (1987), who reported an increase in tumor blood flow.

To rule out the possibility that systemic effects of radiation were responsible for spectral changes, RAJAN et al. (1989) performed experiments in which radiation was administered to only one of two tumors implanted in mice (one tumor per flank). Statistically significant changes (increases in PCr/P_i and pH; decreases in $P_i/\beta NTP$ and tumor volume) occurred only in the treated tumors of each pair, indicating that changes in these spectral parameters were specific indices of tumor response to therapy.

Response to radiation treatment appears to vary according to the tumor and, occasionally, to the dose of radiation administered. SIJENS et al. (1986) and SOSTMAN et al. (1984) found transient increases in high energy phosphates at low doses (10 Gy and 3 Gy) for the NU-82 mammary tumor and BA1112 rhabdomyosarcoma, respectively. At a high dose (20 Gy in each case), reduced ATP and PCr were observed. KOUTCHER et al. (1987) found that ATP levels were elevated in FSaII tumors following radiation in larger, less aerobic tumors, but that no changes were induced in smaller, more aerobic tumors.

6.3.2.3 Hyperthermia

In Fig. 19 the ^{31}P spectral changes resulting from hyperthermic treatment (45 °C for 15 min) of an RIF-1 tumor are presented (GLICKSON et al. 1986, 1987). Hyperthermia produces a rapid and substantial reduction in high energy phosphates, an in-

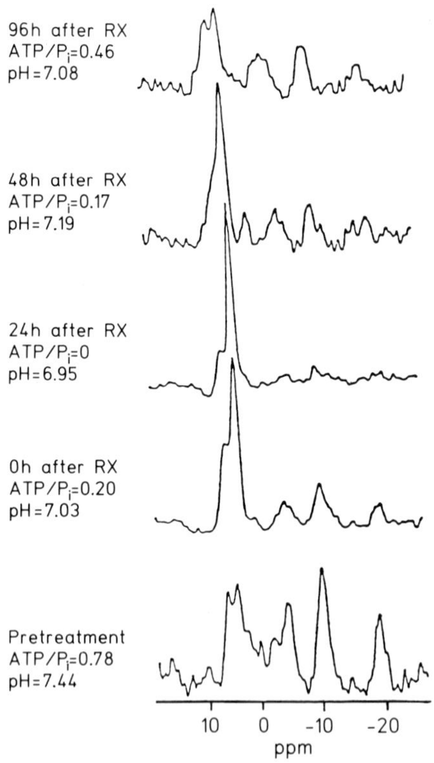

Fig. 19. In vivo ^{31}P NMR spectra (80.96 MHz) of an RIF-1 tumor before and at various times after hyperthermic treatment of 45 °C for 15 min. (GLICKSON et al. 1986)

crease in P_i, and a decrease in pH. These changes, which are opposite of those detected in this tumor after treatment with chemotherapy or γ-irradiation, resemble changes following clamping of the tumor. Twenty-four hours after hyperthermia, the tumor exhibits a spectrum indistinguishable from dead tissue, but 48 h after treatment the reappearance of high energy phosphates is evident. By 96 h after treatment, the spectrum has virtually returned to its pretreatment state. These spectral changes appear similar to those associated with tissue ischemia. LILLY et al. (1985) have demonstrated that changes in pH and NTP/P_i in RIF-1 tumors correlate with reductions in tumor blood flow, consistent with evidence that hyperthermia induces thermal damage to tumor vasculature. SIJENS et al. (1987) observed a decrease in plasma volume, following hyperthermia treatment of the NU-82 mammary tumor, which was correlated with the decrease in ATP/P_i measured by ^{31}P NMR spectroscopy.

Some investigators have proposed possible direct effects of hyperthermia on cellular bioenergetics. NARUSE et al. (1986a) have reported using the rf coil to both monitor and deliver (through rf heating) hyperthermia treatment. MR imaging techniques have recently been introduced to map tissue temperature in the tumor and surrounding tissues (LE BIHAN et al. 1988). Combining this approach with ^{31}P spectroscopy to map both the thermal dose and the metabolic effects of hyperthermia may be possible.

6.3.2.4 Other Therapeutic Modalities

Several other anticancer treatments appear to cause rapid depletion of high energy phosphates, usually accompanied by acidosis. In some cases these treatments have been shown or are suspected to reduce tumor blood flow and induce ischemia. In other cases they are direct metabolic poisons which inhibit ATP production. CECKLER et al. (1986) reported treatment of R3 230AC rat mammary tumors with hematoporphyrin phototherapy. This therapy produced results similar to those obtained by hyperthermia, with a dramatic loss of high energy phosphates and an accumulation of P_i, followed by a rapid recovery of the spectrum after 1–2 days. Similar results were observed by NARUSE et al. (1986b) in a rat glioma model. Administration of the drug flavone acetic acid (EVELHOCH et al. 1988) also produced a dramatic reduction in high energy phosphates, which was also shown to be correlated with a reduction in tumor blood flow. Treatment of various tumors with immunological response modifiers such as tumor necrosis factor (SHINE et al. 1987; PODO et al. 1987) also appears to produce an ischemia-like response.

6.4 NMR Spectroscopic Studies of Humans

In 1983 GRIFFITHS et al. reported the first NMR tumor studies of a human subject. With ^{31}P NMR spectroscopy they examined an alveolar rhabdomyosarcoma on the hand of a 17-year-old female patient, detecting no significant response to chemotherapy. Two years later MARIS et al. (1985) reported on neuroblastoma, a cancer of childhood, which had metastasized to the liver in two female infants. A significant increase in the PME resonance was detected in untreated or unresponsive tumors. Response to radiation and chemotherapy was accompanied by a dramatic decrease in the intensity of the PME peak, and the spectrum became indistinguishable from that of normal liver. ZIMMERMAN et al. (1985), using surface coils, obtained images and spectra of a tumor in the brain.

Many types of human cancer have now been directly examined by ^{31}P NMR spectroscopy. Although no universal characteristics have been identified, many groups have found that tumors tend to have higher ratios of PME/βNTP than are present in normal tissue (OBERHAENSLI et al. 1986). Studies of response to therapy are still largely anecdotal. NG et al. (1987) examined a patient with non-Hodgkin's lymphoma treated with ^{60}Co radiation. The PDE/βNTP ratio decreased during fractionated therapy proportionately with tumor volume. SEMMLER et al. (1988) reported on 23 patients with superficial tumors of several different types. Responses of these tumors to radiation or chemotherapy varied. Response of an osteosarcoma to combined radiation and chemotherapy, as indicated by a 50% reduction in tumor volume, was accompanied by an increase in PCr/P_i. In four patients with squamous cell carcinoma, VOGELE et al. (1988) observed that the PCr/βNTP ratio decreased during untreated tumor growth and increased after radiation therapy, reminiscent of the response of the RIF-1 tumor described in earlier sections of this chapter. In studies of several different tumors, KARCZMAR et al. (1988) reported average decreases in levels of PME/ATP of 55% in patients responding to treatment, while in nonresponders the PME/ATP levels increased 50% during the treatment period.

Studies of tumors in the brain are progressing at a rapid pace. In a surface coil ^{31}P NMR study of six brain tumors, OBERHAENSLI et al. (1986) found that the tumors had a higher pH than normal brain and significantly reduced PCr/ATP ratios. As described earlier, SEGEBARTH et al. (1987) employed image-guided, spatially localized spectroscopy to observe several brain tumors treated with chemotherapy or radiation. In general, response was accompanied by a return towards normal brain spectrum, but currently this response cannot be distinguished from a similar change in the biochemistry of the tumor.

A major recent advance has been the application of ^{1}H NMR spectroscopy to brain tumors. Several groups have been able to show that *N*-acetyl aspartate (NAA), which is the major metabolite resonance in normal brain, is absent or significantly reduced in both primary and metastatic brain tumors (LUYTEN et al. 1988; BRUHN et al. 1988). Because of the high sensitivity of ^{1}H NMR, much smaller volumes can be measured, thereby increasing the resolution of the measurement. A similar approach has been used by IRVING et al. (1987) to noninvasively examine bone marrow. The ^{1}H NMR spectrum of normal bone marrow contains the resonances of lipid (but little water). The presence of a water signal from the marrow region was found only in leukemic patients. Durng remission under therapy the water signal decreased substantially, but just before relapse it returned. Clearly ^{1}H NMR spectroscopy has great potential in the evaluation and monitoring of tumors.

^{19}F NMR spectroscopy has been employed to directly observe the pharmacology of 5FU in the livers of human cancer patients undergoing 5FU therapy (WOLF et al. 1987). As in the murine studies already described, activation of this agent in the liver was detected within minutes of drug administration. HULL et al. (1988) recently employed ^{19}F NMR spectroscopy to monitor 5FU metabolites in the plasma and urine of cancer patients receiving combination chemotherapy. The capabilities of this technique are only beginning to be realized, but its long-term potential in the design of more effective therapy schedules is apparent.

6.5 Status of Cancer Studies

During untreated growth tumors exhibit a consistent pattern of ^{31}P NMR spectral changes, including a progressive increase in P_i, a decrease in high energy phosphates (PCr and occasionally NTP), and either an acid shift in pH or a stable pH. These changes have been attributed to the gradual onset of vascular insufficiency in the tumor. In most cases the spectral characteristics of the tumor appear different from those of surrounding normal tissues, notable exceptions being nephromas and hepatomas in the kidney and liver, respectively. These findings support a significant role for NMR spectroscopy in the diagnosis and staging of many tumors.

Additional studies are required to determine the effect of implantation site on the spectral characteristics of tumors as well as the effects of immunogenicity and presence of metastases in vital organs such as the liver and lung. To establish the diagnostic utility of NMR spectroscopy, studies will need to be performed in which malignant and benign tumors, and nonmalignant abscesses and other pathologies, are compared. No investigations of this kind have yet been reported. Claims have also been made that ^{1}H NMR may provide a basis for determining both the metastatic potential (WRIGHT et al. 1988) and extent of drug resistance (COHEN and LYON 1987) of tumors. Much more work is required to investigate these possibilities.

While ^{31}P NMR spectral changes have generally been detected following administration of antineoplastic agents, few correlations of these changes with reliable indices of therapeutic response have been established. These correlations have been examined in RIF-1 tumors treated with cyclophosphamide (Li et al. 1988) and 5FU (Li et al. to be published), in 9L glioblastoma treated with BCNU (Steen et al. 1988), and in MOPC 104E myeloma treated with cyclophosphamide and BCNU (Ng et al. 1982b).

Because of the systemic toxicity of antineoplastic drugs, therapy-specific effects on the tumor spectrum need to be delineated. Therapeutic specificity of the postchemotherapy spectral changes has been demonstrated in only one instance, the mammary 17/A adenocarcinoma treated with Adriamycin (Evelhoch et al. 1987), for which a comparative study of drug-resistant and drug-responsive cell lines was performed. Another approach was that of Naruse et al. (1985), who examined the NMR spectra of nontumor tissues following chemotherapy and found them unaffected by the agents. This situation does not always occur. The cardiotoxicity induced by the drug Adriamycin can be observed in ^{31}P NMR spectra of rat hearts (Ng et al. 1983).

The data on radiation effects is even more sparse. Only in the RIF-1 tumor has radiation response been quantitatively correlated with spectral changes (Rajan et al.). While distinction between therapy-related and systemic effects has been achieved in this instance, by studies of treated and untreated tumors in the same host (see above), demonstration that changes are therapy specific awaits comparative studies of radiation-sensitive and -resistant sublines of the same tumor. A critical issue is the distinction between the effects of therapeutic response and tumor reoxygenation. Detection of tumor reoxygenation could provide the basis for optimal scheduling of fractionated radiation doses on the basis of NMR measurements. This detection may prove very difficult to accomplish by ^{31}P NMR because levels of detectable phosphate metabolites could be, in many instances, determined by the substrate rather than by oxygen availability (since many tumors are predominantly glycolytic). Therefore, more direct methods for measuring tumor oxygenation may be required for this purpose.

Correlation of tumor response to hyperthermia with an index of tumor response is limited to a single preliminary study based on monitoring a tumor-associated serum marker, alkaline phosphatase, in the murine Nunn osteogenic sarcoma (Lilly et al. 1984). Still, general agreement exists that only one type of spectral change is observed following hyperthermia (i.e., a decrease in signals from all high energy phosphates, an increase in P_i, and an acid shift in pH). Correlation of spectral changes with growth delays and clonogenic cell survival assays is needed. Demonstration that these changes are therapy specific awaits comparative studies between heat-sensitive and heat-resistant tumors. Considerable effort has gone into NMR monitoring of hyperglycemia as a method for sensitizing tumors to hyperthermia (Evelhoch et al. 1984; Hwang et al. 1988). Acidosis and decreased blood flow in the tumor have been detected; both effects may produce thermal sensitization. What is still lacking is a direct correlation of hyperglycemia-induced spectral changes and the extent of thermal sensitization.

A key question remains to be addressed: What is the range of therapeutic response that can be detected by NMR spectroscopy, and how soon after treatment can the magnitude of response be predicted? In complex, overlapping ^{31}P NMR spectra, as seen in tumors, a cell population contributing less than 5%–10% of the signal would likely remain undetected. Consequently, if the extent of cell kill is estimated by comparing spectral contributions of dead and living tumor cells, one to two log orders of cell kill would be all that is detected. This situation applies to hyperthermia and chemotherapy with agents which appear to diminish tumor perfusion. However, for other chemotherapeutic agents and for some kinds of radiation therapy, the NMR response is primarily due to the behavior of the surviving cells, which may be metabolically active even though many are doomed to die as a result of genetic damage. This effect is observed with RIF-1 after treatment with cyclophosphamide.

Reference to Fig. 8 indicates that on the 3rd day after treatment, the spectral perturbations are maximal for a dose of 200 mg/kg. Figure 11 indicates that these doses correspond to approximately 1.5–2.0 log orders of cell kill. The effects of these doses could be detected by monitoring volume changes, but NMR detects these changes much more quickly. Distinguishing between the effects of 100 and 200 mg/kg by volume changes requires at least 10 days. On the 3rd day, no difference is evident in the volumes of tumors treated with 100, 200, or 300 mg/kg, although the ultimate effects of these doses will be quite different (Fig. 12).

Similar evaluation of the data on effects of radiation on RIF-1 tumors indicates that by day 3 after treatment, distinction can be made between the effects of 5 and 15 Gy, but not between 15 and 25 Gy, of radiation. This discrimination corresponds to monitoring approximately 3 log orders of cell kill. Distinction between 15 and 25 Gy is feasible at day 7 after therapy (corresponding to one more log order of cell kill), but by this time volume measurements become competitive with spectral changes in detecting response. Therefore, in monitoring radiation therapy, the chief advantage of NMR spectroscopy will also be detection earlier than is possible by volume measurements. This consideration could be critical for both chemotherapy and radiation therapy; it would allow early modification of ineffectual therapeutic regimens and would spare the patient unnecessary toxicity. Spectroscopy may also provide an early indication of recurrence of disease, as is apparent from inspection of Fig. 19 (compare 24- and 48-h spectra).

Preliminary clinical observations on patients treated with chemotherapeutic agents and/or radiation have produced confusing and often conflicting results. The available data are largely anecdotal on different tumor types, in various locations in the body, and on patients with extensive metastatic disease and different immune capacities. In clinical studies the patient serves as his or her own control, and response is judged by changes relative to pretreatment spectra. However, animal studies indicate that tumor spectra change even in the absence of treatment. The absence of proper control data complicates interpretation of spectral changes. Therapeutic response often is not quantified or is based on subjective criteria. Different therapeutic agents and different doses, sometimes from multiple therapeutic agents, have been employed. All of these factors could affect the spectral characteristics of the tumor both before and after therapy. Spectra attributed to tumors may actually originate in large measure from extraneous tissues both inside and outside the tumor. Some of these problems may arise from imperfect localization techniques, which can lead to sampling of nontumor tissues.

Methods of addressing these problems and validating NMR spectroscopic techniques include the formation of cooperative interinstitutional programs similar to those employed in the evaluation of therapeutic protocols. These programs should involve oncologists, spectroscopists, radiologists, and statisticians. This multidisciplinary approach will not only facilitate the optimization and standardization of methods but will also provide a large enough data base for evaluation of these procedures in the shortest time possible. Improved localization methods and higher spatial resolution should minimize sampling artifacts. Initial studies should be focused on a few tumors that are easily localized and have fairly uniform characteristics among patients; this approach will provide a suitable statistical data base and will be significant clinically. Ideally these studies should be confined to tumors which will be excised or from which biopsy specimens can be readily obtained. The latter may be employed to evaluate histology and assign spectral resonances by high resolution NMR of tumor extracts. Patients with metastatic disease should be excluded from initial studies. Criteria for physiological and nutritional assessment of the patient should also be determined.

Establishing xenografts of human tumors in immunosuppressed animals is highly desirable. Even though the tumor would be exposed to a host environment that differs from that of the human, this model is nevertheless the best and most practical one available. To determine the extent of variability among individuals with similar tumors, studies of these xenografts could be conducted to determine the tumor characteristics during untreated growth. Therapeutic response could be monitored to single and multiple modalities, and response could be quantified on the basis of clonogenic cell survival assays and growth delays. The biochemical characteristics of the tumors (e.g., extent of glycolytic vs oxidative metabolism) could be assessed in vivo and in culture. Such animal and culture data could provide a basis for evaluation of clinical procedures.

6.6 A Look at the Future of NMR Spectroscopy

This section will take a more comprehensive view of future trends in NMR spectroscopy, outlining additional areas of growth which are expected to become increasingly important for expansion of NMR spectroscopic capabilities into the 1990s and beyond.

The driving force behind the development of new NMR spectroscopic methods since its invention in 1946 has been the introduction of higher-field magnets. Theoretically, sensitivity increases with the 7/4 power; practically, it increases with the 1.0–1.75 power of the magnet field strength. This trend towards higher field will have a profound effect on in vivo NMR spectroscopy. Commercial clinical spectrometers currently operate at 1.5 T (15000 gauss, as compared to the earth's field of approximately 0.5 gauss). These high fields require the use of superconducting magnets. A number of 4.0 T whole body spectrometers, currently being tested by commercial manufacturers, should be delivered to academic sites by 1990. Construction of a 10 T whole body spectrometer may possible be achieved within 5 years. The increased field will facilitate the observation of less sensitive nuclei (such as ^{39}K) and will decrease acquisition times and spatial resolution for the more sensitive nuclei. At 4.0 T spatial resolution for spectroscopy by CSI or ISIS should be on the order of 1 and 2 cm for ^{1}H and ^{31}P spectroscopy, respectively. Current operational costs are high because of the cost of liquid helium, which is required to maintain superconductivity. Cryogen costs will diminish if suitable superconductors which operate at liquid nitrogen temperature or higher become available.

At magnetic fields up to 2.3 T, hazards have been limited to the need to avoid ferrous materials and pacemakers. At 4.0 T problems with vertigo have been encountered as subjects moved within the magnet. This condition is believed to result from generation of currents in the inner ear, and ways of overcoming it are being sought. At 4.0 T effects of rf power deposition and static and variable magnetic fields on physiological parameters appears manageable. At higher fields rf heating may pose some problems, but time shared pulsing should minimize this effect.

Next to magnet development, computers have had the greatest technological impact on NMR spectroscopy. The availability of relatively inexpensive, efficient computers was essential for implementation of Fourier transform methods, which are the basis of applications of NMR spectroscopy to the study of biomolecular structure and for both in vivo NMR spectroscopy and NMR imaging. While computers were initially employed exclusively in the acquisition of data, their use in data processing, presentation, and analysis has recently become increasingly important. This trend is likely to continue as computer technology becomes more economical. Supercomputer programs are already available for interpretation of complex isotopic labeling experiments. Sophisticated computers are being employed to overlay imaging data obtained from various modalities and to facilitate planning of radiation therapy. Spectroscopic data will likely be incorporated in multimodality image and function analysis.

In the next few years, the clinical implementation of NMR spectroscopic studies employing isotopically and fluorine-labeled reagents should become more common. This approach, in conjunction with the development of higher-field instruments and indirect detection techniques, is likely to have an enormous impact on medical imaging. These advances will permit monitoring of the flux through key metabolic pathways. Potential applications to oncology include analysis of carbohydrate metabolism, assessment of glycolytic vs oxidative metabolic activity, determination of redox potentials, and pharmacokinetics of isotopically labeled antineoplastic agents.

The cost of ^{13}C-labeled metabolites is currently prohibitive for clinical ^{13}C NMR spectroscopy. However, indirect detection of ^{13}C-labeled carbons by selectively monitoring ^{1}H resonances of directly bonded protons provides a method for detecting carbon flux with sensitivities approaching those of ^{1}H NMR (Freeman et al. 1981; Rothman et al. 1985; Jue 1987). This technique, which is still being refined, should decrease the amount of labeled reagent required for clinical investigation. Increased market demand for these reagents should stimulate the economic synthesis of isotopically labeled compounds and thus lead to a reduced cost for conducting these experiments.

These considerations, as well the increasingly evident utility of these procedures, should make isotopic labeling extremely useful for both clinical and research applications to cancer. The incremental cost of equipping an NMR imager (now considered an essential diagnostic instrument in most institutions) for spectroscopy is negligible in comparison with the cost of equipping an institution for positron emission tomography (PET) scanning, for example. These factors make NMR spectroscopy with isotopically labeled reagents an attractive alternative to PET scanning when sensitivity is not critical. Still, in studies of receptor binding, thymidine incorporation, oxygen uptake, etc., PET will remain the modality of choice.

The ability of NMR spectroscopy to detect therapeutic response will probably be exploited in the development of optimum therapeutic regimens. In the case of hyperthermia, spectral perturbations can be detected virtually immediately after treatment. ^{31}P CSI should become available to monitor the effects of heating on the tumor and on surrounding normal tissue. This capability could be combined with methods for monitoring temperature by intervoxel diffusion imaging (Le Bihan et al. 1988) to monitor and control hyperthermia treatment of tumors. Radiation and chemotherapy effects can be detected within hours of treatment, while tumor reoxygenation may also be detectable in the same time period. Consequently, NMR spectroscopy could be used to devise optimal drug and radiation schedules.

The possibility of detecting Adriamycin-induced cardiotoxicity by ^{13}C NMR spectroscopy was first reported by NG et al. (1983). This study was based on the detection of spectral changes in perfused rat hearts following acute administration of the agent. These studies are now being extended to chronic studies in rats and dogs by both ^{31}P and ^{13}C NMR spectroscopy. The ability to detect both drug toxicity and efficacy by NMR spectroscopy would provide a noninvasive method for determining the overall therapeutic index of antineoplastic agents. NMR spectroscopy would thus be an extremely valuable method for tailoring therapy to the individual patient.

A number of studies employing NMR spectroscopy to analyze excised tissue specimens and body fluids have been reported. The spectral characteristics of breast tumor specimens have been reported to correlate with levels of estrogen receptors (VICTOR et al. 1987). Considerable interest was generated by reports of differences in apparent linewidths of ^{1}H resonances of lipid components of sera from normal and cancer patients (FOSSEL et al. 1986). However, subsequent investigations indicated false positives from hyperlipidemics and considerable overlap with data from normal controls (SAUNDERS et al. 1988). Relaxation times of ^{1}H resonances of glycolipid components of serum from cancer patients have also been reported to reflect metastatic potential and drug resistance (MOUNTFORD and TATTERSALL 1987). Pleiotropic drug resistance has been associated with ^{31}P and ^{13}C NMR spectral differences of perfused tumor cells (COHEN et al. 1986). While some of these initial claims may prove overly optimistic, considerable diagnostic utility appears likely to be derived from analysis of tissue specimens, extracts of tissue specimens, serum samples, and perfused, isolated tumor cells. These data should be of considerable utility to pathologists in the future.

In vivo NMR spectroscopy will clearly provide scientists with a significant new tool for the study of cancer. The unique ability of NMR to observe intracellular biochemistry in a totally noninvasive manner will allow the examination of many questions of solid tumor physiology which were previously unanswerable. Development of the most suitable role for spectroscopy in the clinic, however, will require a substantial amount of additional research. During the next decade NMR spectroscopy is anticipated to become integrated with other imaging modalities and thereby provide biochemical information about the anatomical regions delineated by traditional techniques. The task of researchers at this stage is to identify NMR spectroscopy data which are reliable indicators of tumor characteristics and of the success or failure of therapy. Improvement in the ability of physicians to select a successful treatment, to promptly determine when response is or is not obtained, and to recognize unacceptable toxic effects of therapy promises to have a tremendous impact on the long-term quality of cancer treatment.

References

Ackerman JJH, Grove TH, Wong GG, Gadian DG, Radda GK (1980) Mapping of metabolites in whole animals by P-31 NMR using surface coils. Nature 283: 167–170

Ackerman JJ, Ewy CS, Becker NN, Shalwitz RA (1987) Deuterium nuclear magnetic resonance measurements of blood flow and tissue perfusion employing $^{2}H_2O$ as a freely diffusible tracer. Proc Natl Acad Sci USA 84: 4099–4102

Bottomley PA, Charles HC, Roemer PB, Flamig D, Engeseth H, Edelstein WA, Mueller OM (1988) Human in vivo phosphate metabolite imaging with ^{31}P NMR. Magn Reson Med 7: 319–336

Braunschweiger PG (1988) Effect of cyclophosphamide on the pathophysiology of RIF-1 solid tumors. Cancer Res 48: 4206–4210

Brown JM (1979) Evidence for acutely hypoxic cells in mouse tumours, and a possible mechanism of reoxygenation. Br J Radiol 52: 650–656

Bruhn H, Frahm J, Gyngell ML, Merboldt KD, Hanicke W, Sauter R (1988) Localized proton spectroscopy of tumors in vivo: patients with primary and secondary cerebral tumors. Abstracts of The Society of Magnetic Resonance in Medicine 1: 253

Ceckler TL, Bryant RG, Penney DP, Gibson SL, Hilf R (1986) ^{31}P-NMR spectroscopy demonstrates decreased ATP levels in vivo as an early response to photodynamic therapy. Biochem Biophys Res Commun 140: 273–279

Chen K, Glockner J, Morse PD II, Swartz HM (1988) Oxygen effects on metabolism of nitroxide contrast agents: measurement of redox state in cells. Abstracts of The Society of Magnetic Resonance in Medicine 1: 493

Cohen JS, Lyon RC (1987) Multinuclear NMR study of the metabolism of drug-sensitive and drug-resistant human breast cancer cells. Ann NY Acad Sci 508: 216–228

Cohen JS, Lyon RC, Chen C et al. (1986) Differences in phosphate metabolite levels in drug-sensitive and -resistant human breast cancer cell lines determined by phosphorus-31 magnetic resonance spectroscopy. Cancer Res 46: 4087 – 4090

Daly PF, Lyon RC, Faustino PJ, Cohen JS (1987) Phospholipid metabolism in cancer cells monitored by ^{31}P NMR spectroscopy. J Biol Chem 262: 14875–14878

Damadian R (1971) Tumor detection by nuclear magnetic resonance. Science 171: 1151–1153

Degani H, Horowitz A, Itzchak Y (1986) Breast tumors: evaluation with P-31 MR spectroscopy. Radiology 161: 53–55

Evanochko WT, Ng TC, Glickson JD, Durant JR, Corbett TH (1982) Human tumors as examined by in vivo ^{31}P

NMR in athymic mice. Biochem Biophys Res Commun 109: 1346–1352
Evanochko WT, Ng TC, Lilly MB, Lawson AJ, Corbett TH, Durant JR, Glickson JD (1983) In vivo ^{31}P NMR study of the metabolism of murine mammary 16/C adenocarcinoma and its response to chemotherapy, x-radiation, and hyperthermia. Proc Natl Acad Sci USA 80: 334–338
Evanochko WT, Ng TC, Glickson JD (1984a) Application of in vivo NMR spectroscopy to cancer. Magn Reson Med 1: 508–534
Evanochko WT, Sakai TT, Ng TC et al. (1984b) NMR study of RIF-1 tumors. Analysis of perchloric acid extracts and identification of ^{1}H, ^{31}P, and ^{13}C resonances. Biochim Biophys Acta 805: 104–116
Evelhoch JL, Sapareto SA, Jick DEL, Ackerman JJH (1984) In vivo metabolic effects of hyperglycemia in murine radiation-induced fibrosarcoma: a ^{31}P NMR investigation. Proc Natl Acad Sci USA 81: 6496–6500
Evelhoch JL, Sapareto SA, Nussbaum GH, Ackerman JJH (1986) Correlations between phosphorus-31 NMR spectroscopy and oxygen-15 perfusion measurements in the RIF-1 murine tumor in vivo. Radiat Res 106: 122–131
Evelhoch JL, Keller NA, Corbett TH (1987) Response-specific adriamycin sensitivity markers provided by in vivo phosphorus-31 nuclear magnetic resonance spectroscopy in murine mammary adenocarcinomas. Cancer Res 47: 3396–3401
Evelhoch JL, Bissery MC, Chabot GG, Simpson NE, McCoy CL, Heilbrun LK, Corbett TH (1988) Flavone acetic acid (NSC 347512)-induced modulation of tumor physiology monitored by in vivo nuclear magnetic resonance spectroscopy. Cancer Res 48: 4749–4755
Farrar TC, Becker ED (1971) Pulse and Fourier transform NMR. Academic, New York
Fossel ET, Carr JM, McDonagh J (1986) Detection of malignant tumors: water-suppressed proton nuclear magnetic resonance spectroscopy of plasma. N Engl J Med 315: 1369–1376
Freeman R, Mareci TH, Morris GA (1981) Weak satellite signals in high-resolution NMR spectra: separating the wheat from the chaff. J Magn Reson 42: 341–345
Gadian DG (1982) Nuclear magnetic resonance and its application to living systems. Oxford University Press, Oxford
Gadian DG, Proctor E, Williams SR (1987) Some recent applications of ^{1}H NMR spectroscopy in vivo. Ann NY Acad Sci 508: 241–250
Glickson JD, Evanochko WT, Sakai TT, Ng TC (1986) In vivo NMR studies of RIF-1 tumors. In: Allen PS, Boisvert DPJ, Lentle BD (eds) Magnetic resonance in cancer. Pergamon, Toronto, pp 71–82
Glickson JD, Evanochko WT, Sakai TT, Ng TC (1987) In vivo NMR spectroscopy of tumors. In: Gupta RK (ed) NMR spectroscopy of cells and organisms, vol I. CRC Press, Boca Raton, pp 99–134
Griffey RH, Griffey B, Berghmans K, Wenk R, Gasparovic C, Mann P (1988) Sodium multiple quantum spectroscopy and imaging of tumor cells implanted in nude rats and in cell suspensions. Abstracts of The Society of Magnetic Resonance in Medicine 1: 213
Griffiths JR, Cady E, Edwards RHT, McReady VR, Wilkie DR, Wiltshaw E (1983) P-31 NMR studies of a human tumour in situ. Lancet I: 1435–1436
Griffiths JR, Bhujwalla Z, Coombes RC et al. (1987) Monitoring cancer therapy by NMR spectroscopy. Ann NY Acad Sci 508: 183–199
Gyulai L, Bolinger L, Leigh JS Jr, Barlow C, Chance B (1984) Phosphorylethanolamine – the major constituent of the phosphomonoester peak observed by ^{31}P-NMR in developing dog brain. FEBS Lett 178: 137–142
Hall EJ (1978) Radiobiology for the radiobiologist, 2nd edn. Harper & Row, Philadelphia
Hesketh TR, Moore JP, Morris JDH, Taylor MJ, Rogers J, Smith GA, Metcalfe JC (1985) A common sequence of calcium and pH signals in the mitogenic stimulation of eucaryotic cells. Nature 313: 481–484
Hetherington HP, Avison MJ, Shulman RG (1985) Proton homonuclear editing of rat brain using semiselective pulses. Proc Natl Acad Sci USA 85: 3115–3118
Hoult DI (1979) Rotating frame zeugmatography. J Magn Reson 33: 183–197
Hsieh PS, Balaban RS (1987) ^{31}P imaging of in vivo creatine kinase reaction rates. J Magn Reson 74: 574–579
Hull WE, Port RE, Herrmann R, Britsch B, Kunz W (1988) Metabolites of 5-fluorouracil in plasma and urine, as monitored by fluorine-19 nuclear magnetic resonance spectroscopy, in patients receiving chemotherapy with or without methotrexate pretreatment. Cancer Res 48: 1680–1688
Hwang YC, Kim S-G, Evelhoch JL, Ackerman JJH (1988) Glucose and glucose analog induction of tumor acidification and blood flow modulation in situ: a phosphorus and deuterium NMR investigation. Abstracts of The Society of Magnetic Resonance in Medicine 1: 207
Irving MG, Brooks WM, Brereton IM et al. (1987) Use of high resolution in vivo volume selected ^{1}H-magnetic resonance spectroscopy to investigate leukemia in humans. Cancer Res 47: 3901–3906
Jue T (1987) Winnowing the (carbon-13)-proton resonance in the in vivo NMR spectrum. J Magn Reson 71: 532–538
Karczmar GS, Poole J, Boska MD et al. (1988) ^{31}P MRS study of response of human tumors to therapy. Abstracts of The Society of Magnetic Resonance in Medicine 2: 615
Kim SG, Ackerman JJH (1988) Quantitative determination of tumor blood flow and perfusion via deuterium nuclear magnetic resonance spectroscopy in mice. Cancer Res 48: 3449–3453
Kingsley-Hickman PB, Sako EY, Mohanakrishnan P, Robitaille PML, From AHL, Foker JE, Ûgurbil K (1987) ^{31}P NMR studies of ATP synthesis and hydrolysis kinetics in the intact myocardium. Biochemistry 26: 7501–7510
Koutcher JA, Okunieff P, Neuringer L, Suit H, Brady T (1987) Size dependent changes in tumor phosphate metabolism after radiation therapy as detected by ^{31}P NMR spectroscopy. Int J Radiat Oncol Biol Phys 13: 1851–1855
LeBihan D, Delannoy J, Levin RL (1988) Mapping of temperature using intra-voxel incoherent motion (IVIM) MR imaging-application to hyperthermia. Abstracts of the Society of Magnetic Resonance in Medicine 2: 881
Li SJ, Wehrle JP, Rajan SS, Steen RG, Glickson JD (1988) Response of radiation-induced fibrosarcoma-1 in mice to cyclophosphamide monitored by in vivo ^{31}P nuclear magnetic resonance spectroscopy. Cancer Res 48: 4736–4742
Li SJ, Wehrle JP, Rajan SS, Steen RG, Glickson JD (to be published) Activation and bioenergetic effects of 5-fluorouracil: ^{19}F and ^{31}P nuclear magnetic resonance spectroscopic and tumor blood flow studies of the murine radiation-induced fibrosarcoma-1
Lilly MB, Ng TC, Evanochko WT et al. (1984) Loss of high-energy phosphate following hyperthermia demonstrated by in vivo ^{31}P-nuclear magnetic resonance spectroscopy. Cancer Res 44: 633–638
Lilly MB, Katholi CR, Ng TC (1985) Direct relationship between high-energy phosphate content and blood flow in

thermally treated murine tumors. J Natl Cancer Inst 75: 885–889

Luyten PR, den Hollander JA, Segebarth C, Baleriaux D (1988) Localized ^{1}H NMR spectroscopy and spectroscopic imaging of human brain tumors in situ. Abstracts of The Society of Magnetic Resonance in Medicine 1: 252

Maris JM, Evans AE, McLaughlin AC, D'Angio GJ, Bolinger L, Manos H, Chance B (1985) P-31 nuclear magnetic resonance spectroscopic investigation of human neuroblastoma in situ. N Engl J Med 312: 1500–1505

McCoy CL, Giri BP, Evelhoch JL (1988) A method for direct in vivo measurement of absolute drug concentration from a single ^{2}H NMR spectrum. Abstracts of The Society of Magnetic Resonance in Medicine 2: 820

Mountford CE, Tattersall MH (1987) Proton magnetic resonance spectroscopy and tumour detection. Cancer Surveys 6: 285–314

Naruse S, Harakawa K, Horikawa Y et al. (1985) Measurements of in vivo ^{31}P nuclear magnetic resonance spectra in neuroectodermal tumors for the evaluation of the effects of chemotherapy. Cancer Res 45: 2429–2433

Naruse S, Higuchi T, Horikawa Y, Tanaka C, Nakamura K, Hirakawa K (1986a) Radiofrequency hyperthermia with successive monitoring of its effects on tumors using NMR spectroscopy. Proc Natl Acad Sci USA 83: 8343–8347

Naruse S, Horikawa Y, Tanaka C, Higuchi T, Sekimoto H, Ueda S, Hirakawa K (1986b) Evaluation of the effects of photoradiation therapy on brain tumors with in vivo P-31 MR spectroscopy. Radiology 160: 827–830

Ng TC, Glickson JD (1985) Shielded solenoidal probe for in vivo NMR studies of solid tumors. Magn Reson Med 2: 169–175

Ng TC, Evanochko WT, Glickson JD (1982a) Faraday shield for surface-coil studies of subcutaneous tumors. J Magn Reson 49: 526–529

Ng TC, Evanochko WT, Hiramoto RN et al. (1982b) ^{31}P NMR spectroscopy of in vivo tumors. J Magn Reson 49: 271–286

Ng TC, Daugherty JP, Evanochko WT, Digerness SB, Durant JR, Glickson JD (1983) Detection of antineoplastic agent induced cardiotoxicity by ^{31}P NMR of perfused rat hearts. Biochem Biophys Res Commun 110: 339–347

Ng TC, Glickson JD, Bendall MR (1984) Depth pulse sequences for surface coils: spatial localization and T_1 measurements. Magn Reson Med 1: 450–462

Ng TC, Vijayakumar S, Majors AW, Thomas FJ, Meaney TF, Baldwin NJ (1987) Response of a non-Hodgkin's lymphoma to ^{60}Co therapy monitored by ^{31}P MRS in situ. Int J Radiat Oncol Biol Phys 13: 1545–1551

Oberhänsli RD, Hilton-Jones D, Bore PJ, Hands LJ, Rampling RP, Radda GK (1986) Biochemical investigation of human tumors in vivo with phosphorus-31 magnetic resonance spectroscopy. Lancet II: 8–11

Pedersen PL (1978) Tumor mitochondria and the bioenergetics of cancer cells. Prog Exp Tumor Res 22: 190–274

Podo F, Carpinelli G, DiVito M et al. (1987) Nuclear magnetic resonance analysis of tumor necrosis factor-induced alterations of phospholipid metabolites and pH in friend leukemia cell tumors and fibrosarcomas in mice. Cancer Res 47: 6481–6489

Rajan SS, Wehrle JP, Li SS, Steen RG, Glickson SD (1989) Bioenergetic changes in RIF-1 fibrosarcoma after radiation therapy monitored by ^{31}P NMR spectroscopy (in preparation)

Rodrigues JL, Stevens AN, Wilkinson J, Coombes RC, Griffiths JR (1985) Chemically induced mammary tumours: a ^{31}P nuclear-magnetic-resonance study of growth and therapy. Biochem Soc Trans 13: 887–888

Rothman DL, Arias-Mendoza F, Shulman GI, Shulman RG (1984a) A pulse sequence for simplifying hydrogen NMR spectra of biological tissues. J Magn Reson 60: 430–436

Rothman DL, Behar KL, Hetherington HP, Shulman RG (1984b) Homonuclear proton double-resonance difference spectroscopy of the rat brain in vivo. Proc Natl Acad Sci USA 81: 6330–6334

Rothman DL, Behar KL, Hetherington HP, den Hollander JA, Bendall MR, Petroff OAC, Shulman RG (1985) Proton-observe/carbon-13-decouple spectroscopic measurements of lactate and glutamate in the rat brain in vivo. Proc Natl Acad Sci USA 82: 1633–1637

Saunders JK, Smith ICP, Monck M et al. (1988) A detailed assessment of the recent MRS blood test to detect cancer. Abstracts of The Society of Magnetic Resonance in Medicine 1: 363

Schiffer LM, Braunschweiger PG, Glickson JD, Evanochko WT, Ng TC (1985) Preliminary observations on the correlation of proliferative phenomena with in vivo ^{31}P NMR spectroscopy after tumor chemotherapy. Ann NY Acad Sci 459: 270–277

Segebarth CM, Baleriaux DF, Arnold DL, Luyten PR, den Hollander JA (1987) MR image-guided P-31 MR spectroscopy in the evaluation of brain tumor treatment. Radiology 165: 215–219

Semmler W, Gademann G, Bachert-Baumann P, Zabel HJ, Lorenz WJ, van Kaick G (1988) Monitoring human tumor response to therapy by means of ^{31}P-MR spectroscopy. Radiology 166: 533–539

Shine NJ, Palladino M, Deisseroth A, Karczmar G, Matson G, Weiner MW (1987) Effects of tumor necrosis factor on high-energy phosphates of an experimental mouse tumor. Abstracts of The Society of Magnetic Resonance in Medicine 1: 35

Sijens PE, Bovee WMMJ, Seijkens D, Los G, Rutgers DH (1986) In vivo ^{31}P-nuclear magnetic resonance study of the response of a murine mammary tumor to different doses of γ-radiation. Cancer Res 46: 1427–1432

Sijens PE, Bovee WMMJ, Seijkens D, Koole P, Los G, van Rijssel RH (1987) Murine mammary tumor response to hyperthermia and radiotherapy evaluated by in vivo ^{31}P-nuclear magnetic resonance spectroscopy. Cancer Res 47: 6467–6473

Sillerud LO, Griffey RH, Fegnolio-Preiser C, Shepard S, Halliday KR (1988) In vivo ^{13}C NMR spectroscopy of the human prostate. Abstracts of The Society of Magnetic Resonance in Medicine 1: 250

Skog S, Nordell B, Ericsson A, Tribukait B, Nishida T (1986) Changes in energy metabolism following roentgen irradiation of in vivo growing Ehrlich ascites tumor cells studied by ^{31}P magnetic resonance spectroscopy. Acta Radiol Oncol 25: 63–69

Sostman HD, Armitage IM, Fischer JJ (1984) NMR in cancer I. High resolution spectroscopy of tumors. Mag Reson Imaging 2: 265–278

Steen RG, Tamargo RJ, McGovern KA, Rajan SS, Brem H, Wehrle JP, Glickson JD (1988) In vivo ^{31}P nuclear magnetic resonance spectroscopy of subcutaneous 9L gliosarcoma: effects of tumor growth and treatment with 1,3-bis(2-chlorethyl)-1-nitrosourea on tumor bioenergetics and histology. Cancer Res 48: 676–681

Stevens AN, Morris PG, Iles RA, Griffiths JR (1984) 5-Fluorouracil metabolism monitored in vivo by ^{19}F NMR. Br J Cancer 50: 113–117

Sutherland RM, Franko AJ (1980) On the nature of the radiobiologically hypoxic fraction in tumors. Int J Radiat Onc Biol Phys 6: 117-120

Thomlinson RH, Gray LH (1955) The histological structure of some human lung cancers and the possible implications for radiotherapy. Br J Cancer 9: 539-549

Twentyman PR, Brown JM, Gray JW, Franko AJ, Scoles MA, Kallman RF (1980) A new end point tumor model system (RIF-1) for comparison of end-point studies. J Natl Cancer Inst 64: 595-604

Vaupel PW, Frinak S, Bicher HI (1981) Heterogeneous oxygen partial pressure and pH distribution in C3H mouse mammary adenocarcinoma. Cancer Res 41: 2008-2013

Victor TA, Lawson CA, Wiebolt RC, Nussbaum S, Shattuch MC, Brodin AG, Degani H (1987) Prediction of hormonal response of human breast carcinoma by ^{31}P MR spectroscopy. In: McCarthy S, Haseltine F (eds) Magnetic resonance of the reproductive system. Slack, Thorofare, pp 67-80

Vogele KE, Lenkinski RE, Bilaniuk et al. (1988) An integrated MRI/^{31}P spectroscopy study of head and neck squamous cell carcinomas. Abstracts of The Society of Magnetic Resonance in Medicine 1: 324

Wang Z, Wicklund S, Subramanian VH, Leigh JS (1988) Potassium-39 NMR in vivo studies of humans. Abstracts of The Society of Magnetic Resonance in Medicine 1: 340

Wehrle JP, Li SJ, Rajan SS, Steen RG, Glickson JD (1987) ^{31}P and ^{1}H NMR spectroscopy of tumors in vivo: untreated growth and response to chemotherapy. Ann NY Acad Sci 508: 200-214

Wolf W, Albright MJ, Silver MS, Weber H, Reichardt U, Sauer R (1987) Fluorine-19 NMR spectroscopic studies of the metabolism of 5-fluorouracil in the liver of patients undergoing chemotherapy. Magn Reson Imaging 5: 165-169

Wright LC, May GL, Gregory P, Dyne M, Holmes KT, Williams PG, Mountford CE (1988) Inhibition of metastatic potential by fucosidase: an NMR study identifies a cell surface metastasis marker. J Cell Biochem 31: 49-59

Zimmermann RA, Bottomley PA, Edelstein WA, Hart HR, Redington RW, Bilanink LT, Grossman RI et al. (1985) Proton imaging and phosphorus spectroscopy in a malignant glioma. Am J Neuroradiol 6: 109-110

7 Positron Emission Tomography: Current Achievements and Future Projections

DEAN F. WONG

CONTENTS

7.1 Introduction 117
7.2 Basic Principles of Positron Emission Tomography 117
7.3 Cyclotron vs Generator Produced Isotopes . . . 118
7.4 Role of Kinetic Models 119
7.5 Tissue Perfusion Studies 121
7.6 Regional Glucose and Oxygen Metabolism Studies 121
7.7 In vivo Human Imaging Studies of Neurotransmitter and Receptors 123
7.8 Patient Studies 124
7.9 The Future of PET 125
7.9.1 Introduction 125
7.9.2 Clinical Future 126
7.9.2.1 Early Detection of Disease 127
7.9.2.2 Mapping of Disease Progression 127
7.9.2.3 Monitoring Therapy 127
7.10 Summary 127
References 128

7.1 Introduction

Positron emission tomography (PET) scanning has often been proposed as a basic research tool on the one hand and as a potential clinical imaging modality on the other hand. PET can provide important information about basic physiological mechanisms and identify possible biological markers of disease. There are many future applications, including measurement of biological parameters and therapeutic monitoring of drugs.

In contrast to many radiological procedures which offer anatomical details, PET scanning provides exquisite functional sensitivity. Few imaging techniques provide the breadth of studying topics as diverse as detecting which regions of the brain metabolize glucose differently depending on whether the individual is exposed to music versus language (MAZZIOTTA et al. 1982) or demonstrating the in vivo blockade of brain receptors by therapeutic drugs, which previously could only be measured in blood (WONG et al. 1985a; FARDE et al. 1986). In addition, PET will be instrumental in providing new insights into the metabolism of the maturing brain, the biological basis of neurological/psychiatric disorders (CHUGANI and PHELPS 1986; CHUGANI et al. 1987) and the area of jeopardized ischemic myocardium in cardiac patients (SCHWAIGER et al. 1983, 1984; TILLISCH et al. 1986). Although PET has somewhat lower resolution, complementary studies with X-ray CT and MRI have improved the ability to localize structure with PET. Methods employing lateral X-ray devices (FOX et al. 1985) have been successfully utilized in normal skull anatomy for localizing PET regions. Subsequently, image processing methods such as those of EVANS et al. (1988) have defined anatomically directed PET regions of interest from those of other higher resolution instruments. FOX et al. (1986) have suggested that the functional spatial resolution of structures imaged by PET can be improved by carefully designed behavioral paradigms.

DEAN F. WONG, M.D., Division of Nuclear Medicine, Dept. of Radiology and Radiological Science, The Johns Hopkins University, School of Medicine, 600 North Wolfe Street, Baltimore, MD 21205, USA

7.2 Basic Principles of Positron Emission Tomography

Positron emission tomography scanning and its related technology, single photon emission computed tomography (SPECT), provide tomographic imaging of the regional distribution of radiotracers. An important difference between PET and SPECT is the origin of the radioactivity. In the former, a positron is emitted from the radioisotope labeling the radiotracer; two coincidental gamma rays of 511 keV each and at about 180° from one another are emitted from the annihilation of a positron and local electrons in the biological tissue. In the latter, the radioactive atom emits noncoincident gamma rays directly from the decaying radioactive nucleus. Although the latter method suffers from the lack of coincidence radiation which can improve the quantification, it is much more convenient because most of the isotopes are produced by radioactive generators with relatively long shelf lives. These generators produce the radioisotope of interest from the elution of the daughter from the parent radioisotope. A typical example of this the workhorse of nuclear medicine, the $^{99}Mo/^{99m}Tc$ generator, which produces ^{99m}Tc labeled compounds. Alternatively, other SPECT compounds such as those labeled with ^{123}I are made from commercial cyclotrons and are thus readily available. By contrast, the PET agents are generally made from in-house cyclotrons because of the short half-life of most of the PET radioisotopes of interest.

These radiotracers are labeled to compounds of biological interest and basically attempt to describe the chemistry of the biological process being studied. In all cases the approach is to label a chemical compound with a radioisotope such that the tracer principle is maintained, i.e., the basic pharmacology of the compound is not changed and has not altered the biological process being studied. This often requires low atomic weight isotopes such as ^{11}C, ^{18}F, and ^{13}N. The corresponding stable atoms are prevalent in biological tissues and can often be substituted into ligands to allow the radioactive form of the compound to be imaged. A cyclotron, accelerator, or reactor is usually required in order to produce the short-lived radioisotopes, and a radiochemistry facility is required to carry out the synthetic process. The chemical process may also require considerable nonradioactive chemistry to prepare for the radiolabeling process. This can include precursor work, simulation of radiochemical yields with the unlabeled species, and structure-activity relationships. The latter can be quite complex, especially if a series of potential ligands are being considered for radiolabeling. Once this phase has been undertaken, the next step is to develop the actual radiosynthetic process for the ligand of interest. This may necessitate novel approaches in equipment and procedures, as well as chemical techniques already established at the center. For example, even though ^{11}C may be produced by the cyclotron, a certain chemical radiosynthesis may require a new radiochemical process such as radioactive cyanide production. Another ligand may only require an already established [^{11}C]methyliodide procedure.

The imaging procedures involve the PET scanner which consists of banks of paired detectors to detect the coincidental activity from the annihilation of the positron and negative electron. The physics of the tomographic reconstruction are similar to those of other tomographic procedures, including X-ray CT and MRI imaging. With SPECT, attempts are being made to incorporate iodine (^{123}I) or ^{99m}Tc isotopes. The addition of these radioisotopes (especially the latter) may alter the biodistribution and pharmacology of the labeled ligand. Hence, an attempt has been made to develop unique chemical structures that are lipophilic and neutral, allowing the large ligands to pass biological membranes such as the blood-brain barrier to enter brain tissue from the intravascular space (LEVER et al. 1985).

7.3 Cyclotron vs Generator Produced Isotopes

The advantages of SPECT isotopes become apparent when one considers the ease of synthesis of the ligands for generator produced ^{99m}Tc or ^{123}I ligands which although expensive, are commercially available. The former can be found in practically every nuclear medicine facility in the world. The latter is also easily obtained, but the purer ^{123}I mixtures which are free of high levels of radioactive contaminants such as ^{124}I (which degrade the SPECT images) are produced in only a few sources. The cyclotron produced compounds require a large onsite facility and maintenance, due to the short half-life of the isotopes and the fact that the PET camera must be in close proximity to the radiochemical manufacturing site.

The radiochemical complexities of both SPECT and PET compounds are quite different from those encountered with long half-life compounds, such as tritiated (12 years) and ^{14}C (5000 years). Much higher specific activities are obtained with ^{11}C and ^{18}F labeling (half-lives 20 min and 110 min, respectively). ^{123}I and ^{99m}Tc (half-lives 12 h and 6 h, respectively) require more difficult chemical procedures but tend to have higher specific activities than the isotopes used for nonimaging procedures.

The process by which potential radiopharmaceuticals are identified and subsequently studied for biological appropriateness in animals and finally in man is a complicated and technical matter. It often begins with unlabeled compounds, such as drugs which are known to have biological effects. For example, spiperone, a neuroleptic employed in treating schizophrenia in Japan, has been used to label neurotransmitter receptors (WAGNER et al. 1983; WONG et al. 1984). Other compounds include derivatives of natural substances such as deoxyglucose, which is trapped at the hexokinase step in the glycolytic pathway. The radioactive tracers of carbon, nitrogen, and oxygen replace these common atoms in biological molecules. ^{18}F is sometimes an appropriate substitute for hydrogen atoms. The physiological measurements, which are often uniquely determined by PET (and SPECT in some cases), have been most recently applied to the brain, heart, and lung. These include studies of tissue perfusion, oxygen and glucose metabolism, and neuroreceptor and neurotransmitter distribution and binding (see Tables 1 and 2).

Table 1. Some typical PET radiopharmaceuticals

Tracer	Halflife	Radiopharmaceutical	Typical function
^{11}C	20 min	L-[methyl-^{11}C]methionine	Amino acid transport brain tumors
		[1-^{11}C]2-deoxy-D-glucose	Glucose metabolism
		[^{11}C]*N*-methylspiperone	D_2 dopamine receptors
		[^{11}C]0	Blood volume
		[^{11}C]Sch 23390	D_1 dopamine receptors
		[^{11}]carfentanil	mu opiate receptors
		[^{11}C]Ro 151788	Benzodiazepine receptors
		[^{11}C]raclopride	D_2 dopamine
^{18}F	110 min	2-Deoxy-2-[^{18}F]fluoro-D-glucose	Glucose metabolism
		5-[^{18}F]Fluorodopa	Dopamine metabolism
		[^{18}F][methylspiperone	Dopamine receptors
		[^{18}F]spiperone	Dopamine receptors
^{15}O	2 min	[^{15}O]oxygen	Metabolism
		[^{15}O]H_2	Blood flow
		[^{15}O]C	Blood volume
		[^{15}O]CO	Blood flow
^{13}N	10 min	Ammonia	Perfusion

Table 2. Some typical SPECT radiopharmaceuticals

Tracer	Halflife	Radiopharmaceutical	Typical function
^{99m}Tc	6 h	ECD	Brain perfusion
		HMPAO	Brain perfusion
		Isonitriles (several)	Myocardial perfusion
^{123}I	13 h	Iodoamphetamine	Brain perfusion
		Benzamides (several)	Brain – dopamine receptors

7.4 Role of Kinetic Models

A unique aspect in nuclear medicine is the need for the application of kinetic models to describe the basic quantification in the interpretation of most tomographic images (Figs. 1, 2). The necessity of incorporating the input function (usually from arterial or arterialized venous blood sampling) of the radioactivity, as well as a time course of radioactivity into a form of model (usually a compartmental model) is a key and unique process which is both powerful and controversial for PET and by analogy for SPECT imaging as well. Typical compartmental models, such as the one seen in Figs. 3 and 4, can be used for quantification of glucose metabolism (Huang et al. 1980), receptor binding (Wong et al. 1986a, b), etc. The passage of isotope and the biological flux between these compartments that it represents can be described in mathematical terms. By collecting the appropriate tissue and blood radioactivity data during the imaging studies, these differential equations can be solved for the rate constants between compartments and biological parameters of interest can be derived. Once the rate constants are estimated from normal populations for methods such as the FDG technique for glucose metabolic rate (Huang et al. 1980), some simplifications are plausible under physiological conditions. However, under pathological conditions such simplifications

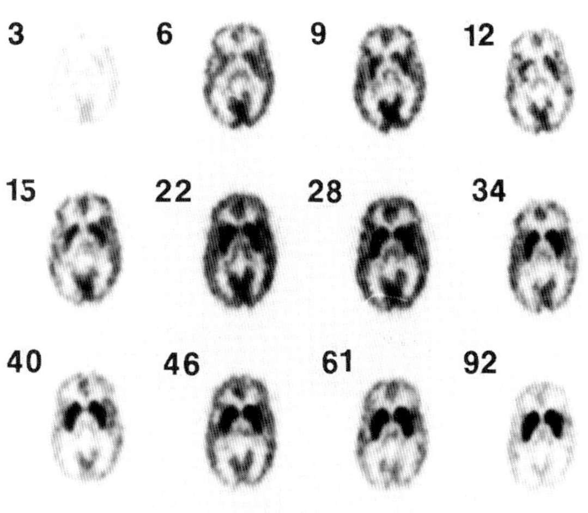

Fig. 1. From *left* to *right, top* to *bottom*, Fig. 1 contains multiple brain images over a 90-min period following the intravenous injection of [^{11}C]*N*-methylspiperone. The images show increasing tracer activity into the caudate and putamen labeling primarily D_2 dopamine receptors, but reversible binding to cortical regions, labeling mainly S_2 serotonin receptors. The *numbers* next to each image represent time (minutes) postinjection of [^{11}C]*N*-methylspiperone

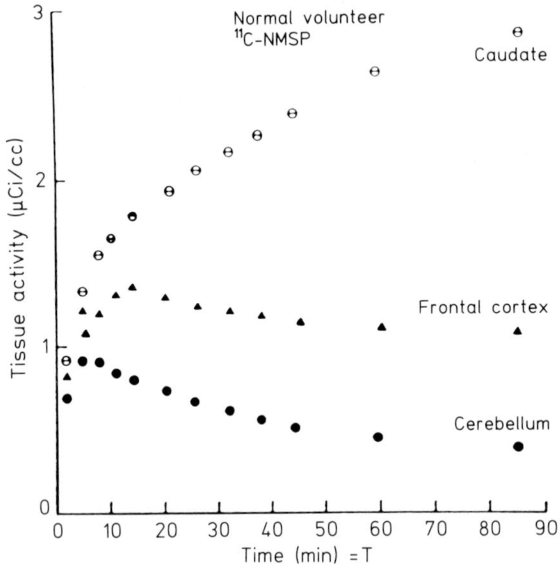

Fig. 2. Time-activity curves following the intravenous injection of [^{11}C]*N*-methylspiperone showing the accumulated activity in three regions in the brain, the caudate nucleus, frontal cortex, and cerebellum. Dynamic curves such as these demonstrate irreversible binding in the case of the caudate nucleus reversible binding in the case of the frontal cortex following a bolus injection of the tracer. Both require different types of kinetics and an appropriate compartmental model as shown in Fig. 3. ⊖ caudate, ▲ frontal cortex, ● cerebellum. (Wong et al. 1986a)

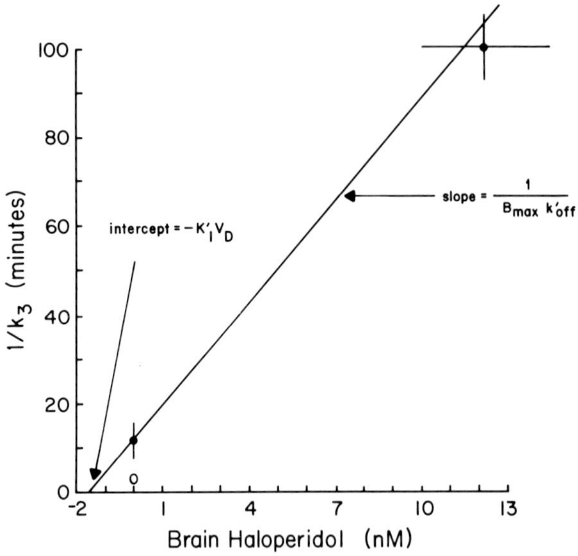

Fig. 4. Relationship between time constant of [^{11}C]*N*-methylspiperone ([^{11}C]NMSP) binding (equal to $1/k_3$) in the caudate nucleus and the tissue content of haloperidol. Tissue content of haloperidol was calculated on the basis of the plasma concentrations of haloperidol and the partition coefficient observed for [^{11}C]NMSP. *Bars* indicate 1 standard deviation. *Abscissa*=tissue content of haloperidol (pmol ml^{-1}); *ordinate*=time constant of [^{11}C]NMSP binding (min). (Wong et al. 1986b)

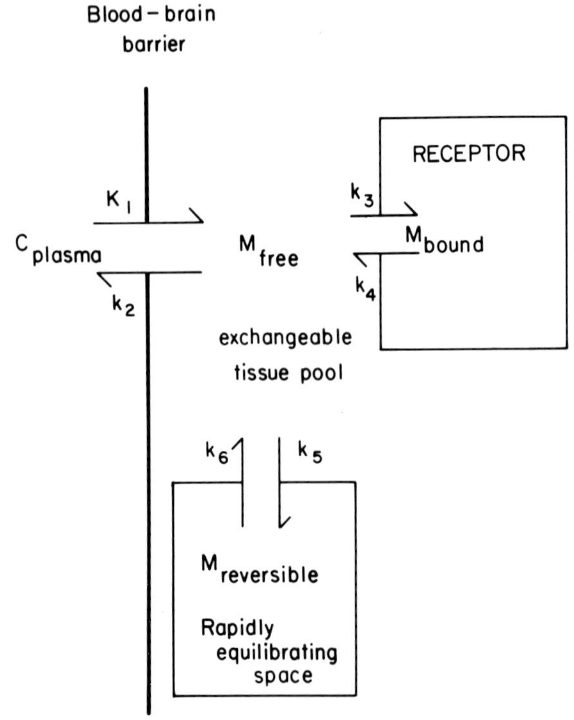

◁ **Fig. 3.** Schematic representation of the three compartment model. The accumulation of [^{11}C]*N*-methylspiperone in the brain occurs in two steps. The ligand crosses the blood-brain barrier, then binds to the receptors. C_{plasma}, concentration of the ligand in arterial plasma; M_{free}, quantity of drug in the exchangeable pool of the tissue; M_{bound}, quantity of ligand bound to the D_2 dopamine receptors; $M_{reversible}$, quantity of drug bound to the secondary or "non-D_2" receptors assumed to be in rapid equilibrium with the free ligand in brain; K_1, clearance from plasma; k_2, rate constant (fractional rate of escape from brain tissues); k_3 and k_4, the rate constants for the association and dissociation of the ligand to and from the D_2 receptors, respectively; k_5 and k_6, rate constants for the lower affinity or secondary, rapidly reversible binding present in the caudate but not the cerebellum. (Wong et al. 1986a)

may not be feasible (HAWKINS et al. 1981, 1986). Quantification will still require the acquisition of an input function from timed radioactive blood samples, but will eliminate the need for dynamic scanning. This method of delayed imaging has been applied widely, mainly for qualitative interpretation, in many forms of clinical nuclear medicine studies, such as in bone scans. Dynamic renal scanning and tissue curve interpretation is more analogous to the PET model approach, but typically lacks the dynamic input function recording necessary for PET.

The consequences of not using a plausible model and analysis can result in erroneous interpretation of the radioactivity distributions and potentially lead to inaccurate conclusions. Some of the important methods requiring mathematical models for proper PET interpretation are listed below.

7.5 Tissue Perfusion Studies

A number of techniques have been developed for the external estimation of regional cerebral blood flow. These have included the continuous and bolus perfusion technique employing $C^{15}O_2$ gas (CELESIA et al. 1983; ALPERT et al. 1977; FRACKOWIAK et al. 1980; ITO et al. 1982; LENZI et al. 1981; LENZI et al. 1982; HOYER 1982; HUANG et al. 1981) or the tissue trapping method such as approximated by [^{13}N]ammonia (KUHL et al. 1980). The latter has been employed in cardiac as well as cerebral blood flow measurements. With the use of short-lived tracers such as oxygen, these measurements can be repeated several times within a few hours. Hence, repeat studies and physiological responses to various stimuli can be directly measured.

Cerebral blood flow (CBF) measurements have been extensively studied using the $^{15}O_2$ technique either as an intravenous bolus of ^{15}O labeled compounds or by continuous inhalation of ^{15}O labeled CO_2. These methods and others involving [^{18}F]fluoromethane (CELESIA et al. 1983) and ^{77}Kr (YAMAMOTO et al. 1977) have generally agreed with the traditional Kety-Schmidt techniques (COLLINS 1978a, b). However, the PET method allows multiple, repeat measures of regional CBF measurements.

Blood-brain barrier (BBB) measurements, including permeability, have been studied with ^{68}Ga-EDTA and ^{82}Rb (YAMAMOTA et al. 1977; YEN et al. 1982). Although these techniques tend to demonstrate BBB abnormalities similar to single photon radionuclide brain scans (as ^{99m}Tc ligands), the PET method allows quantitative measurements of permeability and diffusion rates. Some studies have suggested enhanced sensitivity of PET relative to X-ray for BBB abnormalities because of the larger distribution volume and smaller size of the radionuclides as compared to X-ray contrast media (YEN et al. 1982).

Myocardial blood flow has been examined using a number of positron emitting tracers, including ^{81}Rb and ^{82}Rb (BELLER et al. 1982; BUDINGER et al. 1981) administered intravenously, as well as microspheres radiolabeled with ^{68}Ga or ^{11}C (HNATOWICH 1976; WILSON et al. 1984) given via the left atrium or ventricle. [^{13}N]ammonia was indicated for PET measurements of myocardial blood flow (SCHELBERT et al. 1979, 1980).

7.6 Regional Glucose and Oxygen Metabolism Studies

These studies have provided remarkable insight into normal physiology and pathophysiology of regional cerebral and cardiac metabolism. Pioneering studies were performed in the early 1980s consisting of exploration of metabolic patterns, as a function of age and activation with physiological stimuli.

Numerous studies of the aging effect have shown, at best, mild or possibly insignificant effects of age on glucose and oxygen metabolism (KUHL et al. 1982a, b). However, more recent studies involving PET in children aged from 5 days to 28 months have demonstrated an initially low glucose utilization in the neocortex and striatum, with increasing energy requirements over time, approaching adult values around 8 months of age. In contrast, the pattern of glucose utilization for 2-year-old subjects with mental retardation closely resembles that of infants only a few days old (CHUGANI et al. 1986, 1987).

Pioneering work at UCLA in the 1970s and other centers allowed examination of physiological conditions involving behavioral activation. These studies included visual and auditory stimulation under varying conditions (MAZZIOTTA et al. 1982, 1983). They have provided important insight into anatomical and functional relationships. These investigations have been extended to tasks with hemisphere specialization and glucose metabolic asymmetry.

More recently, physiological measurements with behavioral tasks have revealed potential new insight into tissue metabolism (FOX et al. 1988). The simul-

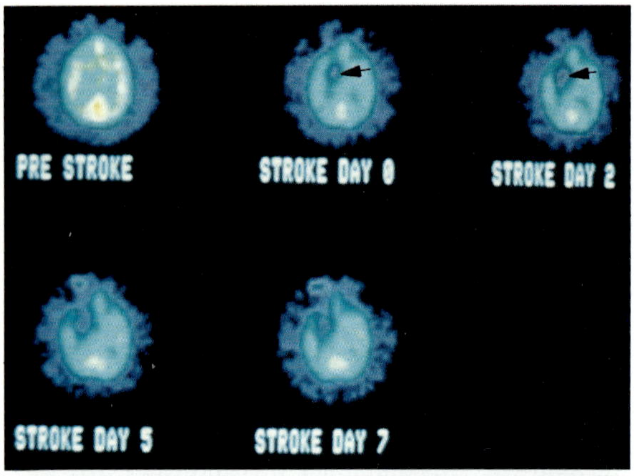

a

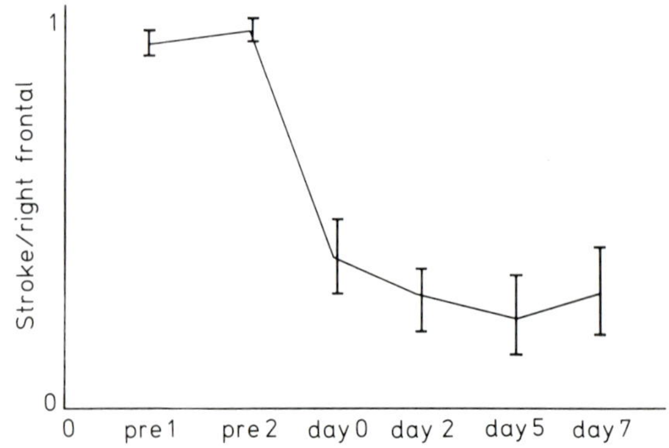

b

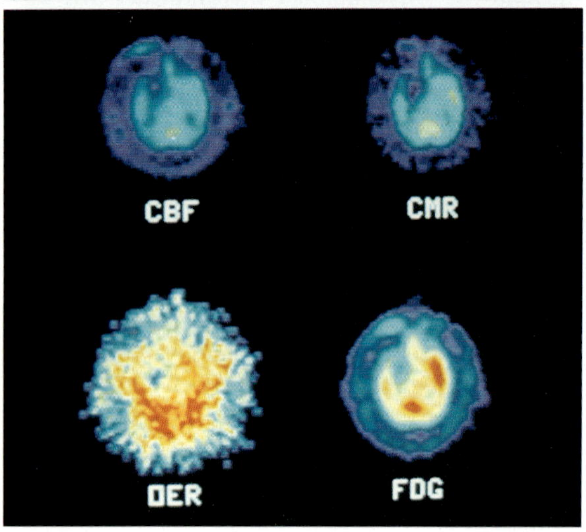

c

Fig. 5. **a** Head images from a baboon brain in baboon stroke model. The cerebral oxygen metabolism in the baboon brain is demonstrated, both prior to and during a 7-day course following permanent left middle cerebral artery ligation. Note the increase in the stroke size *(arrows)* over time. **b** Demonstration of the fall in the ratio of oxygen metabolism of the stroke area to the contralateral normal brain during the stroke. The ratios attempt to normalize for changes in sedation from day to day, assuming that sedation causes general metabolic changes rather than regional ones. **c** Four PET scan modalities taken 7 days after production of stroke. *Left* to *right, top* to *bottom:* the cerebral blood flow image *(CBF),* cerebral oxygen metabolism *(CMR),* oxygen extraction ratio *(OER),* and glucose metabolism *(FDG)* measured by the fluorodeoxyglucose method. These multiple modalities can be used to characterize the stroke and can be used in further testing of various drugs, such as cerebral protective agents. (Wong et al. 1988b)

taneous study of regional oxygen and glucose metabolism in the same individual has provided important information concerning the coupling of these measures. Uncoupling has subsequently been revealed in pathological states such as stroke and tumor (Wise et al. 1983). These studies have provided information about acute and subacute cerebral vascular disorders which may lead to potential improvements in diagnostic or therapeutic modalities. They have also allowed examination of decreased oxygen extraction, hemodynamics, and effects of ischemia and early and late infarction and oxygen metabolism, regional cerebral blood flow, and regional cerebral blood volume (Frackowiak et al. 1980). By examining the effects of acute stroke on the metabolic parameters both in the center of the stroke and the periphery ("penumbra"), the testing of therapeutic modalities on reduction of infarct size will be possible (Marchal et al. 1987). Animal models of stroke are underdeveloped for use with PET measurements of blood flow and metabolism. These models have future applications in evaluating experimental drug therapies (see Fig. 5, Wong et al. 1988b).

One of the most highly developed PET applications for clinical problems is in the area of seizure focus localization and surgical correlation. Much of the attempt is to differentiate benign from more serious seizure foci and to assist in localization for surgery. Although the observed hypometabolism in interictal states and the hypermetabolism in ictal states may not simply be interpreted as inhibition or excitation respectively (Ackerman et al. 1982), the studies may help in further assessing the pathophysiology of seizures. Perturbation studies to reveal abnormal regions also use PET metabolic measurements in combination with anticonvulsants such as thiopental (Engel et al. 1982a, b).

The issue of jeopardized myocardium is another important potential clinical application of PET metabolism studies. Schwaiger et al. (1983, 1984, 1986, 1987), Marshall (1983), and Tillisch et al. (1986), have been studying the metabolic patterns in patients with myocardial infarction and cardiac abnormalities respectively. It appears that combinations of such metabolism studies may be of potential predictive value cardiac disease.

7.7 In Vivo Human Imaging Studies of Neurotransmitter and Receptors

The investigation of the central nervous system has been greatly enhanced by the study of neurotransmitter and receptor sites at the synaptic junction. In the past, techniques such as in vitro receptor binding methods using homogenate brain tissue and autoradiography have given great insight into the location and role of the neurotransmitter/receptor systems in basic physiology, pathophysiology, and drug therapy. The ability to label and image human neurotransmitters and receptors in vivo (GARNETT et al. 1983; WAGNER et al. 1983) using PET has opened a new scientific dimension to the growing field of neuroscience (Fig. 6).

A number of normal physiological studies have been carried out by PET investigations of neurotransmitter receptor. These have included studies involving the effects of age on dopamine receptors. They demonstrated a fall for both men and women but at different rates (WONG et al. 1984). These studies suggest that hormonal effects may be in part important in these different trends. Preliminary studies of dopamine receptor binding in young normal menstruating females at two different phases of the menstrual cycle have shown a trend towards higher rates of binding in the luteal as compared to the follicular phase (WONG et al. 1988a). Studies such as these would not be possible without PET or SPECT imaging.

An important role of PET studies is the testing of drug potency and potential for therapeutic efficiency (Fig. 7). In vitro binding studies are commonly an appropriate first step in screening new drugs for receptor affinity. This screening, however, usually does not take into consideration potential metabolism, nor does it examine the in vivo affinity or nonspecific binding sites in living human brain. In vivo studies with PET allow the comparison of drug levels and dosing protocols of unlabeled new drugs; this is accomplished by using radiolabeled compounds of known specificity (such as [^{11}C]*N*-methylspiperone - [^{11}C]NMSP - for D_2 dopamine and S_2 serotonin, [^{11}C]*N*-methyl bromo LSD (WONG et al. 1987a) for serotonin S_2 sites and [^{11}C]SCH-23390 for D_1 dopamine sites) (WONG et al. 1988a) to compete with the new drugs. The de-

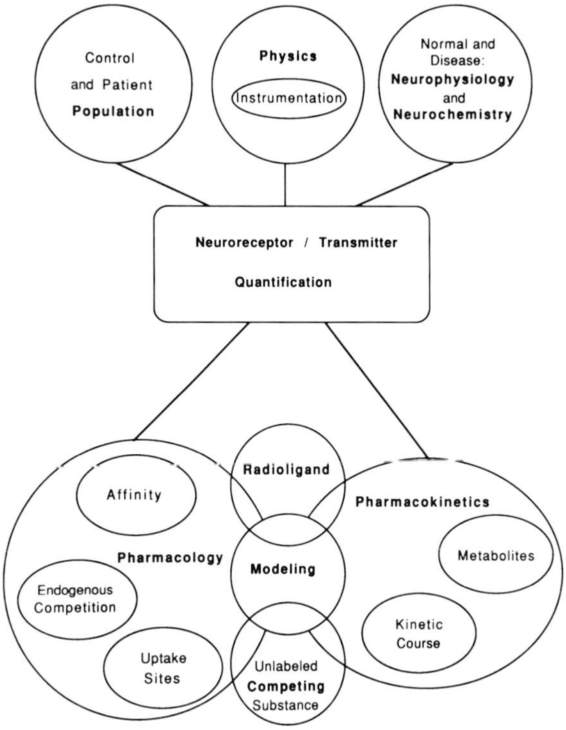

Fig. 6. Illustration of the complexity of neuroreceptor quantification indicating the interrelationship between various aspects of modeling, pharmacology, patient population, neurobiology, physics, and instrumentation

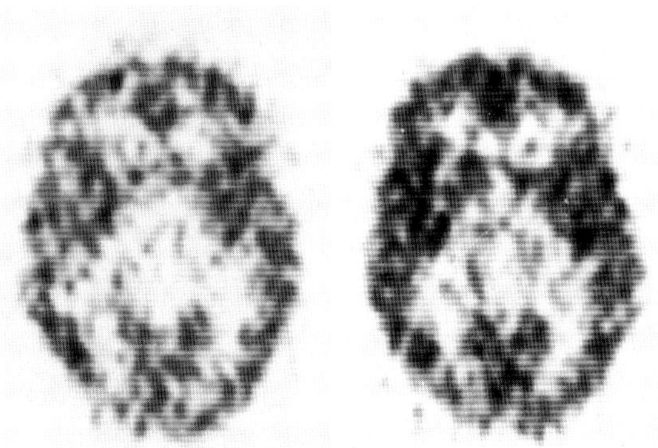

a **b**

Fig. 7 a, b. Two [^{11}C]*N*-methylspiperone ([^{11}C]NMSP) scans done on the same individual after 7.5 mg haloperidol (**a**) and 37.5 mg oral molindone (**b**). These doses are approximately 5:1 in clinical efficaciousness ratio. They demonstrated essentially identical blockade 45 min after the injection of the radioisotope [^{11}C]NMSP. This demonstrates that there is in vivo blockade which is equivalent to the clinically equivalent oral doses of these two neuroleptics. This is an example of how PET scanning can be used to compare receptor occupancy in new drugs. (WONG et al. 1985a) gree of receptor occupancy by the competing unlabeled compounds can be quantified and correlated with other clinical parameters, and with serum levels and oral doses of the unlabeled drug. This holds the promise of extending in vitro screening to another step. Presumably, in vitro binding studies would still be used as the initial screen for new drugs, because many can be efficiently examined for several chemical variations. Once a group of compounds have been identified, they can then be studied in nonhuman primates with PET imaging and a few selected for testing in human beings. With PET, receptor occupancy can then be examined in vivo. In human studies, metabolism in normal volunteers and patients can also be directly quantified regionally. This provides considerable potential for assisting in the prediction of the pharmacological action and efficacy of drugs when administered at therapeutic doses.

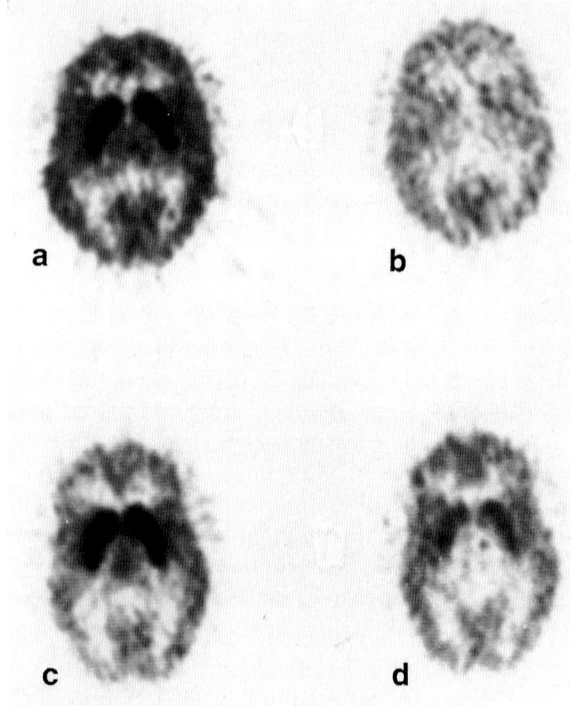

Fig. 8a–d. PET scan images of the radioactivity distribution obtained at the level of the caudate nucleus and putamen 65–95 min after injection of [^{11}C]*N*-methylspiperone ([^{11}C]NMSP) in a normal subject (**a** and **b**) and in a schizophrenic patient (**c** and **d**) in the unblocked (**a** and **c**) and the blocked state (**b** and **d**). Both subjects were males, 24 years of age, and received a single dose of 7.5 mg haloperidol before the second PET scan. This illustrates the more pronounced blockade of [^{11}C]NMSP uptake in the caudate and putamen in the normal subject as compared to the patient, despite the fact that serum haloperidol was lower in the normal (2.5 ng/ml) than in the patient (4 ng/ml). B_{max} values in the normal and the schizophrenic subjects were 11.5 and 35.2 pmol/g, respectively. (Wong et al. 1986c)

7.8 Patient Studies

A large number of studies have been carried out to date in numerous centers throughout the world involving a number of neurological and psychiatric disorders. These have included schizophrenia, manic depressive illness, Tourette's syndrome, Parkinson's disease, seizure disorders, Rett's syndrome, and Lesch-Nyhan syndrome.

An important use of in vivo PET studies is the ability to study drug naive subjects. In these circumstances the certainty of a drug naive state can be ensured by patient and family interviews, as well as drug screening for verification. Recently, a number of studies of diseases have been carried out in drug naive subjects. These have included schizophrenia (Figs. 8, 9) and manic depressive illness (Wong et al. 1986c, 1987b). Initial studies have suggested that drug naive schizophrenics demonstrate some elevations in D_2 dopamine receptors in the caudate nucleus, as do some drug free but previously treated schizophrenics. A subsequent study involving both drug naive and drug treated manic depressive illness has indicated increases in D_2 receptors in some subgroups of patients. In these preliminary studies, increases have been most often associated with patients who have definite psychotic features associated with their illness, regardless of their drug naive or drug treated state. Similar studies are also being carried out with Tourette's syndrome (Wong et al. 1988c).

A number of other investigators have also examined the correlation between receptor occupancy and clinical state. For example Farde et al. (1986) suggested that at least a 90% blockade of receptors was required for effective neuroleptic therapy. Wolf et al. (1987) have examined the haloperidol washout characteristics in plasma and correlated them with the degree of receptor occupancy. These studies and studies in both drug resistant and drug responsive patients, as well as correlations with neuropsychological parameters, will provide important complementary information about these neuropsychiatric disorders.

Studies of Parkinson's disease have examined both the presynaptic dopamine-containing nerve terminal with [^{18}F]fluorodopa and the postsynaptic D_2 dopamine receptor using [^{11}C]NMSP. These

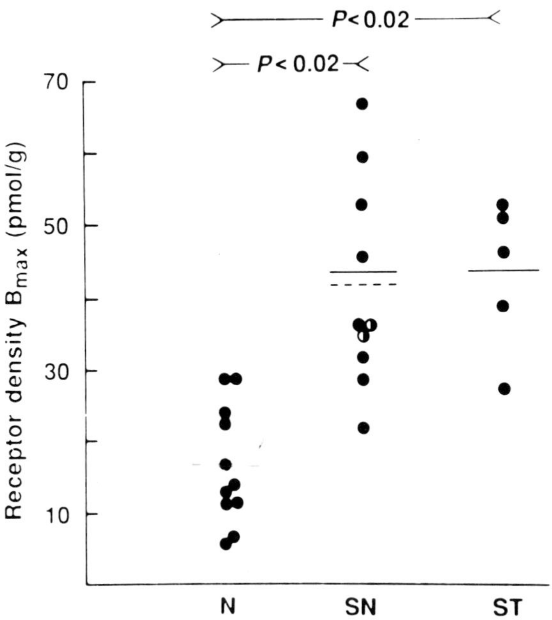

Fig. 9. D_2 dopamine receptor density *(B_{max})* in the caudate nucleus in normal volunteers *(N)* and drug naive *(SN)* and drug treated *(ST)* schizophrenics. The *solid horizontal lines* are the mean values in each group. For the drug naive group this line is the value for the eight subjects who had only a single 7.5 mg dose of haloperidol before their second PET scan [43.3 ± 5.7 pmol/g (SEM)]. The *dotted line* below it is the mean of all ten subjects, including the two who received more than a single dose of haloperidol before their second PET scan (WONG et al. 1986b). The average receptor density of this group was 41.7 ± 4.6 pmol/g. Mean receptor densities for the normal volunteers and the drug treated group were 16.6 ± 2.5 and 43.3 ± 4.7 pmol/g, respectively. There was a significant difference between either the eight or ten drug naive or drug treated schizophrenics and the normal subjects (*t*-test with Bonferroni correction for multiple inference). (WONG et al. 1986c)

studies have also been extended to patients who have been exposed to drugs which give parkinsonism symptoms (LEENDERS et al. 1986).

Positron emission tomography studies of Huntington's chorea with ^{18}FDG have shown definite decreases in affected patients (KUHL et al. 1982a). Some studies also show an intermediate metabolic decrement in at risk subjects relative to normals and affected subjects (HAYDEN et al. 1987; MAZZIOTTA et al. 1987), although one study has not (YOUNG et al. 1987). Furthermore, preliminary studies of D_2 dopamine receptors with [^{11}C]NMSP in Huntington's chorea in affected subjects have suggested a relationship with the duration of illness and have demonstrated considerable decreases in the total number of D_2 dopamine receptors although the local concentrations may in fact not be decreased but actually elevated (WONG et al. 1985b). These patients need to be studied further with appropriate and more sophisticated measures of recovery coefficient corrections.

A closing issue relevant to the status of in vivo neuroreceptor imaging concerns its relationship to behavioral measures. Although only preliminary data exist, some states such as the presence or absence of psychosis have been correlated with higher and lower B_{max} values of D_2 dopamine receptors (WONG et al. 1987b). These measures, together with the ones that were found in schizophrenia, provide encouraging results, which hopefully demonstrate some of the potential of such neuroreceptor binding studies with PET/SPECT imaging. Such dramatic correlations with PET studies have already been shown recently for oxygen metabolism and blood flow as they relate to cognitive functions in the brain (POSNER et al. 1988).

7.9 The Future of PET

7.9.1 Introduction

There are many specific areas where new ligands and new specialized applications will likely ensue within the next 5 years. Although PET scanning is at a very early stage of development, there are several areas of current interest of clinical significance. The future of PET is likely to include:

1. More emphasis on imaging ligands that involve aspects of the nervous system that are both pre- and postsynaptic. The *former* consists of the study of reuptake binding and autoreceptors. These will be important in the study of inhibitory mechanisms and neuronal viability. Such ligands will be important in the identification and detection of the early onset of neuronal degeneration such as in Parkinson's disease. The *latter* will involve a considerable effort to study the next level in the chain of activity in the neuronal pathways – the second messenger system that is initiated by the binding of the neurotransmitter of ligand to the postsynaptic receptor. This will allow the further study of the effects that second messenger systems have on hormonal and other regulatory systems.
2. Cardiac receptor and other neurotransmitter work that will further the relationship between electrophysiology, metabolism, and ischemia.
3. Oncology. A combination of ligands to study various aspects of cell proliferation, including DNA synthesis as well as protein synthesis and more tra-

ditional parameters such as glucose metabolism, will be the subject of future research. The use of various amino acid transport inhibitors such as unlabeled phenylphenalanine will be useful for examining the possibilities of distinguishing radiation necrosis from active tumor. These combinations together with NMR spectroscopy will be helpful in a multiparameter approach to evaluating cancer diagnosis and therapeutic response.

4. Pulmonary studies. Although these studies with PET are only beginning, there is the potential for studying functional aspects of the pulmonary system with PET. Studies with ^{68}Ga microspheres for tomography have been done in the past but now studies with receptors in the lung and investigations of other physiological parameters are possible using the tomographic approach, although some technical problems exist (BRUDIN et al. 1987; NOLOP et al. 1987; MINTUN et al. 1986, 1987; KUMMER, 1987; SCHUSTER and MINTUN, 1987; HUGHES et al. 1987; SCHUSTER et al. 1986).

What about the long-term role of PET and its utilization throughout a well-developed health care system? The first area will continue to be a research application; the characterization of the biochemistry of various diseases, old, such as Alzheimer's disease, or new, such as AIDS related dementia, will continue. The study of various pharmacological and behavioral perturbations and the subsequent response in various disorders will remain an important use of PET/SPECT. PET will likely maintain a prominent position in the research armamentarium as long as pharmacology is an important therapeutic tool since labeled tracers are probably the most sensitive in vivo method for measuring drug action. SPECT will also have an important role in research by providing more logical and convenient tracers such as ^{99}Tc/isotopes which can be labeled to important ligands for flow and function studies involving metabolism and neurotransmitter systems. SPECT will be most useful where large populations of patients might be studied to relate to various clinical parameters. Since SPECT agents traditionally are easier to prepare and have the potential versatility of use "around the clock" without specialized personnel, it is likely that certain research paradigms for large populations (for example screening for a certain disease such as Alzheimer's) will gradually be studied by SPECT over time. This will be true in those situations where time convenience is a factor and where the ultimate relatively lower spatial resolution and quantification of SPECT versus PET are less important as compared to studying large populations. This will allow research to be carried out at multiple centers quite distant from cyclotrons such as in rural areas. Multicenter research, such as in the central nervous system, could be carried out with the appropriate isotopes at a very sophisticated level once the SPECT quantification models have been worked out. In contrast PET studies will then focus more on specific diseases and improving quantification to a high precision and accuracy where subtle differences or absolute quantification is more desirable. As PET scanners grow in their technical sophistication and reach the resolution limits of a few millimeters and as models become more sophisticated and developed, there will be a concomitant great expansion of the use of PET by both basic and clinical scientists.

In the research area, we are currently in a phase of "taste testing" where some investigators are fully committed, others are partly committed, and still others are somewhat unfortunately disillusioned by the controversies that surround any new technology. Because the tracer principle is so fundamental and because the basic physics and mathematics of the tracer methodology are deeply rooted in the fundamental scientific principles, PET and SPECT have a very firm foundation as research tools. Over the next 10–20 years, we will see a tremendous improvement in machines and methods and most importantly, personnel committed to the improvements of techniques. As this is achieved, PET will become a research tool perhaps not unlike other moderately sophisticated tools, such as electron microscopes.

7.9.2 Clinical Future

The future of PET in clinical studies will depend on several factors. First upon the success of research in PET and SPECT to develop methods that are clinically relevant. Although this process has already begun in many areas, wide-spread and clinical application of PET will depend heavily on these research developments. A second key factor is the availability of these techniques to the general population. Given current growth patterns, it is likely that PET and SPECT will grow in major metropolitan areas. By the year 2000 it is likely that most major cities in the United States will be within a reasonable distance from a major PET facility. Furthermore, the development of SPECT instrumentation and the simultaneous strong interest in new commercially available SPECT agents, especially for the brain (^{123}I and ^{99m}Tc), assure the continued growth of SPECT. Thus, major medical centers such as those associated with universities and even large community medical centers will have PET facilities and probably most nuclear medicine departments of moderate size or larger will have at least one SPECT camera. The continuing interest in small radioisotope/radiochemical production facilities such as radiochemical delivery systems and improvements in camera design and efficient use of crystal and concomitant electronics will allow economic growth of PET for intermediate sized medical centers, such as community hospitals and small university settings. If commercial development of these "package PET centers" is successful in producing more routine synthesis such as that of ^{18}FDG, then some degree of PET imaging will be practical. This, together with the development of generator produced radioisotopes such as existing rubidium and gallium and perhaps future ones such as copper isotopes, will extend the radiopharmaceutical capabilities of these small PET centers.

Thus, assuming successful research demonstration of the clinical utility of PET and SPECT and with widespread availability of the instrumentation, what are the likely areas of research?

7.9.2.1 Early Detection of Disease

Certainly some of the goals for future tomographic applications include the early detection of a disease process. As is true of many areas of diagnostic medicine, there is great hope for techniques to detect disease processes at an early stage. Although it is unclear to what degree certain tomographic procedures may be specific for certain diseases, certainly functional abnormalities might be detected at an early stage. For example, subtle early changes in regional blood flow of glucose or oxygen metabolism might be demonstrated in diseases such as AIDS related dementia, cocaine abuse, and Alzheimer's disease. Currently, large studies are ongoing in multiple centers which correlate early Huntington's disease with decrease glucose metabolism. Recent studies involving receptor abnormalities from schizophrenia and mania give rise to speculation that early changes in neurotransmitter function might herald disease onset (WONG et al. 1986c, 1987b).

7.9.2.2 Mapping of Disease Progression

Functional changes in disease states have already been demonstrated, such as in the relationship between glucose metabolism and the grade of the tumor (DICHIRO et al. 1982).

7.9.2.3 Monitoring Therapy

One of the most likely applications for functional PET and SPECT imaging is in monitoring therapeutic regimes, including drug and other therapies. For example, the issue of radiation necrosis versus recurrent tumor following brain tumor radiotherapy is an important area for the application of various PET functional ligands such as [^{11}C]methionine (LAFRANCE et al. 1987; BERGSTROM et al. 1983, 1985). Another area is the use of receptor occupancy studies using PET receptor binding radioligands. A classic example is that of monitoring D_2 receptor blockade as it relates to clinical course. For example, patients who are totally blocked on a given neuroleptic but have persistent symptoms might be changed to another drug where the receptor occupancy is lower. Correlation of this receptor blockade, which is measured in vivo in brain, with serum neuroleptic levels and clinical course will provide better insight into all these modalities in following the course of patients. Recently, the development of simple dual detection probes (BICE et al. 1987) has allowed the possibility for measurement of this receptor occupancy in sites several miles away from a cyclotron. These probes require much lower doses of injected radioactivity for the mapping of a time-activity curve as well as for transport. Hence, a clinical PET center could develop isotopes such as ^{11}C or ^{18}F ligands and transport them by car to a peripheral site where probe devices could be used to measure potentially clinically important variables such as receptor occupancy. This method, not unlike other procedures, may be useful in tracking therapy or disease course.

7.10 Summary

The exciting events with PET and SPECT studies are just at the beginning of a tremendous expansion in basic science and clinical applications for the study of human physiological processes. There is no technique currently available that has the sensitivity or potential specificity of chemical mechanism in vivo in various organs as the brain, heart, lung, and elsewhere in the body. The next few years will undoubtedly yield rapid advances in new ligand development, providing an understanding of both physiological and pathophysiological processes that could never be studied by any other method. Studies of second messenger systems in the brain (WORLEY et al. 1987) probably will be the next frontier in brain imaging. The use of biological markers in concert with the new genetic markers of neuropsychiatric illness provides a spectacular potential for improving our understanding of the etiology, possible diagnosis, and optimal treatment of these diseases. The demonstration of changes in diseases such as cancer and the examination of function in common diseases, such as cardiopulmonary diseases, are also likely future areas of PET studies. This, together with great improvements in anatomical imaging and the coordination and correlation of these features with PET scanning, promises to be one of the most exciting areas in radiological imaging developments.

References

Ackermann RF, Finch DM, Babb TL et al. (1982) Increased glucose metabolism during long-duration recurrent inhibition of hippocampal pyramidal cells. J Neuroscience 4: 251-264

Alpert NM, Ackerman RH, Correia JA et al. (1977) Measurement of rCBF and $rCMRO_2$ by continuous inhalation of ^{15}O-labeled CO_2 and O_2. Acta Neurol Scand 56 (Suppl 72): 186-187

Beller GA, Cochavi S, Smith TW et al. (1982) Positron emission tomographic imaging of the myocardium with ^{81}Rb. J Comput Assist Tomogr 6: 341-349

Bergstrom M, Collins VP, Ehrin E et al. (1983) Discrepancies in brain tumor extent as shown by computer tomography and positron emission tomography using [^{68}Ga] EDTA, [^{11}C] glucose and [^{11}] methionine. J Comput Assist Tomogr 7: 1062-1066

Bergstrom M, Mosskin M, Ericson K et al. (1985) Accumulation kinetics of ^{11}D-D-glucose, (methyl-^{11}C)-L-methionine and ^{68}Ga-EDTA in brain tumors measured with positron emission tomography. In: Lilja A (ed) Radiological aspects of the diagnosis of supratentorial gliomas. Uppsala University, pp 2-17

Bice AN, Wong DF, Wagner HN Jr (1987) On estimating the loss of quantification in PET due to finite detector resolution. Eur J Nucl Med 13: 1-6

Brudin LH, Rhodes CG, Valind SO et al. (1987) Regional lung density and blood volume in nonsmoking and smoking subjects measured by PET. J Appl Physiol 63: 1324-1334

Budinger TF, Derenzo SE, Huesman RH et al. (1981) Quantitative myocardial flow extraction data using gated ECT (abstract). J Nucl Med 21: P16

Celesia G, Polcyn R, Holden J et al. (1983) 18-F-fluoromethane positron emission tomography determination of regional cerebral blood flow in cerebral infarction. J Cereb Blood Flow Metab 3 (Suppl 1): 523-524

Chugani HT, Phelps ME (1986) Maturational changes in cerebral function in infants determined by ^{18}FDG positron emission tomography. Science 231: 840-843

Chugani HT, Phelps ME, Mazziotta JC (1987) Positron emission tomography study of human brain functional development. Ann Neurol 4: 487-497

Collins RC (1978a) Kindling of neuroanatomic pathways during recurrent focal penicillin seizures. Brain Res 150: 503-518

Collins RC (1978b) Use of cortical circuits during focal penicillin seizures: An autoradiographic study with ^{14}C-deoxyglucose. Brain Res 150: 487-502

Dichiro G, DeLaPaz RL, Brooks RA et al. (1982) Glucose utilization of cerebral gliomas measured by [^{18}F]fluorodeoxyglucose and positron emission tomography. Neurology 32: 1323-1329

Engel J Jr, Kuhl DE, Phelps ME (1982a) Patterns of human local cerebral glucose metabolism during epileptic seizures. Science 218: 64-66

Engel J Jr, Kuhl DE, Phelps ME et al. (1982b) Interictal cerebral glucose metabolism in partial epilepsy and its relation to EEG changes. Ann Neurol 33: 400-413

Evans AC, Beil C, Marrett S et al. (1988) Anatomical-functional correlation using an adjustable MRI-based region of interest atlas with positron emission tomography. J Cereb Blood Flow Metab 8: 255

Farde L, Hall H, Ehrin E et al. (1986) Quantitative analysis of dopamine D_2 dopamine receptor binding in the living brain by PET. Science 231: 258-261

Fox PT, Perlmutter JS, Raichle ME (1985) A stereotactic method of anatomical localization for positron emission tomography. J Comput Assist Tomogr 9: 141-153

Fox PT, Mintun MA, Raichle ME et al. (1986) Mapping human visual cortex with positron emission tomography. Nature 323: 806-809

Fox PT, Raichle ME, Mintun MA et al. (1988) Nonoxidative glucose consumption during focal physiologic neural activity. Science 241: 462-464

Frackowiak RS, Lenzi G, Jones T et al. (1980) Quantitative measurement of regional cerebral blood flow and oxygen metabolism in man using ^{15}O and positron emission tomography: Theory, procedure, and normal values. J Comput Assist Tomogr 4: 727-736

Garnett ES, Firnau G, Nahmias C (1983) Dopamine visualized in the basal ganglia of living man. Nature 305: 137-138

Hawkins RA, Phelps ME, Huang SC et al. (1981) Effect of ischemia on quantification of local cerebral glucose metabolic rate in man. J Cereb Blood Flow Metab 1: 37-51

Hawkins RA, Phelps ME, Huang SC (1986) Effects of temporal sampling, glucose metabolic rates, and disruptions of the blood-brain barrier on the FDG model with and without a vascular compartment: Studies in human brain tumors with PET. J Cereb Blood Flow Metab 6: 170-183

Hayden MR, Hewitt J, Stossl AJ et al. (1987) The combined use of positron emission tomography and DNA polymorphysms for preclinical detection of Huntington's disease. Neurology 37: 1441

Hnatowich DJ (1976) Labeling of human albumin microspheres with Ga-68. J Nucl Med 17: 57-60

Hoyer S (1982) Normal and abnormal circulation and oxidative metabolism in the aging human brain. J Cereb Blood Flow Metab 2 (Suppl 1): 510-513

Huang SC, Phelps ME, Hoffman EJ et al. (1980) Noninvasive determination of local cerebral metabolic rate of glucose in man. Am J Physiol 238: E69-E82

Huang SC, Phelps ME, Hoffman EJ et al. (1981) Error sensitivity of fluorodeoxyglucose method for measurement of cerebral metabolic rate of glucose. J Cereb Blood Flow Metab 1: 391-401

Hughes JM, Brudin LH, Valind SO et al. (1987) Positron emission tomography in the lung. J Thorac Imaging 1: 79-88

Ito M, Lammertsma AA, Wise RJ et al. (1982) Measurement of regional cerebral blood flow and oxygen utilization in patients with cerebral tumors using ^{15}O and positron emission tomography: Analytical techniques and preliminary results. Neuroradiology 23: 63-74

Kuhl DE, Phelps ME, Kowell AP et al. (1980) Mapping local metabolism and perfusion in normal and ischemic brain by emission computed tomography of ^{18}FDG and $^{13}NH_3$. Ann Neurol 8: 47-60

Kuhl DE, Metter EJ, Riege WH et al. (1982a) Effects of human aging on patterns of local cerebral glucose utilization determined by the [^{18}F] fluorodeoxyglucose method. J Cereb Blood Flow Metab 2: 163-171

Kuhl DE, Phelps ME, Markham M et al. (1982b) Cerebral metabolism and atrophy in Huntington's disease determined by ^{18}FDG and computed tomographic scan. Ann Neurol 12: 425

Kummer F (1987) Nuclear medicine in diseases of the lung - present status and future. Introduction - clinical aspects. Eur J Nucl Med 13 (Suppl): 2-5

LaFrance ND, Tuama L, Villemagne V et al. (1987) Quantitative imaging and follow-up experience of C-11-L-methionine accumulation in brain tumors with positron emission tomography. J Nucl Med 28: 645

Leenders KL, Poewe WH, Palmer AJ et al. (1986) Inhibition of L-[^{18}F] fluorodopa uptake into human brain by amino acids demonstrated by positron emission tomography. Ann Neurol 20: 258

Lenzi GL, Frackowiak RS, Jones T et al. (1981) $CMRO_2$ and CBF by the oxygen-15 inhalation techniques: Results in normal volunteers and cerebrovascular patients. Eur Neurol 20: 285-290

Lenzi GL, Frackowiak RS, Jones T (1982) Cerebral oxygen metabolism and blood flow in human cerebral ischemic infarction. J Cereb Blood Flow Metab 2: 321:335

Lever SZ, Burns HD, Kervitsky TM et al. (1985) Design, preparation, and biodistribution of a technetium-99-m triaminedithiol complex to assess regional cerebral blood flow. J Nucl Med 26: 1287-1294

Marchal G, Evans A, Dagher A et al. (1987) The evolution of cerebral infarction with time: A PET study of the ischemic penumbra. J Cereb Blood Flow Metab 7 (Suppl): 599

Marshall RC, Tillisch JH, Phelps ME et al. (1983) Identification and differentiation of resting myocardial ischemia and infarction in man with positron computed tomography, ^{18}F-labeled fluorodeoxyglucose and N-13 ammonia. Circulation 67: 766-778

Mazziotta JC, Phelps ME, Carson PE et al. (1982) Tomographic mapping of human cerebral metabolism: auditory stimulation. Neurology 32: 921-937

Mazziotta JC, Phelps ME, Halgren E (1983) Local cerebral glucose metabolic response to audiovisual stimulation and deprivation: Studies in human subjects with positron CT. Human Neurobiol 2: 11-23

Mazziotta JC, Phelps ME, Pahl JJ et al. (1987) Reduced cerebral glucose metabolism in asymptomatic subjects at risk for Huntington's disease. N Engl J Med 316: 357

Mintun MA, Ter-Pogossian MM, Green MA et al. (1986) Quantitative measurement of regional pulmonary blood flow with positron emission tomography. J Appl Physiol 60: 317-326

Mintun MA, Dennis DR, Welch MJ et al. (1987) Measurements of pulmonary vascular permeability with PET and gallium-68 transferrin. J Nucl Med 28: 1704-1716

Nolop KB, Rhodes CG, Brudin LH et al. (1987) Glucose utilization in vivo by human pulmonary neoplasms. Cancer 60: 2682-2689

Posner MI, Petersen SE, Fox PT et al. (1988) Localization of cognitive operations in the human brain. Science 240: 1627-1631

Schelbert HR, Phelps ME, Hoffman EJ et al. (1979) Regional myocardial perfusion assessed with N-13 labeled ammonia and positron emission computerized axial tomography. Am J Cardiol 43: 209-218

Schelbert HR, Henze E, Phelps ME (1980) Emission tomography of the heart. Semin Nucl Med 10: 355

Schuster DP, Marklin GF (1986) Effect of changes in inflation and blood volume on regional lung density - a PET study: 2. J Comput Assist Tomogr 10: 730-735

Schuster DP, Mintun MA (1987) Pulmonary circulation, extravascular water, and solute flux as determined by positron emission tomography. Lymphology 20: 25-35

Schuster DP, Marklin GF, Mintun MA et al. (1986) PET measurement of regional lung density: 1. J Comput Assist Tomogr 10: 723-729

Schwaiger M, Huang SC, Krivokapich J et al. (1983) Myocardial glucose utilization measured noninvasively in man by positron tomography (abstract). J Am Coll Cardiol I: 688

Schwaiger M, Brunken RC, Grover M et al. (1984) Regional metabolism in patients with acute myocardial infarction determined by positron tomography (PET) (abstract). Circulation 70 (Suppl II): 249

Schwaiger M, Brunken R, Grover-McKay M et al. (1986) Regional myocardial metabolism in patients with acute myocardial infarction assessed by positron emission tomography. J Am Coll Cardiol 8: 800-808

Schwaiger M, Brunken RC, Krivokapich J et al. (1987) Beneficial effect of residual anterograde flow on tissue viability as assessed by positron emission tomography in patients with myocardial infarction. Eur Heart J 8: 981-988

Tillisch J, Brunken R, Marshall R et al. (1986) Reversibility of cardiac wall-motion abnormalities predicted by positron tomography. N Engl J Med 314: 884-888

Wagner HN, Burns HD, Dannals RF et al. (1983) Imaging dopamine receptors in the human brain by positron tomography. Science 22: 1264-1266

Wilson RA, Shea MJ, De Landsheere CH et al. (1984) Validation of quantitation of regional myocardial blood flow in vivo with ^{11}C-labeled human albumin microspheres and positron emission tomography. Circulation 70: 717-723

Wise R, Rhodes C, Gibbs J et al. (1983) The relationship between oxygen metabolism and glucose utilization in early cerebral infarcts. J Cereb Blood Flow Metab 3 (Suppl 1): S580-S581

Wolf AP, Shiue CY, Fowler JS et al. (1987) The relationship between dopamine D-2 receptor occupancy by antipsychotic drugs and plasma drug levels as determined by ^{18}F-N-methyl-spiroperidol (^{18}F-NMS) and positron emission tomography (PET). J Cereb Blood Flow Metab 7: S361

Wong DF, Wagner HN Jr, Dannals RF et al. (1984) Effects of age on dopamine and serotonin receptors measured by positron tomography in the living human brain. Science 226: 1393

Wong DF, Wagner HN Jr, Coyle J et al. (1985a) Assessment of dopamine receptor blockade by neuroleptic drugs in the living human brain. J Nucl Med 26: 52

Wong DF, Links J, Wagner HN Jr et al. (1985b) Dopamine and serotonin receptors measured in vivo in Huntington's disease with C-11 N-methylspiperone PET imaging (abstract). J Nucl Med 26: P107

Wong DF, Gjedde A, Wagner HN Jr (1986a) Quantification of neuroreceptors in the living human brain. I. Irreversible binding of ligands. J Cereb Blood Flow Metab 6: 137-146

Wong DF, Gjedde A, Wagner HN Jr et al. (1986b) Quantification of neuroreceptors in the living human brain. II. Inhibition studies of receptor density and affinity. J Cereb Blood Flow Metab 6: 147–153

Wong DF, Wagner HN Jr, Tune LE et al. (1986c) Positron emission tomography reveals elevated D_2 dopamine receptors in drug-naive schizophrenics. Science 234: 1558–1563

Wong DF, Lever JR, Hartig PR et al. (1987a) Localization of serotonin 5-HT_2 receptors in living human brain by positron emission tomography using N1-([^{11}C]-Me)-2-Br-LSD. Synapse 1: 393–398

Wong DF, Pearlson G, Tune LE et al. (1987b) In vivo measurement of D2 dopamine receptor abnormalities in drug naive and treated manic-depressive patients. J Nucl Med 28: 611

Wong DF, Broussolle EP, Wand G et al. (1988a) In vivo measurement of dopamine receptors in human brain by positron emission tomography: age and sex differences. In: Joseph JA (ed) Central determinants of age-related declines in motor function. Ann NY Acad Sci, New York, 203–214

Wong DF, Solomon H, Natarajan TK et al. (1988b) Cerebral blood flow, oxygen and glucose metabolism in jeopardized cerebrum after experimental stroke. J Nucl Med 29: 852–853

Wong DF, Singer H, Pearlson G et al. (1988c) D2 dopamine receptors in Tourette's syndrome and manic depressive illness. J Nucl Med 29: 820

Worley PF, Baraban JM, Snyder SH (1987) Beyond receptors: Multiple second-messenger systems in brain. Ann Neurol 21: 217–229

Yamamoto YL, Thompson CJ, Meyer E et al. (1977) Dynamic positron emission tomography for study of cerebral hemodynamics in a cross section of the head using positron-emitting ^{68}Ga-EDTA and ^{77}Kr. J Comput Assist Tomogr 1: 43–55

Yen CK, Yano Y, Budinger TF et al. (1982) Brain tumor evaluation using Rb-82 and positron emission tomography. J Nucl Med 23: 532–537

Young AB, Penney JB, Starosta-Rubinstein S et al. (1987) Normal caudate glucose metabolism in persons at risk for Huntington's disease. Arch Neurol 44: 254

8 Interventional Radiology

JAMES H. ANDERSON

CONTENTS

8.1 Introduction 131
8.2 Intraarterial Chemotherapy 132
8.2.1 Clinical Acceptance 132
8.2.2 Pharmacokinetics 133
8.2.3 Drug Streaming 134
8.3 Valvuloplasty and Balloon Catheter Applications in Treating Congenital Cardiopulmonary Disease. 135
8.4 Intravascular Use of Lasers 138
8.5 Biliary Applications 141
8.6 Thrombolysis 143
8.7 Intravascular Stents 144
8.7.1 Introduction 144
8.7.2 Palmaz Stent 145
8.7.3 Gianturco Zig-zag Stent 145
8.7.4 Wallstent 146
8.7.5 Thermal Memory Alloy Stents 146
8.8 Atherectomy Catheters 147
8.9 Evaluating Interventional Procedure Efficacy Using Functional Parameters 150
References 150

8.1 Introduction

Interventional radiology has rapidly emerged to represent one of the most dynamic specialties in radiology and one which plays a significant role in attracting young physicians into radiology residency and fellowship programs. Many of the procedures used routinely today were considered highly experimental just a few years ago. The future of interventional radiology is no longer in question and there is no doubt that it will contribute significantly to the future growth of academic radiology. Special fellowships in interventional radiology are available, a journal devoted to laboratory and clinical interventional studies has been published, and both a European and an American society have been formed to support this rapidly growing and stimulating specialty.

JAMES H. ANDERSON, Ph. D., Dept. of Radiology and Radiological Science, The Johns Hopkins University, School of Medicine, 600 North Wolfe Street, Baltimore, MD 21205, USA

As the applications of interventional radiology reach beyond the visceral and peripheral vascular beds and into the heart and nonvascular areas, new opportunities for investigation and patient care application will become apparent. The future of interventional radiology is bright, and is limited only by the imagination of the clinicians and researchers.

The applications of interventional radiology have grown considerably during the past 10 years and it is impossible to do justice to all areas within the confines of a single book chapter. The procedures presented in this chapter have been chosen because the author feels that they represent emerging areas that are of current interest. These areas should also receive intense clinical and research attention in the near future. This is not meant to imply that other areas of interventional radiology that are not discussed in this chapter will not experience growth and development. However, some of these procedures are more well established and their research and developmental future will largely involve refinement.

As with other areas of medical imaging, recent technological advancements in both the physical and biological sciences will find applications in interventional radiology. The success of these new applications will depend on a combined multidisciplinary effort that emphasizes both controlled clinical and basic research. Although most new interventional procedures originate as ideas generated from clinical problems and observations, the new techniques are perfected and refined to an accepted clinical procedure through practical laboratory and clinical research and development. This has been the history of the development of well accepted techniques such as transluminal angioplasty and embolotherapy. A similar approach must be taken in developing and applying new techniques as well as in reevaluating those procedures that have not received such widespread clinical acceptance.

8.2 Intraarterial Chemotherapy

8.2.1 Clinical Acceptance

Intraarterial chemotherapy has both cancer and noncancer applications. Noncancer applications include local infusions of: (1) vasoconstricting and vasodilating agents to decrease or increase local blood flow for both diagnostic and therapeutic purposes and (2) thrombolytic agents to stimulate or increase the rate of thrombolysis in occluded vessels or grafts. Cancer applications include intraarterial administration of radioactive "seeds" or antineoplastic drugs either in solutions or emulsions, as well as those physically or chemically bound to inert or dissolvable particulate embolic materials.

Intraarterial cancer chemotherapy represents one of the most potentially important, but yet least understood and controversial, areas of interventional radiology. Conceptually, the ability to administer a drug superselectively into the vascular bed of a tumor is very appealing. Superselective arterial administration should provide high levels of drug to the tumor and ideally very low levels to the systemic circulation. The latter is particularly important since systemic toxicity is often the dose limiting factor in chemotherapy. Clinical studies have focused on therapeutic response as measured by tumor regression or prolongation of life span. Tumors involving the liver, brain, bone, pelvis, and extremities have received the greatest attention. The liver has been particularly appealing since liver tumors receive their blood supply almost exclusively from the hepatic artery whereas the normal liver tissue receives both hepatic arterial and portal venous blood (HEALY 1965). Because of the dual blood supply to the lung, ZIGIANG et al. (1986) have used a similar rationale (bronchial artery infusion) for bronchogenic carcinoma.

Unless intraarterial delivery provides a very significant advantage over more conventional forms of drug administration, the approach cannot be expected to receive widespread clinical acceptance. The time, expense, and potential complications of long-term indwelling arterial catheters, as well as the potential complications of delivering high concentrations of drugs into local vascular territories, necessitate justification based on significant improvement in clinical response. The current lack of enthusiasm that many interventional radiologists have for intraarterial cancer chemotherapy is related to equivocal results in clinical efficacy and to potential complications. Preliminary results of a randomized study comparing hepatic artery infusions with central venous infusions confirmed only a modest improvement in hepatic tumor control by the arterial treatment route (KEMENY and DALY 1986). On the other hand, using the intraarterial route in nonrandomized trials, investigators reported tumor response in as many as 88% of patients compared with the much lower response rates known from intravenous bolus drug administration (STAGG et al. 1984). This apparent variation in response is largely responsible for the confusion regarding the value of intraarterial chemotherapy for cancer.

Recent attention has been given to procedures that improve drug/blood mixing and provide more uniform delivery of drug especially to liver and brain tumors. Another major area of clinical investigation involves combining chemotherapy with embolotherapy (sometimes called chemoembolotherapy) using particulate embolic materials or chemotherapy laden microspheres, polymers, starches, etc. (OHNISHI et al. 1987; MAYHEW 1988). The goal of this approach is to provide a more sustained release of drug over time or to impede flow and increase the concentration or contact time of the drug within the tumor.

Future research in intraarterial chemotherapy for tumors should concentrate on issues other than the straight-forward approach of measuring tumor regression following the intraarterial or intravenous administration of the same drug at the same dose over the same period of time. The design of intraarterial chemotherapy protocols must consider factors other than the route of administration. Examples of these other factors include the biochemical and antitumor properties of the drugs being infused as well as the optimal dose, frequency, and duration of infusions. In addition, local physiological alterations related to intraarterial delivery must be considered relative to therapeutic efficacy and toxicity. In order to properly consider these factors, basic research studies must be designed to properly evaluate drug pharmacokinetics and to design research protocols to take maximal advantage of both the biological and pharmacokinetic parameters of the drug and method of delivery. It is only under these conditions that data can be provided that may be useful in designing clinical protocols. Very few attempts have been directed at evaluating pharmacokinetic properties that are essential in understanding the application of intraarterial chemotherapy for tumors.

8.2.2 Pharmacokinetics

Very little information is available regarding the pharmacokinetics of intraarterial vs intravenous chemotherapy. However, such information is essential if clinical chemotherapy protocols are to be designed to maximize the potential advantages of intraarterial chemotherapy. For example, BCNU is a nitrosourea chemotherapeutic agent that has physical-chemical properties (low molecular weight, favorable lipophilicity, and relatively rapid body clearance) that make it theoretically ideal for brain tumors. Although some investigators have found improved response rates following intraarterial BCNU chemotherapy (CASCINO et al. 1983; GREENBERG et al. 1984; FOO et al. 1985), interest in the intraarterial administration of the drug has waned. This decline in interest for intraarterial BCNU chemotherapy is largely related to the equivocal therapeutic results (SHAPIRO et al. 1987) and the reported ocular and neurological complications (SHINGLETON et al. 1982; GEBARSKI et al. 1984).

Although the ocular and neurological complications have been linked to drug streaming, very few data are available relating to how much BCNU actually reaches tumor following intraarterial and intravenous chemotherapy. Theoretical considerations (COLLINS 1984) predict that internal carotid artery (ICA) delivery should provide 3–5 times as much BCNU to brain tumors as would be expected following intravenous administration of the same dose. Common carotid arterial (CCA) delivery of BCNU in monkeys achieved 1.5–2.5 times higher brain nucleic acid-bound drug levels in the infused hemisphere than with intravenous infusion (LEVIN and KABRA 1975). Positron emission tomography scanning suggested that ^{11}C-BCNU can accumulate to higher concentrations in tumor areas of blood-brain barrier breakdown than in normal brain (DIKSIC et al. 1984). Quantitative autoradiography in the C-6 rat glioma brain tumor after ICA C^{14}-labeled PCNU [1-(2-chloroethyl)-3-(2,-6)dioxo-1-piperidyl)1-nitrosourea] has shown a total exposure of normal brain cortex 400% greater after intraarterial compared to intravenous delivery while that of tumor was only 115% greater in the same comparison (HIESIGER et al. 1985). Studies of hepatic artery infusions with the fluorinated pyrimidines by ENSMINGER et al. have been encouraging (ENSMINGER et al. 1978a, b; ENSMINGER and GYVES 1983a, b, 1984). Information comparing the theoretical predictions with actual tissue concentrations of these drugs in a uniform model is needed.

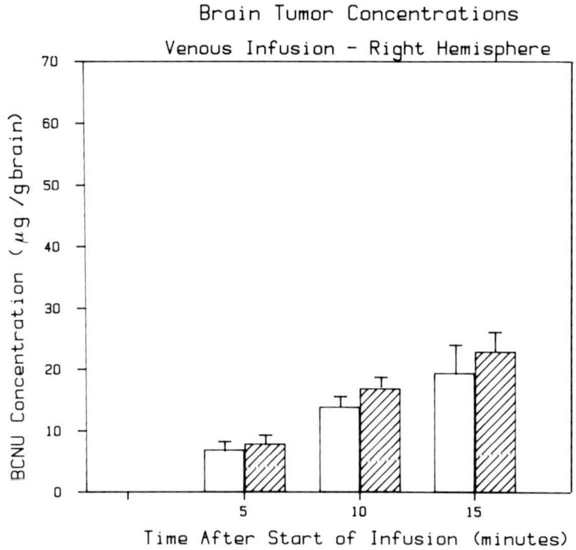

Fig. 1. BCNU levels in rabbit brain tumors following intravenous delivery of BCNU. BCNU concentrations (in µg/g tissue) are shown at 5-, 10-, and 15-min time points following initiation of 15-min infusions. BCNU levels were determined at two tumor locations – tumor center and tumor edge. Note that the concentration of BCNU in the tissues increases as a function of time during the 15-min infusion period. *Bars* indicate ±2 standard errors of the mean (SEM). *Open bars*, tumor center; *hatched bars*, tumor edge

Our recent laboratory studies have concentrated on quantitating BCNU levels following either intraarterial or intravenous delivery in rabbits bearing VX-2 brain tumors. For these studies, BCNU was administered at a dose of 300 mg/m^2 and delivered as an infusion (3.6 mg/ml) at 1.5 ml/min for 15 min into either the right common carotid artery or the right femoral vein. The animals had 10-day-old VX-2 tumors in the anterior right cerebral hemisphere. The tumors were induced using techniques developed in our laboratory (CARSON et al. 1982). Animals were sacrificed at 5, 10, and 15 min into the infusion. Within 60 s following sacrifice, the brains were removed and frozen in liquid nitrogen. Tumor tissue was assayed for BCNU using gas chromatography techniques. Figure 1 shows the concentration of BCNU in tumor tissue at 5-, 10-, and 15-min time points into the infusion when the drug was given by the intravenous route. As expected, and as predicted from theoretical considerations, BCNU concentrations in tumor increased as a function of time during the infusion, i.e., the 15-min level was higher than the 10-min level, which was in turn higher than the 5-min level. During intraarterial administration (Fig. 2), BCNU levels in tumor at 5 min into the infusion were 5–6 times higher than at 5 min following intravenous administration. This

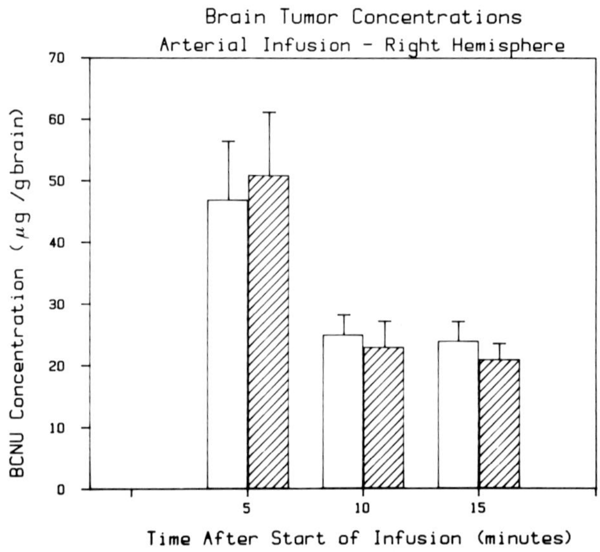

Fig. 2. BCNU levels in rabbit brain tumor following intraarterial administration of BCNU. As in Fig. 1, animals were sacrificed at 5, 10, or 15 min following initiation of a 15-min infusion. Note how BCNU levels at the 5-min time point are much higher than for the 5-min time point of intravenous treated animals (see Fig. 1). Also note that the BCNU levels decrease at 10 and 15 min instead of increasing as was seen in the intravenous group of animals. *Open bars*, tumor center; *hatched bars*, tumor edge

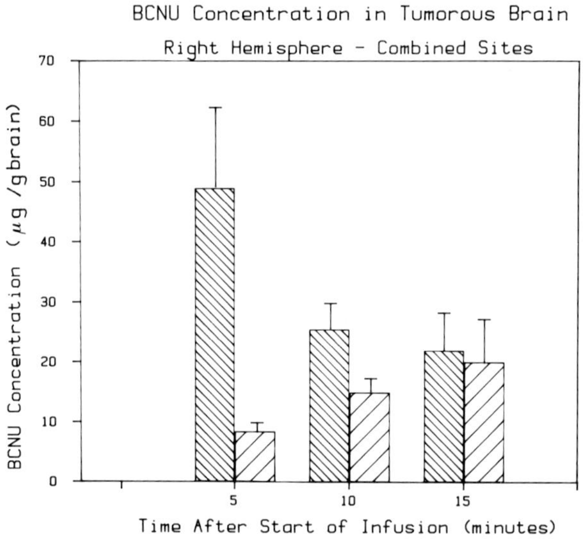

Fig. 3. The relationship between BCNU tumor levels in intravenous and in intraarterial treated animals. Data from the tumor center and tumor edge samples have been combined. The differences in tumor BCNU levels as a function of time following intraarterial and intravenous delivery of the drug are clearly evident from this figure. *Heavily hatched bars*, arterial infusion; *lightly hatched bars*, venous infusion

increase (sometimes called the Rd or arterial advantage) is close to theoretical predictions. However, at 10 and 15 min into the intraarterial infusion, tumor BCNU levels decrease instead of increasing. At the 15-min time point, tumor BCNU levels during intraarterial infusion were similar to levels obtained during intravenous administration. This comparison is clearly evident in Fig. 3, which shows tumor BCNU levels for both intraarterial and intravenous administration at 5, 10, and 15 min into the infusion. These data suggest that some process is occurring during the intraarterial infusion to decrease the advantages of intraarterial delivery. These data could help explain the equivocal clinical results of intraarterial vs intravenous BCNU chemotherapy for brain tumors.

We are currently evaluating the possible cause for this decrease in tumor tissue drug level seen during intraarterial infusion. Preliminary results suggest that the decrease may be related to local vasodilatation produced during the arterial administration of BCNU. Vasodilatation would be expected to decrease the concentration gradient of drug presented to the tumor and therefore decrease the amount entering the tumor. It is of interest to note that although vasodilatation associated with intraarterial BCNU delivery has never been previously documented, it has been suggested as a possible cause for the ocular toxicity often associated with intraarterial use of the drug (Gebarski et al. 1984).

The results of our preliminary studies with BCNU confirm the need for more research into basic pharmacokinetics of intraarterial vs intravenous chemotherapy. Such studies will provide valuable information that may be used to better design human chemotherapy infusion protocols.

8.2.3 Drug Streaming

A major problem that must be overcome in intraarterial chemotherapy is drug streaming (layering of the drug infusate in the arterial blood without adequately mixing with the blood). For intraarterial chemotherapy, most drugs are infused into arteries at rates far below the blood flow rate in the vessel. Miller et al. (1984) assessed perfusion patterns during hepatic artery infusion chemotherapy and showed that infusion rates compatible with those employed for intraarterial hepatic artery chemotherapy provided a variety of perfusion patterns in the liver. Uneven intrahepatic distribution of the infusate can account for inadequate treatment of tumors or undue toxicity to normal liver (MILLER et al. 1984; WALLACE et al. 1984). Infusion catheter position within the artery may be quite variable due to factors which may alter the geometrical relationship or position of the catheter tip within the artery. Such factors may include patient body position, bowel peristalsis, and respiratory movements.

The most prevalent example of local toxic effects of streaming has been ocular damage and blindness as well as local neurological injury following internal carotid artery administration of BCNU (SHINGLETON et al. 1982; GEBARSKI et al. 1984). Streaming can best be eliminated by providing complete drug-blood mixing immediately distal to the catheter tip (BARTH et al. 1988; WRIGHT et al. 1986; LUTZ et al. 1986). The most practical method of achieving mixing is to increase the velocity of the infusate relative to blood flow or to use infusion parameters or catheters with tip designs that induce turbulence or disruption of blood flow around the catheter tip. Increasing the velocity of the infusate relative to blood flow may lead to volume overloading problems. Several methods can be used to overcome this, including decreasing the rate of blood flow in the vessel by using partially inflated balloon infusion catheters (BARTH et al. 1988). The partially inflated balloon also facilitates turbulence at the catheter tip, which improves drug/blood mixing. Other techniques include diastolic administration of drugs using cardiac gated injector systems (ANDERSON et al. 1982) and the use of pulsed low volume, high velocity drug injection techniques. In addition, catheters have been designed with flexible tips which are intended to provide better drug/blood mixing. All clinical and research studies relating to efficacy of intraarterial chemotherapy must consider drug streaming problems.

Selective infusion of chemotherapeutic agents beyond the ophthalmic artery has been made easier with the introduction of soft calibrated-leak microcatheters (KERBER and HEILMAN 1985) and the recently introduced Tracker catheter (KIKUCHI et al. 1987). The Tracker catheter was designed specifically for superselective angiography, embolization, and controlled infusions of drugs. The catheter is made of a composite construction of polyethylene and is graded in thickness and outer diameter from a 2.7-French radiopaque tip to a 3.0-French diameter proximal portion. The catheter can be passed coaxially through a 5-French delivery catheter and it can be passed to intracranial arteries without the use of either an injection chamber or repeated balloon inflation (KIKUCHI et al. 1987).

8.3 Valvuloplasty and Balloon Catheter Applications in Treating Congenital Cardiopulmonary Disease

One of the very first applications of interventional radiology was for a congenital heart defect. In 1967, PORSTMANN reported a transcatheter nonthoracotomy technique for closures of patent ductus arteriosus (PORSTMANN et al. 1967). The procedure involved passing a sponge plug over a guide wire that crossed the patent ductus. Catheter access was gained through a cutdown and entry into the femoral artery. The plug was sized and shaped from previous angiographic studies to fit snugly into the congenital communication. Although PORSTMANN reported long-term success and low morbidity, the procedure has never gained acceptance in the United States as a standard or accepted form of treatment for patent ductus arteriosus. Still, WIERNY et al. (1986) reported that since 1967, 800 patients have been successfully treated with the technique in Europe and Japan. Another early, major cardiac interventional procedure was balloon catheter septostomy introduced by RASHKIND and MILLER in 1966. This transcatheter, nonthoracotomy procedure proved very effective in reducing right ventricular hypertension and improving blood oxygenation in patients suffering from pulmonary atresia, transposition of the great vessels, and total anomalous pulmonary venous return. The procedure gained clinical acceptance and is still used today.

The use of balloon dilatation catheters to treat pulmonary valvular stenosis by KAN et al. (1982) at Johns Hopkins ushered in a new era in transcatheter balloon therapy and stimulated an interest that had not been experienced since the early pioneering work of RASHKIND and MILLER (1966) and PORSTMANN et al. (1967). The work of KAN et al. (1982) was revolutionary because unlike the approaches of RASHKIND or PORSTMANN, pulmonary valvular dilatation required the use of an angioplasty balloon catheter, the temporary cessation of venous return, and significant alterations in cardiac hemodynamics. The success of pulmonary valvuloplasty since 1982 makes it the treatment of choice over surgery and stimulated investigations into the use of balloon dilatation catheters to treat peripheral pulmonary stenosis as well as aortic and mitral valve stenosis and coarctation. This renewed interest in these cardiac interventional procedures along with the application of percutaneous transluminal angioplasty for coronary artery stenosis and the use of thrombolytics for coronary artery thrombosis will certainly continue and stimulate new approaches for the future. Such activity will be fitting tribute to the pioneering work of RASHKIND and PORSTMANN.

The most successful valvuloplasty procedure, and the one that has been used to treat the largest number of patients, has been for stenotic pulmonary valves (Fig. 4). BASS (1988) summarizes the success of this procedure by stating that it is a significant improvement over surgical valvotomy in terms of cost and patient convenience. There have been no reported deaths associated with the procedure; pulmonary regurgitation, if present at all, is mild and hemodynamically insignificant, and late follow-up has shown persistent or further improvement (KVESELIS et al. 1985). MULLINS et al. (1988) reported long-term (2 years) follow-up on 63 patients, ranging in age from 3 months to 76 years, and concluded that the data confirm that balloon dilatation angioplasty for pulmonary valve stenosis is safe and effective and stenoses do not return. ROBERTS (1987) also considers valvuloplasty the treatment of choice for patients with pulmonary valve stenosis except in those cases involving dysplastic pulmonary valves. These more recent articles reflect similar observations made earlier (KAN et al. 1984a, b; LABABIDI and WU 1983; WALLS et al. 1984; ROCCHINI and KVESELIS 1984).

Fig. 4. **a** Angiography shows a very narrow channel through the pulmonary artery valve *(arrow)* in a child with pulmonary valve stenosis. **b** A balloon angioplasty catheter has been placed across the stenotic valve and inflated. Note balloon indentations at the level of the stenotic valve. **c** Further inflation of the balloon relieves the stenosis, as indicated by the uniform diameter of the inflated balloon. **d** Postvalvuloplasty angiography indicates a much larger opening through the pulmonary valve

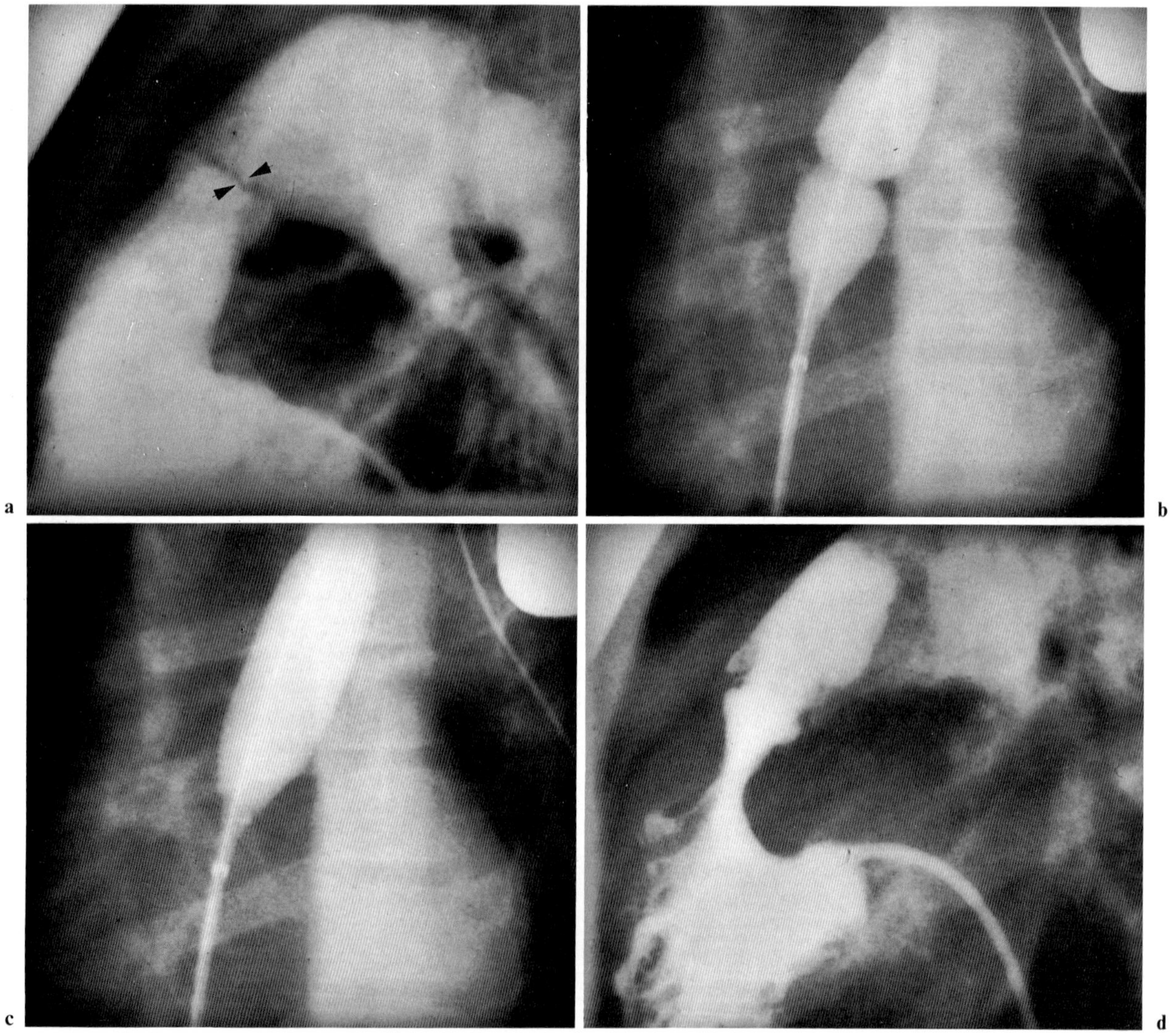

Since it is important to minimize the duration of pulmonary artery inflow obstruction during valvuloplasty, the inflation-deflation times of the balloon should be as short as possible. It was for this reason that MITCHELL et al. (1984) introduced balloon catheters with a larger lumen supplying the balloon. This modification in conjunction with larger balloons extended the application and safety of valvuloplasty procedures.

The extension of valvuloplasty procedures to the mitral and aortic valves came after the initial application for the pulmonary valve. It is still too early to predict whether mitral and aortic valvuloplasty will be as successful and clinically acceptable as for the pulmonary valve and more time is needed to evaluate long-term results. However, it is apparent that anatomical and physiological factors are more of a concern with regards to dilating the aortic or mitral valve. LABABIDI et al. (1984a) reported on the first large series (23 patients) receiving aortic valvuloplasty. Although this initial report was encouraging, it was obvious that many problems were presented that were not encountered with pulmonary valve dilatation. More research is needed to better understand the effect of transient aortic outflow tract obstruction on left ventricular hypertension, coronary artery perfusion, and overall cardiac hemodynamics. In order to minimize the potential for aortic rupture, LABABIDI et al. (1984a) stressed the use of balloons with a maximal inflation diameter of 1 mm smaller than the aortic valve annulus. The fear of a tear in the aortic wall during balloon inflation is magnified by the high pressure generated in the vessel during the cardiac cycle. Left ventricular hypertension associated with temporary balloon occlusion of the aortic valve cannot be significantly reduced by using the central lumen of the valvuloplasty catheter to create a left ventricular central venous shunt (WHITE et al. 1986b). The only way to decrease left ventricular hypertension during aortic outflow tract obstruction is to concomitantly reduce pulmonary artery inflow by use of a pulmonary artery occlusion balloon (WHITE et al. 1986b).

Valve insufficiency and regurgitation is more of a problem with aortic valve dilatation than with that of the pulmonary valve. BASS (1988) feels that this factor alone has caused some institutions to limit the candidates for aortic valvuloplasty to those who have failed surgical aortic valvotomy without developing significant aortic regurgitation or to patients who would be a great risk during cardiopulmonary bypass. Also, aortic valvuloplasty may not be as effective in patients with significantly thickened valves and where obstruction results from the bulk of leaflet tissue rather than from commissure fusion (BASS 1988). The encouraging results experienced by LABABIDI et al. (1984a) and those reported by HELGASON et al. (1985) and WALLS et al. (1984) need to be updated with longer term follow-up.

Mitral valve dilatation can be approached from either the antegrade or retrograde approach. LOCK et al. (1985) reported on eight patients receiving mitral valvuloplasty for rheumatic valve stenosis. They reported a 52% fall in pressure gradient following the procedure and a persistence of this gradient in all but one patient at 2-8 weeks follow-up. BABIC et al. (1988) reported mitral valve dilatation using a retrograde approach. The technique consisted of using a transseptal catheter to place a 0.035-in. diameter exchange guide wire into the ascending aorta. The wire was then grasped with a snare wire passed to the ascending aorta from the femoral artery. The original exchange wire was then retrieved through the femoral artery and a balloon catheter was passed over it to straddle the stenotic mitral valve. Either approach requires some form of transseptal entry and this adds to potential complications. As with aortic valve dilatation, long-term follow-up studies are needed to evaluate future clinical applications.

Aortic coarctation is another condition potentially amenable to balloon catheter dilatation procedures (LABABIDI et al. 1984b). Thus far, the results of coarctation dilatation are mixed. Restenosis often occurs and gradients often return shortly after dilatation (WHITE et al. 1986a). The procedure may have more application in infants, where the surgical approach is not as good as in adults. As with aortic valvular stenosis, overinflation of the balloon can lead to major complications.

The use of large angioplasty balloon catheters to relieve valvular stenosis led to the use of similar techniques to create adequate interatrial openings in conditions which necessitated relief of increased right heart pressure or improved blood oxygenation (MITCHELL et al. 1986). Septostomy using a large diameter angioplasty balloon catheter provided interatrial communication using stationary radial applied force as opposed to the more conventional balloon pull through technique that occasionally results in vena caval injury and complications. Atrial septostomy using angioplasty techniques is still in the developmental stage and has received very limited clinical attention. Much more work needs to be done in comparing the long-term results of the procedure with those obtained by the Rashkind technique. An immediate extension of balloon angioplasty septostomy involves the development of a nonthoracotomy approach to left ventricular assistance as an emergency procedure in patients who require immediate reduction in left ventricular workload. Large bore catheters percutaneously placed in the left atrium could be used to shunt blood away from the left side of the heart. The large bore catheter could be connected to a pump that would reroute the blood (via a second catheter) to the lower abdominal aorta.

The future for both clinical and basic science research in cardiac interventional procedures is very encouraging. Although the radiologist's approach has essentially been in research related to technique development, future studies must begin to focus on more precise physiological measurements relating to the effects of the procedures. Animal research preceded the first valvuloplasty procedure and provided important information relating to hemodynamic changes associated with temporary occlusion of the pulmonary inflow tract. Major research efforts in valvuloplasty now center on both hemodynamic and electrophysiological studies related to the procedure and the development of new or modified balloon catheters that may be more amenable to aortic valvuloplasty. The clinical utilization of these procedures is increasing and more information is needed relating to the structural and physiological consequences.

8.4 Intravascular Use of Lasers

The successful utilization of lasers in dermatology (Apfelberg et al. 1981) and ophthalmology (Zaret et al. 1963) has stimulated increased attention for their use in other medical disciplines, including interventional radiology. Although the potential use of lasers for both vascular and nonvascular interventional applications is very substantial, most work has centered on vessel recanalization. In dermatologic and ophthalmologic applications, the clinician can directly observe the effects of the laser treatment and has complete directional control of the energy beam (Spears 1986). However, the luxury of direct visualization and laser energy controllability is not available to the radiologist who wishes to remove plaque or thrombus from an artery in situ. These limitations contribute to the complications associated with intravascular laser therapy, limit its widespread acceptance, and represent major areas of intense research.

Interventional radiologists are accustomed to progressing through several "generations" of equipment and device modifications before widespread clinical acceptance of a technique or procedure is guaranteed. The use of lasers will be no exception to this rule. Industry realizes the vast market available if lasers can be used safely and effectively for vascular recanalization. These are tremendous financial incentives to stimulate industry in research and development to improve the efficacy and safety of intravascular laser therapy. There is no doubt that within the next 10 years, laser research will provide the interventional radiologist with a product that will make the lasers of today appear crude. Interventional radiologists must actively participate in this laser application research. The major problems associated with the intravascular use of lasers and the areas where research must focus include problems relating to (Choy 1986):

1. Vessel perforation
2. Distal embolization of debris
3. Reocclusions
4. Vascular spasm
5. Selectivity in target tissue ablation

The above problems can only be answered through research directed at (Bowker 1986):

1. Determining the optimal type, power, exposure, duration, and wavelength required for ablating various biological and inorganic materials deposited within vessels
2. Evaluating the best methods of delivering and guiding the laser engery
3. Developing methods to enhance tissue selectivity to absorb the energy
4. Improving methods to discriminate target tissue from normal tissue
5. Improving alignment of the energy beam within the vessel
6. Eliminating unwanted thermal injury and reducing "burnback" or tissue injury due to tip temperature increasing to ignition point (when in contact with the lesion) and burning the fibers

The visible beam of the argon laser and the invisible infrared radiation of the neodymium-"doped" yttrium-aluminium-garnet (Nd:YAG) and the carbon dioxide (CO_2) lasers produce thermal injury resulting in a vaporized crater with contiguous charring and disruption of adjacent cellular and molecular material (Lee et al. 1986). Nd:YAG lasers produce the deepest tissue penetration and affect the largest tissue volume (Lee et al. 1986). Argon laser energy is absorbed by hemoglobin and its penetration in blood is not as great as for the Nd:YAG laser. Both Nd:YAG and argon laser heat accumulation and tissue damage can be minimized by using extremely short pulses and saline flushing to provide long thermal relaxation times (CHOY 1986).

The most appealing potential use of lasers in interventional radiology would be for atherosclerotic obstructions. The opportunity to physically remove the plaque from the vessel as opposed to compressing it into the vessel wall provides a new and potentially important treatment approach. However, the use of lasers for this application is hindered by the heterogenous nature of plaque. Target tissue properties affect the degree of laser energy absorption, and at the present time, no laser beam wavelength is absorbed specifically by plaque (LEE et al. 1986). In addition, there is no evidence to indicate that reocclusion rates would be less following laser therapy as opposed to percutaneous transluminal angioplasty. Although a clean smooth walled lumen can be created through low density lipid plaques, high density deposits of calcified salts are very resistent to thermal ablation and temperatures of greater than 1000 °C must be achieved to photoablate heavily calcified plaque (LEE et al. 1985). This may damage surrounding normal tissue. ABELA et al. (1984) reported that laser therapy does not accelerate the atherosclerotic process in rhesus monkeys and that laser induced arterial injuries in dogs stimulated reendothelialization (ABELA and CONTI 1983). Much more work is needed to define the advantages of laser therapy versus angioplasty. At the present time lasers and angioplasty procedures are often used sequentially to recanalize vessels.

Confining the laser energy heat production to a focal tip attached to the end of the fiberoptic bundle helps to reduce the occurrence of vessel wall perforation that is so common with bare tip fiberoptic lasers. The "hot tip" laser (Fig. 5) has been accepted as a compromise until technology advances the state of the art using the more exotic excimer laser or devising a nontoxic fiberoptic system to guide the CO_2 laser beam. Hot tip lasers are not used alone to treat obstructive vascular lesions, but are employed in combination with angioplasty or fibrinolytic therapy. LABS et al. (1987b, 1988) have recently shown that thrombus dissolution by urokinase is greatly enhanced when the clot is first "lased" with an argon hot tip device to increase the surface area of the clot exposed to the chemical thrombolytic.

Hot tip argon lasers have found their greatest application in patients with long occlusions and multiple stenoses mainly of the femoropopliteal arteries. Treatment of these patients with standard angioplasty techniques often meets with failure since it is

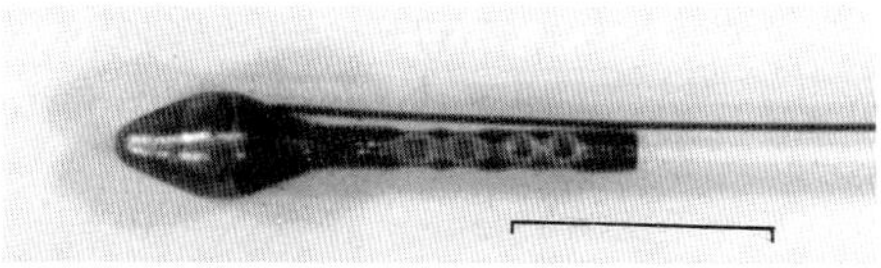

Fig. 5. An argon hot tip laser. The metallic tip is connected to the fiberoptic laser fiber. Scale = 5 mm

difficult to position the angioplasty balloon catheter because of mechanical problems in passing a guide wire across the obliterated lumen without causing subintimal dissections. With the hot tip laser, argon light is transmitted down the quartz fiber and heats the metallic probe tip to temperatures up to 400 °C. Some angiographers feel that passage of the hot tip laser through the obstruction to create a 2 mm diameter path (which will subsequently accept an angioplasty balloon catheter) is much easier and safer than when regular guide wires are employed (Fig. 6). Perforation still occurs when the hot tip comes in contact with the vessel wall, but surprisingly, such perforation is almost always self-sealing. It should be pointed out that most interventional radiologists use the hot tip laser for creating an initial channel through the lesion, when more conventional use of a guide wire is of no value. In order to minimize vessel perforation, attention has been directed towards the use of short duration pulses of energy and saline flushing to dissipate heat from the normal vessel wall (LABS et al. 1987a). Although many angiographers feel the heat generated at the tip is valuable in recanalizing a small lumen through the obstruction, some question the need for a laser system to provide the heat source. Many feel that the bullet shape of the probe tip by itself facilitates passage through obstructions, and some angiographers will attempt passing a "cold" nonenergized probe through the lesion prior to attempting a similar approach using the argon energy (VANBREDA, personal communication, 1988). The degree of heating that is necessary to recanalize various stenotic lesions has not been adequately addressed and more work needs to be done in evaluating laser energized probes where the degree of heat production can be variably controlled.

LAMMER et al. (1988) recently reported on the use of a hot sapphire tip argon laser system. They concluded that the use of the sapphire tip probe (in contrast to the metal tip) overcame the initial clinical limitation caused by the high perforation rate with bare fibers (LAMMER et al. 1987; GINSBURG et al. 1985) and the thermal damage caused by the metal cautery cap of conventional hot tip lasers

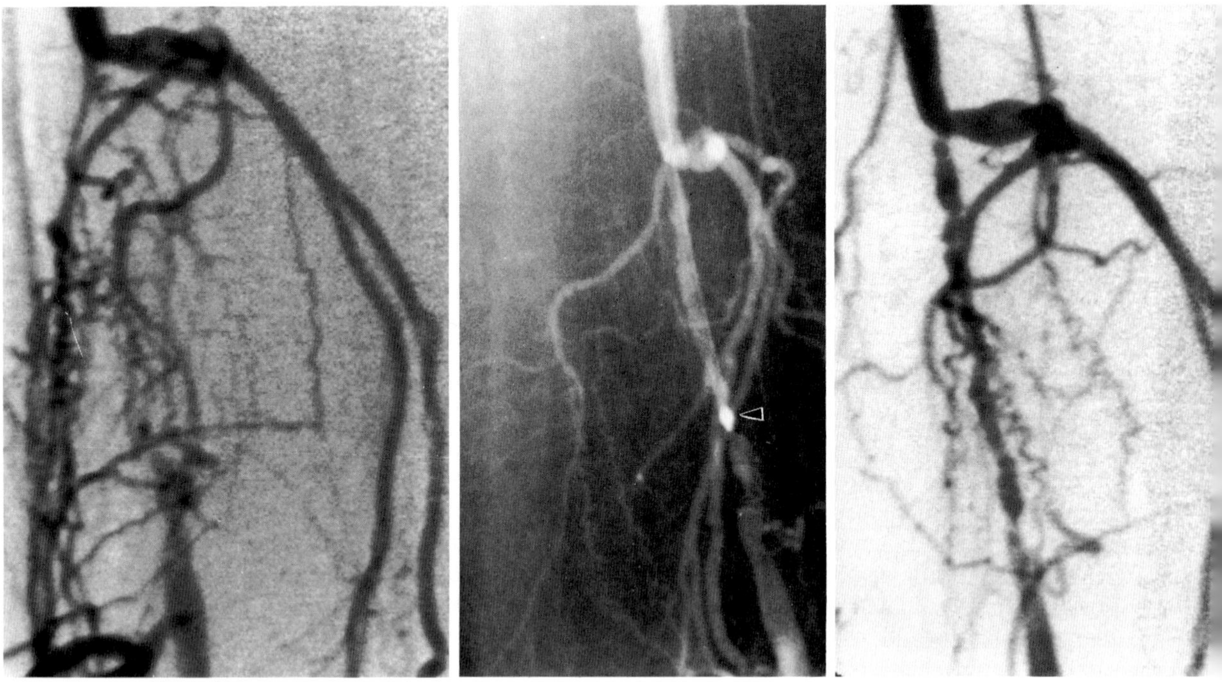

a b c

Fig. 6. **a** A 12-cm long femoral artery occlusion is seen in this arteriogram of a 31-year-old male with osteomyelitis. Note the extensive collaterial circulation developed around the occluded femoral artery. **b** Contrast media injection shows a recanalized channel forming during passage of the argon hot tip laser (*arrows* indicates laser hot tip). **c** Postlaser angiography reveals recanalized channel through the previously occluded vessel. The channel provided an avenue for an angioplasty balloon catheter which was subsequently used to enlarge the vessel lumen

(LEE et al. 1984; SANBORN et al. 1985). The sapphire tip required lower energies for tissue ablation, resulted in a decreased perforation risk, and provided larger diameter recanalized channels (because of its shape); moreover, because sapphire has a melting point of 2000 °C, the tip is not damaged as are quartz glass fibers if a layer of coagulated blood and tissue surrounds it and increases local temperature above the melting point of glass (LAMMER et al. 1988).

Excimer lasers emit ultraviolet light and have the advantage of producing photochemical ablation without generation of thermal energy (LEE et al. 1986). The excimer laser energy breaks protein molecular structures, resulting in controllable disintegration of tissue rather than burning or charring (GRUNDFEST et al. 1985). The depth of penetration varies with the cumulative number of pulses while the diameter of the laser channel and its surroundings remain largely unchanged (LEE et al. 1986; GRUNDFEST et al. 1984; ISNER et al. 1984a, b). Although the excimer may appear to be the laser of choice, it has only been recently introduced into the clinical setting for intravascular use and more time is needed to evaluate its efficacy and safety.

Carbon dioxide laser energy is converted to heat in a very small volume of 1.0 mm^3 and could be used for more precise destruction of lesions. The CO_2 laser efficiency is high and the cost of the apparatus is relatively low, but CO_2 lasers are limited to open procedures because no nontoxic fiberoptic has yet proven satisfactory to guide the laser beam in closed areas (GREATBATCH 1986).

One potential advantage of the tremendous amount of money and effort expended by the defense industry in the current Star Wars research is the medical "spin off" of research and development into lasers. Work with shorter wavelength laser systems in the ultraviolet and X-ray range could be valuable for medical applications (THOMSEN 1983). The practicality of creating small units capable of generating free-electron laser energy (MARSHALL 1985) and research into photoreactive dyes that could be attached to monoclonal antibodies to localize in specific tissue locations are areas of future work (GREATBATCH 1986).

8.5 Biliary Applications

The role of interventional radiologists in managing and treating biliary disease has increased significantly over the past 5 years. This trend should continue as both clinical and research interests in gallbladder therapy are aimed at more aggressive nonsurgical approaches. The introduction of biliary lithotripsy, advances in guide wire and catheter technology, and the use of percutaneous techniques to dissolve and/or remove gallstones are major factors in the increased application of interventional radiology in biliary disease. These factors, coupled with the economic pressures to reduce hospital patient care costs, are attractive incentives to further extend the role of the interventional radiologist beyond the traditional vascular system. The economic incentives alone are tremendous when one considers that the prevalence of gallstones in the United States alone is 20 million people with an incidence of 1 million/year. Over 500000 cholecystectomies are performed in the United States per year at a cost of over 2 billion dollars (SCHOENFIELD et al. 1981). The mortality of cholecystectomy in patients between 50 and 64 is 3% and this increases to 10% in patients over 65. The protean manifestations of gallstone disease account for it being one of the most common causes of hospitalization for surgery (LUFT et al. 1979).

The interventional radiologist has always maintained a high profile in managing patients with biliary disease. Percutaneous catheterization of the bile ducts to establish temporary biliary drainage prior to surgery has been employed for many years (RING et al. 1978; RING 1984; MORI et al. 1977). Catheter access through drainage tube tracts has allowed the interventionalist the opportunity to remove ductal stones that persist after surgery (RING 1984), provide catheter aided drainage into the duodenum (HARBIN and FERRUCCI 1980), place stents and drainage tubes (MCLEAN et al. 1982), and dilate strictures originating from benign disease or those produced following choledochojejunostomy anastomosis (BURHENNE 1973).

Extracorporal shockwave lithotripsy (ESWL) is currently (1989) being introduced into the United States as a nonsurgical approach to removing gallstones. This follows substantial successful clinical experience with the procedure in Europe. The interventional radiologist's involvement in ESWL stems from a history of involvement in similar therapy for urinary stones, an active involvement in managing patients using transcatheter biliary decompression procedures, the need for imaging support in association with biliary lithotripsy, and the potential applications of combining ESWL with nonsurgical transcatheter interventional procedures.

Extracorporal shockwave lithotripsy is a relatively new procedure, with the first human prototype unit being supplied in Europe in 1985. Various manufacturers are now involved in producing ESWL equipment and by the end of 1988, 50–60 sites in the United States were evaluating the clinical use of this new procedure. Ultrasonography is used to localize gallstones, and shockwave energy is translated to the stones using spark gap, electromagnetic, or piezoelectric principles. Stone fragmentation is thought to be produced via cavitation on the surface of the stones. Lithotripsy appears to be most successful for cholesterol stones or stones with a small amount of calcium. Stones with diameters less than 2 cm are most amenable to this procedure.

SACKMANN et al. (1988) reported successful initial ESWL fragmentation of gallstones in 174 of 175 patients with negligible complications. They treated only 28% of referred patients because of their strict protocol entrance requirements that included presence of three or fewer noncalcified stones with no stone greater than 3 cm in diameter. The patients were required to have a functioning gallbladder on oral cholecystography and no other medical complications such as acute biliary obstruction, cholecystitis, pregnancy, or arrhythmias (SACKMANN et al. 1988). The principal criterion for success was sonographic clearance of fragments from the gallbladder on follow-up imaging. Clearance approached 30% at 2 months, 48% between 2 and 4 months, and 91% at 12–18 months.

FERRUCCI (1988) stresses the importance of utilizing oral bile acid adjuvant therapy for dissolving fragments of cholesterol gallstones. He emphasizes that a correlation exists between gallstone size and the role of dissolution and that the mechanical effects of fragmentation by ESWL serve to increase the surface area exposed to the dissolving process (FERRUCCI 1988). Oral agents that have received the most attention include chenodeoxycholic acid and ursodeoxycholic acid. Ursodeoxycholic acid is reported to have less side-effects (VAN SONNENBERG and HOFMANN 1988), but more work is needed in evaluating either agent alone or both in combination. At the present time, dissolution is only applicable for cholesterol calculi (VAN SONNENBERG and CASOLA 1988). As long as the cystic duct remains patent and the gallbladder mucosa remains functional in the presence of supersaturated bile, stone recurrence is a high probability (BECKER and KOPECKY 1988).

From the point of view of future interventional radiological applications, the combined use of ESWL and transcatheter interventions is most promising and an area of important research consideration. The overall goal of such an approach would be to not only rid the gallbladder of stones, but to prevent further stone formation. This approach involves several steps which are at the present time quite experimental in nature. As a first step, studies are underway to evaluate transcatheter stone dissolution either alone or in combination with ESWL. The two agents receiving most attention for transcatheter stone dissolution are monooctanoin and methyl-tert-butyl-ether (MTBE). BECKER and KOPECKY (1988) suggest that instillation of MTBE into the gallbladder should be considered an alternative form of therapy for select patients, such as those with radiolucent gallstones and those who strongly object to cholecystectomy (FROMM 1986) or represent poor anesthetic or surgical candidates (THISTLE 1987). Although monooctanoin has been the preferred agent (BUTCH et al. 1984; TEPLICK and HASKIN 1984), MTBE is rapidly becoming the agent of choice for contact gallstone dissolution (VAN SONNENBERG et al. 1986; ALLEN et al. 1985a, b). ALLEN showed that cholesterol gallstones rapidly dissolve in vitro with MTBE (ALLEN et al. 1985a, b), and reported the first successful case of gallstone dissolution using MTBE (ALLEN et al. 1985a).

However, as with oral bile acids, the use of transcatheter stone dissolution agents or ESWL either alone or in combination with orally administered agents will not prevent recurrence of stone formation (BECKER and KOPECKY 1988; RUPPIN and DOWLING 1982). The only way to guarantee no stone re-formation is with surgery or by means of transcatheter ablation of the gallbladder. This latter approach is not without its problems and has yet to be shown to be successful. In order to replace cholecystectomy, transcatheter gallbladder ablation must equal the surgical procedure in its efficacy and surpass it in safety (BECKER and KOPECKY 1988). Although the concept of combined ESWL and transcatheter therapy to first rid the gallbladder of stones and then to totally ablate the gallbladder is very appealing, many problems must be overcome. These problems include: (1) proving that combining ESWL with transcatheter assisted stone dissolution is more effective than either one of the procedures alone (the concept that ESWL will potentiate chemical dissolution by increasing the contact surface areas of stones subjected to chemical action needs stronger support), (2) safe accomplishment of total gallbladder ablation, and (3) the possibility of short- or long-term complications being produced by gallbladder ablation itself.

The first major obstacle to be overcome in ablating the gallbladder involves providing permanent occlusion and destruction of the cystic duct. Patency of the cystic duct poses the threat of recurrent cholecystolithiasis, because the free flow of bile into the gallbladder will likely interfere with obliteration (BECKER and KOPECKY 1988) and reepithelialization following successful gallbladder mucosal obliteration in animals has been shown to be due most likely to ingrowth of epithelium from the intact mucosa of the cystic duct (GETRAJADMAN et al. 1986). In addition, cystic duct occlusion is necessary in order to prevent gallbladder sclerosing agents from entering the duodenum or bile ducts. Because of the nature of the mucosal lining of the cystic duct, mechanical devices such as coils or balloons do not provide permanent occlusion as they so successfully do in blood vessels. However, recent studies in animals report successful transcatheter occlusion of the cystic duct using endoluminal radiofrequency coagulation (C. D. BECKER et al. 1988), laser energy (SULLIVAN, personal communication, 1988), and installation of chemical sclerosing agents (WIDLUS, personal communication, 1988) (Fig. 7). The use of chemical agents to sclerose and permanently occlude the cystic duct requires balloon catheter techniques to prevent passage of the sclerosing agent in-

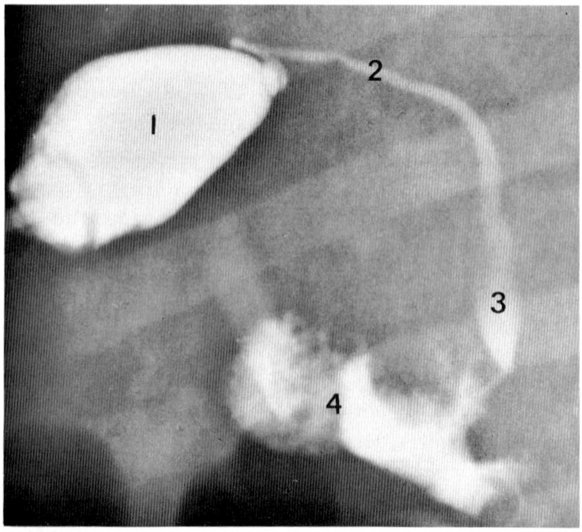

Fig. 7. Cholecystogram in a pig model developed for gallbladder ablation studies. The gallbladder *(1)*, cystic duct *(2)*, common bile duct *(3)*, and duodenum *(4)* are clearly seen. Catheter access to the biliary system is gained through a surgically placed tube in the gallbladder

to the common duct. Further research is needed to perfect cystic duct occlusion and all of the above techniques need independent verification by additional research groups.

Even if safe and permanent cystic duct occlusion can be achieved, total destruction of cystic duct and gallbladder epithelium must be achieved. Attempts at percutaneous gallbladder ablation in large animals have not been successful (REMLEY et al. 1986; GETRAJADMAN et al. 1986; SALOMONOWITZ et al. 1984). Attempts in small animals have also not been successful except in the rabbit (GETRAJADMAN et al. 1986). However, recently described animal models using pigs (McGAHAN et al. 1987; C. D. BECKER et al. 1988) may help to accelerate this important area of research. Important questions that need answering include:

1. What agent or combination of agents is most useful in destroying the gallbladder mucosa?
2. Is it necessary to extensively wash the gallbladder mucosa of its contents prior to chemical contact ablation attempts?
3. If an appropriate sclerosing chemical is found, what should be the parameters of its use, i.e., duration of contact, single vs repeat contact times?
4. Can chemical agents provide a complete destruction of the mucosa?
5. What are the real and potential short- and long-term complications of gallbladder ablation procedures?

8.6 Thrombolysis

For the interventional radiologist, thrombolytic therapy can be used for thrombosis when present alone or in conjunction with atheromatous disease. In the latter case, percutaneous transluminal angioplasty or thrombectomy may be employed if applicable. Converting occlusions to stenoses using thrombolytic therapy prior to angioplasty is becoming very popular. Until recently, streptokinase and urokinase have been the primary agents utilized. However, the relatively recent clinical introduction of recombinant tissue type plasminogen activator presents new opportunities that will be heavily investigated over the next several years.

CHARLES DOTTER was instrumental in the initial conception of many present-day clinically accepted interventional procedures. Until 1974, most thrombolytic therapy was given by the intravenous route. It was DOTTER who suggested using a low dose intraarterial approach (KERLAN 1984). Today some consider the use of low dose intraarterial fibrinolytic therapy in acute and subacute arterial occlusion to be a well established method of treatment. Urokinase and streptokinase have received the most clinical attention and of the two, urokinase is the most popular because it appears to produce fewer systemic fibrinogenolytic disturbances (TENNANT et al. 1984, McNAMARA and FISCHER 1985) and does not show allergic type reactions that are occasionally associated with streptokinase (MAIZEL and BOOKSTEIN 1986; SASAHARA 1988).

Streptokinase and urokinase activate the fibrinolytic system by converting both circulating and fibrin bound plasminogen to plasmin, which in turn digests fibrin (RISIUS et al. 1987). Because both agents convert both circulating and fibrin bound plasminogen, there is a tendency to precipitate a systemic fibrinolytic state characterized by depletion of fibrinogen, plasminogen, antiplasmin, factor V, and factor VIII (RISIUS et al. 1987). Essentially, both agents activate the body's natural fibrinolytic system (SASAHARA 1988), which may potentially precipitate systemic hemorrhagic episodes. Because of this problem, most recent work with urokinase and streptokinase has centered on optimizing drug administration protocols. GARDINER et al. (1986) studied intraarterial thrombolytic therapy in occluded femoropopliteal grafts employing urokinase in 22 cases and streptokinase in 22. Urokinase bolus injections followed by infusions had better results (77% vs 41%) and fewer complications (23% vs 50%) than streptokinase (GARDINER et al. 1986). The optimal treatment followed that recommended by (McNAMARA and FISCHER 1985), which consisted of an intravenous bolus of 30000-60000 IU followed by 4000 IU/min given intraarterially for the first 2 h, 2000 IU/min intraarterially for the next 2 h, and 1000 IU/min until complete local thrombolysis. GARDINER et al. (1986) suggested this protocol to be performed concomitant with 500-1000 IU/h intravenous heparin. The infusion should not go beyond 48 h unless clear evidence of thrombolysis is occurring.

Tissue type plasminogen activator (t-PA) is a serine protease with a high affinity for fibrin (ALLEN and PEPPER 1981; THORSEN et al. 1972; BACHMAN and KRUITHOF 1984; RIJKEN and COLLEN 1981) and a low affinity for circulating plasma plasminogen (COLLEN and VERSTRAETE 1983). Results employing t-PA in patients with thrombosed peripheral arteries and bypass grafts suggest it is a potent, relatively fibrin specific thrombolytic agent that avoids the fibrinogenolysis seen with streptokinase and urokinase (GRAOR et al. 1986a, b; RISIUS et al. 1986, 1987). The agent is relatively clot specific, converting fibrin bound plasminogen to plasmin on the clot surface (RANBY 1982; HOYLAERTS et al. 1982), and produces rapid thrombolysis without activating a systemic lytic state (VANDEWERF et al. 1984; GOLD et al. 1984). However, this does not preclude the fact that t-PA may lyse thrombi located in areas outside the primary site of concern. This may contribute to systemic bleeding.

BECKER and HOLDEN (1988) call t-PA a magic bullet that may replace the use of urokinase and streptokinase. The fibrinogenolytic-fibrinolytic ratio of t-PA is markedly lower than that of urokinase in vitro (MATSUO and COLLEN 1981).

Because of its apparent advantages, t-PA holds great promise for both intraarterial and intravenous use. However, despite the accelerated thrombolysis produced by intraarterial fibrinolytic agents, the intravenous approach is most ideal and most practical for immediate administration to cardiac patients prior to the time when they can be transported to the hospital and angio suite for intraarterial catheterization (MAIZEL and BOOKSTEIN 1986). The concept of intravenous administration of thrombolytic agents as soon as possible after the onset of a myocardial thrombotic episode is gaining acceptance, especially when the potential for systemic fibrinolysis is minimized, as may be the case with the use of t-PA. The approach of providing intravenous thrombolytic therapy as soon as possible after a heart attack (most likely administered by paramedics at the scene of the episode or on the way to the hospital) was the initial idea of CHARLES DOTTER. Although some were initially critical of this suggestion, the availability of t-PA may revive the Dotter principle.

Other potential fibrinolytic agents that are still very much in their initial research development stage include:

1. Acrylated streptokinase-plasminogen complex, which binds to fibrin and activates fibrin bound plasminogen (BECKER and HOLDEN 1988)
2. Prourokinase – has little or no activity while circulating but activates plasminogen in the presence of fibrin clot (BECKER and HOLDEN 1988)
3. Urokinase coupled to a fibrin specific monoclonal antibody (BODE et al. 1985)

8.7 Intravascular Stents

8.7.1 Introduction

One of the most promising interventional radiological devices currently being evaluated is the intravascular stent (Figs. 8, 9). Except in a few cases where angioplasty is ineffective, stents are being developed to help maintain vessel patency (prevent restenosis) following angioplasty by providing a supportive endoprosthesis (PALMAZ et al. 1986b). In some cases, the stent is delivered over an angioplasty balloon such that balloon dilatation and stent placement occur simultaneously. In other instances, stents are placed as a separate procedure following successful balloon angioplasty. Stents are designed to oppose vascular elastic recoil, especially in lesions that are usually refractory to balloon dilatation (PALMAZ et al. 1986a). Once in place across a dilated stenotic lesion, the stents become incorporated into the wall of the blood vessel by the process of endothelialization and intimal proliferation. An ideal stent is one that can easily be introduced into the vascular treatment area, possesses a predictable, controllable, and permanent degree of expansion, does not migrate, produces minimal biological rejection reaction, is nonthrombogenic, and quickly becomes endothelialized and incorporated as an integral part of the vessel wall. Stent research and development focus on the above properties.

The concept of transcatheter delivery of a vascular endoprothesis is not new. CHARLES DOTTER first recognized the need for such a device during his early research in transluminal angioplasty (DOTTER and JUDKINS 1964). Five years later, DOTTER was the first to describe the experimental use of a tubular coilspring stent (DOTTER 1969). During the next decade, most stent research centered around the use of thermal expansion (Nitinol) metallic alloy materials. SIMON et al. (1977) pioneered this work and centered attention on Nitinol's use for both vascular stents and vena caval filters.

Intense active interest in stent research was reinitiated in the early and mid 1980s. The period of relative inactivity since DOTTER's first report on stents was probably related to the active development and clinical utilization of percutaneous transluminal angioplasty.

At the present time (1988), intravascular stent research and clinical evaluation are directed towards four basic stent designs: (1) the Palmaz balloon expandable stent, (2) the Gianturco zig-zag design device, (3) the self-expanding Wallstent, and (4) the thermal memory alloy stent.

8
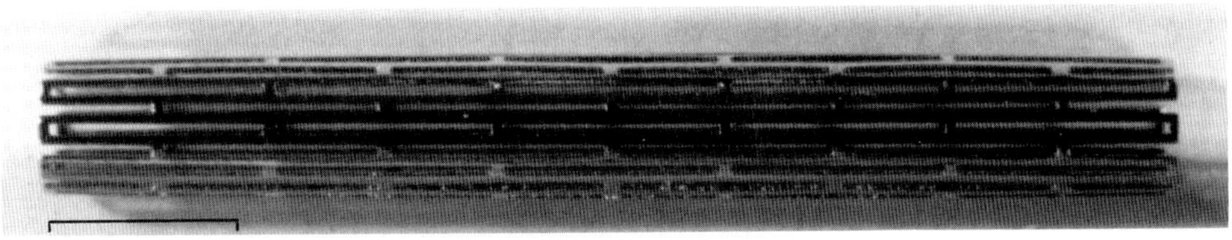

9a b
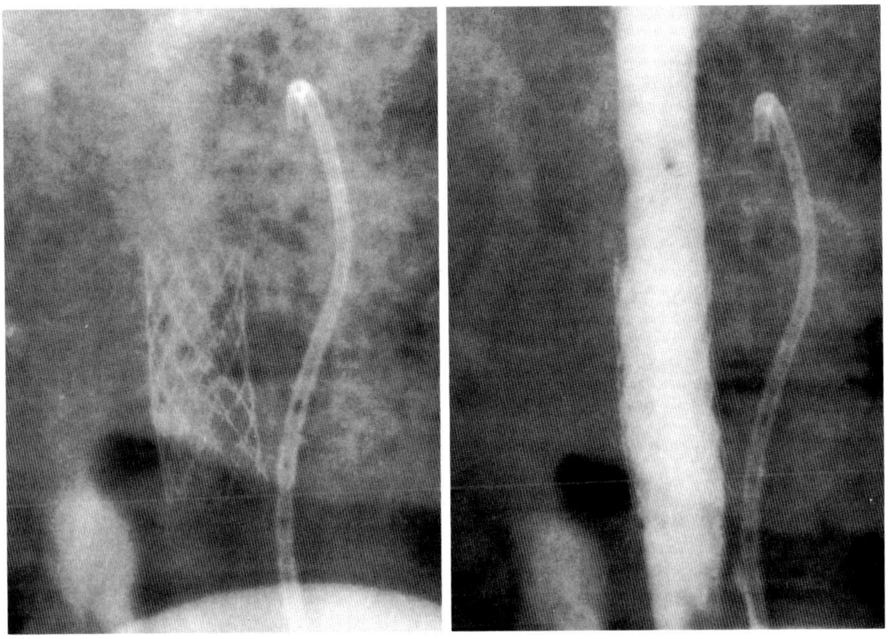

Fig. 8. A Palmaz stent in its nonexpanded form. Scale = 5 mm

Fig. 9. a A 12-mm diameter Palmaz stent placed in the inferior vena cava of a 16-week-old pig. The stent was placed via the femoral vein. **b** Illustration of patency of the stented area. Note that in **a** and **b**, a catheter is present in the aorta. This catheter is unrelated to the stent placement procedure. Scale = 5 mm

8.7.2 Palmaz Stent

PALMAZ originally made his wire mesh stent by manually weaving 0.015 mm diameter stainless steel under a low power microscope (PALMAZ et al. 1985a, b). The cross points of the mesh were soldered with low temperature silver solder. The stents were introduced over an angioplasty balloon and had a collapsed to expanded diameter of 1:3 (PALMAZ et al. 1985b). The mesh retained its shape after the balloon was inflated and kept the diameter of the vessel as large as the maximum diameter of the inflated balloon (PALMAZ et al. 1986b). The more recent Palmaz stents employ 6–8 rows of staggered offset slots formed by stainless steel wire struts (PALMAZ 1988; PALMAZ 1988). In the expanded position, the stent has the ability to oppose maximum hoop stress because of the favorable distribution of the stress along the stent struts (PALMAZ et al. 1987). The stent will expand to the diameter of the inflated delivery balloon or to its limit of expansion (MULLINS et al. 1988).

8.7.3 Gianturco Zig-zag Stent

The Gianturco expandable wire stents are cylindrical wire structures 0.5–3.5 cm in diameter. The name zig-zag relates to the overall appearance and configuration of the stent. They are constructed of tempered stainless steel wire bent into a zig-zag pattern; the two ends of the wire are then joined to form a cylinder (FALLONE et al. 1988). The dilating force of the stent can be controlled by the wire size, the number of angles of wire bends, and the stent length (WRIGHT et al. 1985). FALLONE et al. (1988) recently described the force, tension, and pressure exerted by the stent on vessels and predicted that once the pressure exerted by the vessels under abnormal situations could be measured, the appropriate stent could be chosen quantitatively.

UCHIDA et al. (1988) and ROSCH et al. (1987) described modifications of the Gianturco stent. These modifications included adding monofilament line to the wire skirts of the stent to help control expansion, facilitate stent placement, and prevent dislodgement.

8.7.4 Wallstent

The Wallstent consists of surgical-grade stainless steel alloy filaments woven in a tubular fashion (ZOLLIKOFER et al. 1988). This self-expanding microporous stent has a major advantage of being pliable and having longitudinal flexibility. Flexibility is imparted to the stent because the wire filaments are not soldered together. The expandable force and flexibility of the stent may be varied by altering the closeness of the wire mesh weave and thickness of the wire filaments (0.08–0.20 mm) (ZOLLIKOFER et al. 1988). This self-expanding stent is delivered over a special catheter that has a thin membrane that covers the stent and prevents expansion of the stent until it is in proper position. The Wallstent is self-expanding once the membrane is retracted.

8.7.5 Thermal Memory Alloy Stents

Thermal memory alloy stents are made of Nitinol or Nitinol-like nickel-titanium materials. The basic design is of a lightly coiled spring. The shape is preformed by heating. When cooled, the wire can be straightened and introduced into the body through a catheter. The wire is passed from the catheter and is exposed to 10 ml of 60°–65 °C saline flush injected rapidly by hand through the catheter side port. This restores the coil spring shape and presses the stent against the vessel wall. A recent report on 2-year follow-up of the stents in the iliac and femoral arteries of dogs revealed 100% patency in 12 stents with no migration, erosion, inflammation, surface thrombus, or side branch stenosis (SUTTON et al. 1988). Neointima covered the stents and provided complete endothelialization without change in thickness over time.

As previously mentioned, intravascular stents find their major current application when used in conjuction with angioplasty to prevent recurrent stenosis. PALMAZ (1988) indicates that the stent is not intended to replace the well-established role of angioplasty but rather to compensate for its limitations. Long-term patency of balloon dilated vessels if often limited by thrombus formed on irregular cracked atheromatous surface which is likely to be replaced by smooth muscle and fibrous tissue (DOUBILET and ABRAMS 1984; KALMAN and JOHNSTON 1985). The smooth and regular lumen obtained with the placement of stents should decrease or prevent irregularities after angioplasty (PALMAZ 1988).

In addition, stents will prove useful in other conditions not amenable to angioplasty. Such applications include peripheral pulmonary stenoses, systemic venous stenoses, and vessel lumens narrowed by dissection, tumorous processes, postoperative edema, or hematoma. Stents may also find application for "patching" aneurysms. Incomplete relief has been noted after angioplasty of peripheral pulmonary artery and vein stenoses (DRISCOLL et al. 1982; LOCK et al. 1981). Venous structures are elastic in nature and while dilating the vessel is usually easily done, once the balloon is deflated, the lumen may return to the predilatation diameter. Late restenosis occurs most commonly from fibrosis and atherosclerosis. Also, patients may not be able to withstand occlusion of a vital vessel for the time necessary to obtain adequate balloon dilatation. This may occur in ductus dependent infants with congenital heart disease who cannot tolerate 5- to 10-min balloon occlusion of the ductus arteriosus (CORWIN et al. 1981; LUND et al. 1984). These problems may possibly be better managed through the use of intravascular stents. Relatively little work has been directed towards the use of vascular stents in congenital heart diseases. This is an area very much in need of research.

ZOLLIKOFER et al. (1988) used stents to provide a safe means of preventing recurrent stenosis for the fibrous elastic narrowings seen in postoperative venous lesions or graft anastomoses and hemodialysis shunts where the effects of percutaneous transluminal angioplasty are often of short duration. CHARNSANGAVEJ et al. (1986) evaluated the use of stents in the stenotic inferior vena cava of dogs. They subsequently used stents to successfully treat 12 patients with inferior vena cava syndrome and one with retroperitoneal fibrosis obstructing the inferior vena cava. In all cases, the stents provided immediate relief of the caval stenosis (CHARNSANGAVEJ et al. 1986). ROSCH et al. (1987) used modified Gianturco stents to create intrahepatic portocaval shunts in animals. PALMAZ et al. (1985b) employed his stent in similar experimental procedures.

CHARNSANGAVEJ et al. (1985) studied the value of intravascular stents in aortic dissections. They simulated aortic dissection by injecting normal saline and contrast medium into the walls of aortic specimens from human cadavers. Successful stent dilatation of the narrowed aortic lumens was demonstrated in all the specimens. They felt placement of an endovascular stent at the site of an intimal tear may push the intima against the outer layer and thus prevent further extension or recurrence of the dissection (CHARNSANGAVEJ et al. 1985). MULLINS et al. (1988) evaluated the efficacy and safety of the Palmaz stent in the pulmonary arteries and systemic veins in dogs. Of 13 stents, 11 were placed successfully in pulmonary arteries and 11 of 14 were successfully placed in tributaries of the vena cava. Three inadvertent embolizations occurred. The dogs were recatheterized at intervals ranging from 56 to 278 days. Twelve stents were patent and nonobstructive; two were malpositioned. Patent stents were completely covered with neointima and showed no thrombus.

In the coronary circulation or in areas of high motion (knee area), flexible stents are needed. The first clinical study of self-expanding flexible stents in the coronaries was reported by SIGWART et al. (1987). Early assessment immediately after stent placement showed an additional morphological improvement over the percutaneous transluminal angioplasty results affecting both the stenotic and nonstenotic segments. This demonstrated the intrinsic dilating properties of the stent. Dilatation continues until an equilibrium is achieved between the circumferential elastic resistance of the arterial wall and the dilating force of the stent (SIGWART et al. 1987). The stent used for these studies was the Wallstent. This device has been reported to induce limited intimal proliferation and low occlusion rates (ZOLLIKOFER et al. 1988). These features may be related to its small wire size, self-expansion properties, and inherent pliability. PUEL et al. (1988) placed the self-expanding stent in the left anterior descending artery in nine patients and in the circumflex in two others. Stent placement followed successful angioplasty. Angiographic studies 3 months later in six patients showed a decrease in the minimal luminal cross-sectional area but no hemodynamically significant repercussions (PUEL et al. 1988).

SCHATZ et al. (1987) also studied acute and chronic biological response to balloon expandable intracoronary stents in adult dogs. Twenty stents were placed in the left anterior descending, left main, or circumflex artery. All dogs survived the stent placement procedure with no evidence of myocardial infarction, spasm, rupture, or aneurysm of the vessels. Neointimal proliferation reached maximal thickness by 8 weeks and all stents were covered with endothelium by 1 week.

STRECKER et al. (1988) described another flexible wire mesh stent made from either stainless steel alloy or stainless steel containing copper or tantalum. The steel copper and tantalum stents produced a severe inflammatory response while the stainless steel alloy stents showed no tissue reaction in dogs. The stent was constructed of 0.06–0.10 mm diameter wire and required balloon expansion for placement. The most important feature of this stent was its flexibility. DUPRAT et al. (1987b) also described an experimental flexible balloon expanded stainless steel stent that has potential application in small peripheral, visceral, and coronary arteries. Again, flexibility is the main advantage of this stent.

Compared with surgical grafts, early spread of endothelium over the stented surface is a unique feature (PALMAZ 1988). Because of the antithrombogenic properties of endothelium, a completely endothelialized prosthetic conduit is protected from thrombus formation that may occur in situations of slow or turbulent flow (PALMAZ 1988).

The process of complete endothelialization depends on many factors, including the location of the stent (artery or vein), flow characteristics within the vessel, the conformity of stent apposition to the intimal wall, and structural characteristics of the stent itself. The thickness of the metal struts has been reported to be of major importance in determining the time interval for complete endothelialization (ZOLLIKOFER et al. 1988). The amount of intimal hyperplasia is increased in rigid stents (DUPRAT et al. 1987a, b; DOTTER et al. 1983). DUPRAT (1987a) showed the occlusion rate is related to the correct sizing of the stent, with stent/artery ratios greater than 1.2 leading to increased intimal proliferation and thrombosis.

8.8 Atherectomy Catheters

Atherectomy catheters have recently been introduced into the armamentarium of the interventional radiologist. The main application for atherectomy catheters will be for heavily calcified or eccentric lesions which may not be suitable for balloon angioplasty (HOFLING et al. 1988). The Simpson and Kensey atherectomy catheters have received the greatest laboratory and clinical attention although it must be emphasized that the work is very preliminary at the time of this writing. The Simpson ather-

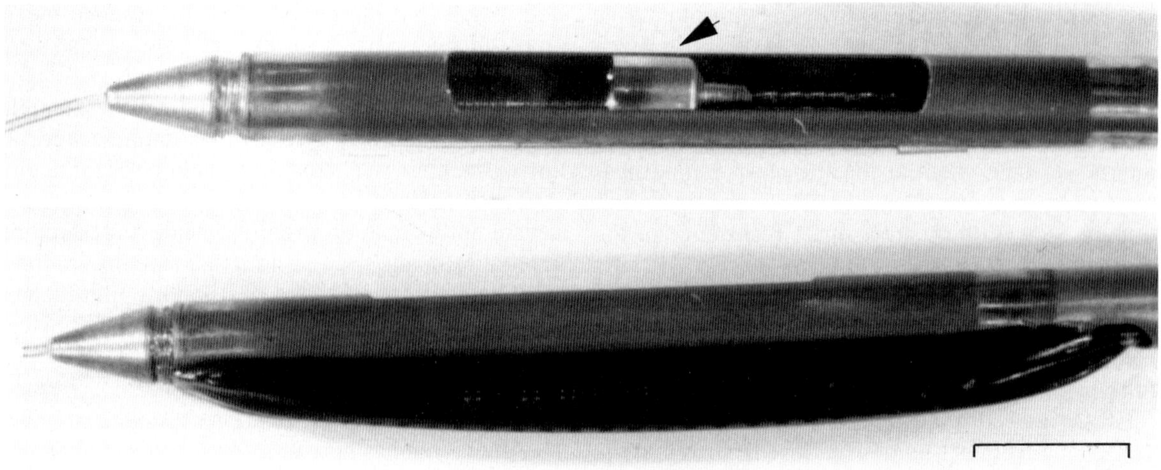

a

b

Fig. 10a, b. The Simpson atherectomy catheter. The longitudinal groove and cutting blade of the catheter can be seen *(arrow)*. **b** shows the catheter with its balloon inflated. Scale = 5 mm

Fig. 11. a Angiography reveals intraluminal plaque in the lower abdominal aorta of a 57-year-old male with life-style altering claudication. The plaque occludes approximately 80% of the right common femoral artery. **b** The atherectomy catheter is pressed up against the plaque. Note that because of the large diameter of the aorta, an angioplasty balloon catheter *(arrow)* was placed (via the opposite femoral artery) to facilitate positioning of the atherectomy catheter against the plaque. **c** Postatherectomy angiogram reveals a much larger channel created through the lesion. This channel facilitated a subsequent balloon angioplasty procedure to further enlarge the vessel lumen

ectomy catheter contains a metallic tip with a biopsy-like longitudinal opening on one side and a balloon on the other side (Figs. 10, 11). When the tip of the instrument is placed in a region of plaque, the balloon is inflated. This pushes the longitudinal opening against the plaque. With the balloon inflated, a cutting blade is advanced across the longitudinal opening to shave off pieces of the plaque. The cutting blade's forward motion is powered by a hand held rotary motor device connected to the catheter blade mechanism. The plaque material that is shaved off is supposedly trapped in the longitudinal opening of the catheter tip. When the balloon is deflated, the catheter can be repositioned for additional cuts until the catheter tip cup housing is filled with plaque material. The catheter is then withdrawn and the cup emptied. This process is repeat-

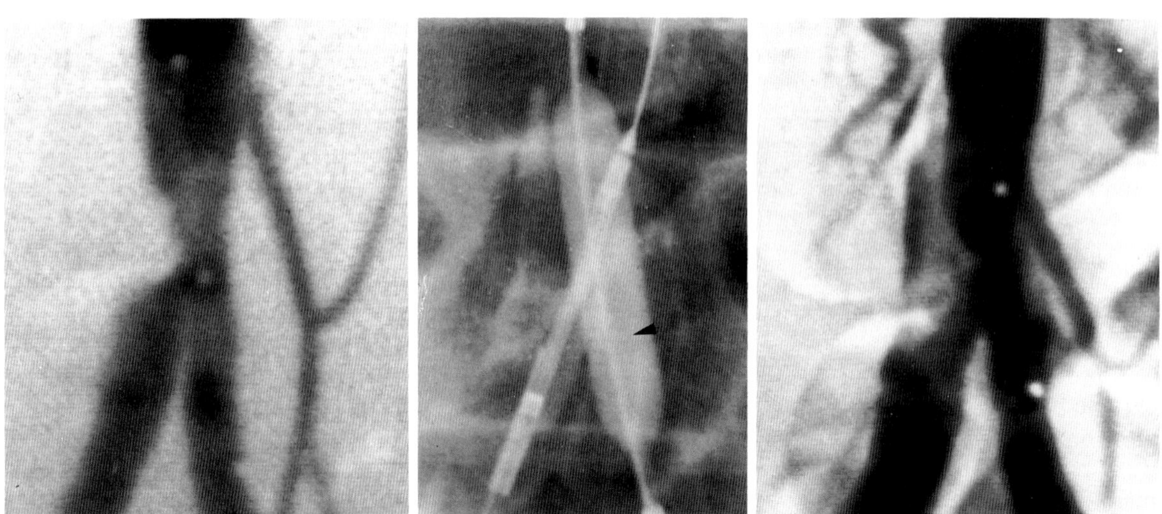

a b c

ed until enough of the plaque is removed to reestablish the vascular lumen.

HOFLING et al. (1988) reported on 41 stenotic lesions in 21 patients treated with the Simpson atherectomy catheter. The lesions included 5 iliac, 35 superficial femoral, and 1 popliteal. Four of the lesions were totally occluded and 16 were calcified. The mean degree of obstruction was reduced from 82% to 21% and maintained this level at 6-month follow-up (HOFLING et al. 1988). SIMPSON et al. (1986) reported on 27 patients with lesions similar to those reported by HOFLING et al. (1988) and noted a stenosis reduction from 79% to 22%. No vascular perforations, significant angiographic dissections, or acute occlusions were noted. Angiography showed the vascular luminal outlines to be smoother than are normally seen with angioplasty. SIMPSON's earlier work in cadaver vessels showed improved lumen size with histologically smooth vessel margins and no evidence of intimal flaps or dissections (SIMPSON et al. 1985). Only one perforation in 410 passes of the catheter was noted in the cadaver study. Calcified or eccentric lesions were as effectively treated as concentric or noncalcified lesions (SIMPSON et al. 1985). SCHWARTEN et al. (1988) indicated that the technique is more time consuming than angioplasty but that primary success (residual stenosis less than 30%) had been achieved in 80% of his patients. Supplemental balloon angioplasty has resulted in a 100% primary success rate and no complications occurred (SCHWARTEN et al. 1988). SIMPSON et al. (1988) recently reported on 61 patients with occlusive peripheral vascular disease who were treated with transluminal atherectomy. Mean percent diameter stenosis was reduced from 71% to 23%. Complications included one thrombus which resolved after intraarterial streptokinase and one probable distal embolization without sequelae. There were no instances of acute occlusion, vascular spasm, or vessel perforations. Six-month follow-up showed that patients with residual stenoses less than 30% after initial atherectomy had a lower restenosis rate (18%) than patients with initial residual stenoses greater than 30% (52%) (SIMPSON et al. 1988).

The Kensey atherectomy catheter operates on a principle much different than that of the Simpson device. In the Kensey catheter, the distal tip contains a miniature cam that rotates at speeds up to 150000 rpm (KENSEY et al. 1987). The cam is driven by an internal torsion-drive wire connected to an external motor/power source. The catheter also contains a channel through which fluid flows under pressure. At the base of the cam, the fluid exits as fine jet sprays that are directed laterally against the vessel wall. The jet cools and lubricates the rotating cam, dilates the artery, and serves to keep the cam centered in the lumen (KENSEY et al. 1987). The combination of the injected saline and rotating cam produces a vortex which is designed to pulverize (5- to 10-μm diameter particles) the atheromatous material. KENSEY first tested his device in diseased (atherosclerotic) superficial femoral artery segments taken from cadavers and xenografted into femoral arteries of dogs. The xenografts were recanalized by advancing the rotating tip gently in a to-and-fro manner through the plaque. Recanalization was successful in all attempts (24 vessels) with only one perforation. The animals were sacrificed within 1–11 days following the procedure. Although small emboli were found in the brain and kidneys, the animals showed no apparent neurological or limb ischemic symptoms. Further studies are needed to better define the degree and potential complications of emboli released during the recanalization process. Embolization of the pulverized material may present a problem, especially since soft tissues (clot, fibrin, vessel wall fragments) do not pulverize into small 5- to 10-μm diameter particles as seems to be the case with harder more calcified materials (COLEMAN, personal communication, 1988). Obviously, more work needs to be completed in evaluating the extent and ramifications of emboli released during intravascular catheter atherectomy. It is of interest to note that WHOLEY and SMOOT (1988) have utilized the Kensey high speed rotational catheter to pulverize and fragment gallstones in the common duct. The catheter is placed through existing T-tubes. This example illustrates the ingenuity of interventional radiologists in applying techniques and devices to multiple clinical conditions.

Other prototype atherectomy devices include a rotating guide wire device with an abrasive (30- to 40-μm diamond particles partially embedded in a nickel substrate head) bullet shaped head (HANSEN et al. 1987), a rotational wire with a blunt tip (designed to wind fibrin around the shaft) (HANSEN et al. 1987), and a rotating atherolytic wire with a distal tip (WHOLEY and SMOOT 1988). The rotating guide wire with the abrasive bullet shaped head (HANSEN et al. 1987) is more amenable for calcified lesions which are more subject to the cutting effect. Preferential cutting of the calcified lesions is analogous to the ability of the vibrating saw to remove an orthopedic cast without cutting skin (HANSEN et al. 1987).

8.9 Evaluating Interventional Procedure Efficacy Using Functional Parameters

Interventional radiologists have often relied on morphological information to access transcatheter therapy. In some instances, this may be sufficient, as is the case for evaluating results following large vessel occlusion of an arteriovenous fistula or embolization to control a major internal bleeding vessel. However, in other instances, functional evaluation may be the best indicator of success. ATHANASOULIS (1983) emphasized the need to combine morphological and functional data in evaluating patients with suspected vascular disease. With the introduction of nuclear magnetic resonance spectroscopy (NMRS) and positron emission tomography (PET), the opportunity exists for using metabolic and functional parameters as indicators of response to therapy. At the present time, investigators are evaluating how these modalities can be used not only to evaluate therapeutic response, but also to monitor delivery of therapy. Future work needs to be directed at evaluating how to make best use of this functional information. In terms of peripheral vascular disease, the endpoint in successful therapy, whether it be vascular surgery, angioplasty, atherectomy, or thrombolytic therapy, is relief of ischemia. ^{31}P-NMR spectroscopy provides a sensitive means to evaluate the metabolic status of limb musculature (TROPP et al. 1988) and its use would complement morphological data obtained from angiography. Limbs are particularly suited for this application, since the high energy phosphate metabolism of muscle provides important information relating to ATP levels, tissue pH, and aerobic-anaerobic metabolism. Since the clinical manifestations of peripheral vascular disease can be expressed as the result of alterations in tissue energy metabolism, ^{31}P-NMR may be a powerful tool to evaluate transcatheter techniques aimed at improving circulation and improving the energy supply/demand status of the tissue.

The use of ^{31}P-NMR to monitor response to therapy for tumors has been proposed by many investigators, including WEHRLE and GLICKSON (1986). In studies performed with subcutaneous rodent tumors, ^{31}P-NMR served as a sensitive indicator to predict metabolic changes related to response following either irradiation or chemotherapy. Information is lacking as to how these rodent studies can be translated to deep seated tumors in humans. Future studies need to be designed to more closely match those that are practical from a clinical point of view. More specific information regarding the use of NMR spectroscopy in monitoring tumor response to therapy is provided in Chap. 6.

Positron emission tomography offers a unique opportunity to evaluate functional data from images. Although concern remains over the degree of availability of PET centers and the significant costs of PET studies, the potential for quantitating blood flow, glucose utilization, and oxygen consumption as monitors of postinterventional procedures is available today. More information on PET application is provided in Chap. 7.

The application of functional evaluations of interventional procedures provides the radiologist with the opportunity to become more involved in the overall care and management of the patient. Interventional radiologists must become more involved in the disease process. "If the tools rather than the disease process becomes our major goal, we will lose credibility and may even suffer erosion of our specialty by nonradiology specialists interested more in the biology of disease. By concentrating on the disease process, we go a long way to dispel any notion that the radiologist is a technician rather than a clinician" (WHITE 1987).

Other potential areas of research combining NMR spectroscopy and interventional radiology include: (1) evaluating efficacy of intraarterial embolization to control tumor growth; (2) evaluating intraarterial vasodilator therapy to relieve localized ischemia, including cardiac ischemia; (3) evaluating improved regional perfusion following vascular occlusion interventions to correct arteriovenous malformations and congenital heart defects.

References

Abela GS, Conti CR (1983) Laser revascularization: what are its prospects? J Cardiovasc Med 8: 977-984
Abela G, Franzini D, Crea F, Pepine CJ, Conti CR (1984) No evidence of accelerated atherosclerosis following laser radiation (abstract). Circulation 70 (Suppl II): 323
Allen MJ, Borody TJ, Bugliosi TF, May GR, LaRusso NF, Thistle JL (1985a) Rapid dissolution of gallstones by methyl tert-butyl ether. N Engl J Med 312: 217-220
Allen MJ, Borody TJ, Bugliosi TF, May GR, LaRusso NF, Thistle JL (1985b) Cholelitholysis using methyl tertiary butyl ether. Gastroenterology 88: 122-125
Allen RA, Pepper DS (1981) Isolation and properties of human vascular plasminogen activator. Thromb Haemost 45: 43-50
Anderson JH, Gianturco C, Wallance S et al. (1982) Preferential coronary arterial drug delivery. Tex Heart Inst J 9: 407-414
Apfelberg DB, Maer MR, Lash H, Rivers J (1981) The argon laser for cutaneous lesions. JAMA 245: 2073-2078

Athanasoulis CA (1983) Morphology vs function: Imaging vs hemodynamic analysis. Vasc Lab Review 1: 2

Babic UU, Dorros G, Pejcic P et al. (1988) Percutaneous mitral valvuloplasty: Retrograde transarterial double balloon technique utilizing the transseptal approach. Cathet Cardiovasc Diagn 14: 229-237

Bachmann F, Kruithof IE (1984) Tissue plasminogen activator: chemical and physiological aspects. Semin Thromb Hemost 10: 6-17

Barth KH, Lutz RJ, Kremers PW et al. (1988) Mixing problems of low flow hepatic artery infusion. Improvement with small caliber double lumen balloon catheters. Invest Radiol 23: 519-523

Bass JL (1988) Catheter-directed interventional procedures in children. In: Castaneda-Zuniga WR, Tadavarthy SM (ed) Interventional radiology. Williams & Wilkins, Baltimore, p 336

Becker CD, Quenville NF, Burhenne HJ (1988) Long-term occlusion of the porcine cystic duct by means of endoluminal radio-frequency electrocoagulation. Radiology 167: 63-68

Becker GJ, Holden RW (1988) Fibrinolytic therapy. In: Castaneda-Zuniga WR, Tadavarthy SM (ed) Interventional radiology. Williams & Wilkins, Baltimore, p 359

Becker CJ, Kopecky KK (1988) Can the newer interventional procedures replace cholecystectomy for cholecystolithiasis? The potential role of percutaneous cystic duct ablation. Radiology 167: 275-279

Bode C, Matsueda GR, Hui KY, Haber E (1985) Antibody-directed urokinase: a specific fibrinolytic agent. Science 229: 765

Bowker TJ (1986) Laser-tissue interaction and arterial perforation thresholds in laser angioplasty. Semin Intervent Radiol 3: 39-46

Burhenne HJ (1973) Nonoperative retained biliary tract stone extraction: A new roentgenologic technique. AJR 117: 388

Butch RJ, MacCarty RL, Mueller PR et al. (1984) Monooctanoin perfusion treatment of intrahepatic calculi. Radiology 153: 375-377

Carson BS, Anderson JH, Grossman SA et al. (1982) An improved rabbit brain tumor model amenable to diagnostic radiographic procedures. Neurosurgery 11: 603-608

Cascino TL, Byrne TN, Deck MDF et al. (1983) Intra-arterial BCNU in the treatment of metastatic brain tumors. J Neurooncol 1: 211-218

Charnsangavej C, Wallace S, Wright KC, Carrasco CH, Gianturco C (1985) Endovascular stent for use in aortic dissection: an in vitro experiment. Radiology 157: 323-324

Charnsangavej C, Carrasco CH, Wallace S, Wright KC, Ogawa K, Richli W, Gianturco C (1986) Stenosis of the vena cava: Preliminary assessment of treatment with expandable metallic stents. Radiology 161: 295-298

Choy DSJ (1986) Laser applications in cardiovascular disease. Semin Intervent Radiol 3: 1-9

Collen D, Verstraete M (1983) Systemic thrombolytic therapy of acute myocardial infarction? Circulation 68: 462-465

Collins JM (1984) Pharmacologic rationale for regional drug delivery. J Clin Oncol 2: 498-504

Corwin RD, Singh AK, Karlson KE (1981) Balloon dilatation of ductus arteriosus in a newborn with interrupted aortic arch and ventricular septal defect. Am Heart J 3: 446-447

Diksic M, Sako K, Feindel W et al. (1984) Pharmacokinetics of positron-labeled 1,3-bis(2-chloroethyl)nitrosourea in human brain tumors using positron emission tomography. Cancer Res 44: 3120-3124

Dotter CT (1969) Transluminally-placed coilspring endarterial tube grafts. Long term patency in canine popliteal artery. Invest Radiol 4: 327-332

Dotter CT, Judkins MP (1964) Transluminal treatment of arteriosclerotic obstruction. Circulation 30: 654-670

Dotter CT, Buschmann RW, McKinney MK, Rosch J (1983) Transluminal expandable and Nitinol coil stent grafting: preliminary report. Radiology 147: 259-260

Doubilet P, Abrams HL (1984) The cost of underutilization: percutaneous transluminal angioplasty for peripheral vascular disease. N Engl J Med 310: 95-102

Driscoll D, Hussleen P, Mullins C (1982) Congenital stenosis of individual pulmonary veins: Clinical spectrum and unsuccessful treatment by transvenous balloon dilatation. Am J Cardiol 49: 1767-1772

Duprat G, Wright KC, Charnsangavej C, Wallace S, Gianturco C (1987a) Self-expanding metallic stents for small vessels: An experimental evaluation. Radiology 162: 469-472

Duprat G, Wright KC, Charnsangavej C, Wallace S, Gianturco C (1987b) Flexible balloon-expanded stent for small vessels. Radiology 162: 276-278

Ensminger WD, Gyves JW (1983a) Regional chemotherapy of neoplastic diseases. Pharmacol Ther 21: 277-293

Ensminger WD, Gyves JW (1983b) Clinical pharmacology of hepatic arterial chemotherapy. Semin Oncol 10: 176-182

Ensminger WD, Gyves JW (1984) Regional cancer chemotherapy. Cancer Treat Rep 68: 101-115

Ensminger WD, Thompson M, Come S et al. (1978a) Hepatic arterial BCNU: A pilot clinical-pharmacologic study in patients with liver tumors. Cancer Treat Rep 62: 1509-1512

Ensminger WD, Rosowsky A, Raso V et al. (1978b) A clinical-pharmacological evaluation of hepatic arterial infusions of 5-fluo 2′-deoxyuridine and 5-fluorouracil. Cancer Res 38: 3784-3792

Fallone BG, Wallace S, Gianturco C (1988) Elastic characteristics of the self-expanding metallic stents. Invest Radiol 23: 370-376

Ferrucci JT (1988) Gallstone ESWL - the first 175 patients. AJR 150: 1231-1233

Foo S, Randohoff J, Berenstein A et al. (1985) Intra-arterial BCNU chemotherapy for malignant gliomas. J Neurosurg 62: 458-459

Fromm H (1986) Gallstone dissolution therapy: current status and future prospects. Gastroenterology 91: 1560-1567

Gardiner GA Jr, Koltun W, Kandarpa K et al. (1986) Thrombolysis of occluded femoropopliteal grafts. AJR 147: 621-626

Gebarski SS, Greenberg HS, Gabrielsen TO et al. (1984) Orbital angiographic changes after intracarotid BCNU chemotherapy. AJNR 5: 55-58

Getrajadman GI, O'Toole K, Laffey KJ, Martin EC (1986) Cystic duct occlusion and transcatheter sclerosis of the gallbladder in the rabbit. Invest Radiol 21: 400-403

Ginsburg R, Wexler L, Mitchell RS, Profitt D (1985) Percutaneous transluminal laser angioplasty for treatment of peripheral vascular disease. Radiology 156: 619-624

Gold HK, Fallon JT, Yasuda T et al. (1984) Coronary thrombolysis with recombinant human tissue-type plasminogen activator. Circulation 70: 700-707

Graor RA, Risius B, Young JR et al. (1986a) Peripheral artery and bypass graft thrombolysis with recombinant human tissue-type plasminogen activator. J Vasc Surg 3: 115-124

Graor RA, Risius B, Lucas FV et al. (1986b) Thrombolysis with recombinant human tissue-type plasminogen activator in patients with peripheral artery and bypass graft occlusions. Circulation 74 (Suppl I): 1-20

Greatbatch W (1986) Engineering aspects of laser irradiation in medicine: An introduction for radiologists. Semin Intervent Radiol 3: 21–25

Greenberg HS, Ensminger WD, Chandler WF et al. (1984) Intra-arterial BCNU chemotherapy for treatment of malignant gliomas of the central nervous system. J Neurosurg 61: 423–429

Grundfest W, Litvack F, Forrester J et al. (1984) Pulsed ultraviolet lasers provide precise control of atheroma ablation (abstract). Circulation 70 (Suppl II): 35

Grundfest WS, Litwack F, Forrester JS et al. (1985) Laser injury of human atherosclerotic plaque without adjacent tissue injury. J Am Coll Cardiol 5: 929–933

Hansen DD, Auth DC, Vracko R et al. (1987) Mechanical thrombectomy: A comparison of two rotational devices and balloon angioplasty in subacute canine femoral thrombosis. Am Heart J 114: 1223–1231

Harbin WP, Ferrucci JT (1980) Nonoperative management of malignant biliary obstruction: a radiologic alternative. AJR 135: 103–107

Healey JE (1965) Vascular patterns in human metastatic liver tumors. Surg Gynecol Obstet 120: 1187

Helgason H, Keane JF, Kulik TJ, Lock JE (1985) Balloon dilation of aortic root in lambs and of valvar aortic stenosis in children (abstract). Circulation 72 (Suppl II): 260

Hiesiger EM, Basler GA, Lipschutz L et al. (1985) Quantitative autoradiographic (QAR) determination of ^{14}C-PCNU concentration [^{14}C-PCNU] in C_6 rat glioma after intracarotid (IC) administration. Proc Am Assoc Cancer Res 26: 349

Hofling B, Backa D, Lauterjung L, Polnitz AV et al. (1988) Percutaneous removal of atheromatous plaques in peripheral arteries. Lancet 1: 384–386

Hoylaerts M, Rijken DC, Lijnen HR, Collen D (1982) Kinetics and the activation of plasminogen by human tissue plasminogen activator: role of fibrin. J Biol Chem 257: 2912–2919

Isner JM, Clarke RH, Donaldson RF et al. (1984a) The excimer laser: gross, light microscopic, and ultrastructural analysis of potential advantages for use in laser therapy of cardiovascular disease (abstract). Circulation 70 (Suppl II): 35

Isner JM, Clarke RH, Pardian NG et al. (1984b) Laser myoplasty for hypertrophic cardiomyopathy: in vitro experience in human postmortem hearts and in vivo experience in a canine model (transarterial) and human patient (intraoperative). Am J Cardiol 53: 1620–1626

Kalman PG, Johnston KW (1985) Outcome of a failed percutaneous transluminal dilatation. Surg Gynecol Obstet 161: 43–46

Kan JS, White RI Jr, Mitchell SE, Gardner TJ (1982) Percutaneous balloon valvuloplasty: A new method for treating congenital pulmonary valve stenosis. N Engl J Med 307: 540–542

Kan JS, White RI Jr, Mitchell SE, Anderson JH, Gardner TJ (1984a) Percutaneous transluminal balloon valvuloplasty for pulmonary valve stenosis. Circulation 69: 554–560

Kan JS, White RI Jr, Mitchell SE, Anderson JH (1984b) Transluminal balloon valvuloplasty for the treatment of pulmonary and aortic valvular stenosis. Semin Intervent Radiol 1: 217–223

Kemeny N, Daly J (1986) Preliminary results of a randomized study of intrahepatic infusions versus systemic infusion of 5-fluoro-21-deoxy-uridine for metastatic colorectal carcinoma. Recent Results Cancer Res 100: 171–178

Kensey KR, Nash JE, Abrahams C, Zarins CK (1987) Recanalization of obstructed arteries with a flexible, rotating tip catheter. Radiology 165: 387–389

Kerber CW, Heilman CB (1985) New calibrated leak microcatheters for cyanoacrylate embolization and chemotherapy. Am J Neuroradiol 6: 434–436

Kerlan RK Jr (1984) Selective fibrinolytic therapy. In: Moss A, Ring E, Higgins C (ed) NMR, CT and interventional radiology. Univ of California Printing Dept, San Francisco, p 133

Kikuchi Y, Strother CM, Boyer M (1987) New catheter for endovascular interventional procedures. Radiology 165: 870–871

Kveselis DA, Rocchini AP, Snider AR et al. (1985) Results of balloon valvuloplasty in the treatment of congenital valvar pulmonary stenosis in children. Am J Cardiol 56: 528

Lababidi Z, Wu J-R (1983) Percutaneous balloon pulmonary valvuloplasty. Am J Cardiol 52: 560–562

Lababidi Z, Wu J-R, Walls JT (1984a) Percutaneous balloon aortic valvuloplasty: Results in 23 patients. Am J Cardiol 53: 194–197

Lababidi ZA, Daskalopoulos DA, Stoeckle H Jr (1984b) Transluminal balloon coarctation angioplasty: Experience with 27 patients. Am J Cardiol 54: 1288–1291

Labs JD, White RI, Anderson JH, Williams GM (1987a) Thermodynamic correlates of hot tip laser angioplasty. Invest Radiol 22: 954–959

Labs JD, White RI, Anderson JH, Perler BA, Williams GM (1987b) Laser thrombectomy and arterial prosthetic graft recanalization. Surg Forum 38: 326–328

Labs JD, Caslowitz PL, Anderson JH et al. (1988) Experimental treatment of thrombotic vascular disease. J Vasc Surg (in press)

Lammer J, Pilger E, Kleinert R, Ascher PW (1987) Laserangioplastic peripherer arterieller Verschlüsse. Roentgenstr 147: 1–5

Lammer J, Pilger E, Kleinert R (1988) Laser angioplasty by sapphire contact probe. Experimental and clinical results. J Intervent Radiol 3: 53–58

Lee G, Ikeda RM, Chan ML (1984) Dissolution of human atherosclerotic disease by fiberoptic laser-heated metal cautery cap. Am Heart J 107: 777–778

Lee G, Ikeda RM, Chan MC et al. (1985) Limitations, risks and complications of laser recanalization: a cautious approach warranted. Am J Cardiol 56: 181–185

Lee G, Chan MC, Ikeda RM et al. (1986) The status and future of laser angioplasty. Semin Intervent Radiol 3: 11–19

Levin V, Kabra P (1975) Brain and tumor pharmacokinetics of BCNU and CCNU following I.V. and intracarotid artery (I.C.A.) administration. Proc Am Assoc Cancer Res 16: 19

Lock JE, Niemi T, Einzig S, Amplatz K, Burke B, Bass JL (1981) Transvenous angioplasty of experimental branch pulmonary artery stenosis in newborn lambs. Circulation 64: 886–893

Lock JE, Khalilullah M, Shrivistava S, Bahl V, Keane JF (1985) Percutaneous catheter commissurotomy in rheumatic mitral stenosis. N Engl J Med 313: 1515

Luft HS, Bunker JP, Enthoven AC (1979) Should operations be regionalized? The empirical relation between surgical volume and mortality. N Engl J Med 301: 1364–1369

Lund G, Rysavy J, Cragg A, Salomonowitz E, Vlodaver Z, Castaneda-Zuniga W, Amplatz K (1984) Long-term patency of the ductus arteriosus after balloon dilatation: An experimental study. Circulation 69: 772–774

Lutz RJ, Dedrick RL, Boretos JW et al. (1986) Mixing studies during intracarotid artery infusions in an in vitro model. J Neurosurg 64: 277–283

Maizel AS, Bookstein JJ (1986) Streptokinase, urokinase, and tissue plasminogen activator. Pharmacokinetics, relative advantages, and methods for maximizing rates and consistency of lysis. Cardiovasc Intervent Radiol 9: 236-244

Marshall TC (1985) Free electron lasers. Macmillan, New York, pp 1-5

Matsuo O, Collen DC (1981) Comparison of the relative fibrinogenolytic, fibrinolytic and thrombolytic properties of tissue plasminogen activator and urokinase in vitro. Thromb Haemost 45: 225

Mayhew E (1988) Selective drug delivery systems. Invest Radiol 23: 229-231

McGahan JP, Lester LL, Tesluk H (1987) Dissolution of gallstones using cholecystectomy in the pig. Invest Radiol 22: 201-205

McLean GK, Ring EJ, Freiman DB (1982) Therapeutic alternatives in the treatment of intrahepatic biliary obstruction. Radiology 145: 289-295

McNamara TO, Fischer JR (1985) Thrombolysis of peripheral arterial and graft occlusions: improved results using high-dose urokinase. AJR 144: 769-775

Miller DL, Schneider PD, Gianola FJ et al. (1984) Assessment of perfusion patterns during hepatic artery infusion chemotherapy: EOA-13CT and ^{99m}Tc-MAA scintigraphy. AJR 143: 827-831

Mitchell SE, White RI, Kan JS et al. (1984) Improved balloons for large vessel and valvular angioplasty. AJR 142: 571-572

Mitchell SE, Kan JS, Anderson JH et al. (1986) Atrial septostomy: Stationary angioplasty balloon technique. Pediatr Res 20: 173 A

Mori K, Misumi A, Sugiyama M et al. (1977) Percutaneous transhepatic bile drainage. Ann Surg 185: 111

Mullins CE, O'Laughlin M, Vick W et al. (1988) Implantation of balloon-expandable intravascular grafts by catheterization in pulmonary arteries and systemic veins. Circulation 77: 188-199

Ohnishi K, Shiyiro S, Nomura F et al. (1987) Arterial chemoembolization followed by transcatheter hepatic artery embolization for hepatocellular carcinomas. Am J Gastroenterol 82: 876-879

Palmaz JC (1988) Balloon expandable intravascular stents. AJR 150: 1263-1269

Palmaz JC, Sibbitt RR, Reuter SR, Tio FO, Rice WJ (1985a) Expandable intraluminal graft: a preliminary study. Radiology 156: 73-77

Palmaz JC, Sibbitt RR, Reuter SR, Garcia F, Tio FO (1985b) Expandable intrahepatic portocaval shunt stents: early experience in the dog. AJR 145: 821-825

Palmaz JC, Sibbitt RR, Tio FO, Reuter SR, Peters JE, Garcia F (1986a) Expandable intraluminal vascular graft: A feasibility study. Surgery 99: 199-205

Palmaz JC, Windeler SA, Garcia F, Tio FO, Sibbitt RR, Reuter SR (1986b) Atherosclerotic rabbit aortas: Expandable intraluminal grafting. Radiology 160: 723-726

Palmaz JC, Kopp DT, Hayashi H et al. (1987) Normal and stenotic renal arteries: Experimental balloon-expandable intraluminal stenting. Radiology 164: 705-708

Palmaz JC, Richter GM, Noeldge G et al. (1988) Intraluminal stents in atherosclerotic iliac artery stenosis: Preliminary report of a multicenter study. Radiology 168: 727-731

Porstmann W, Wierny L, Warnke H (1967) Der Verschluß des Ductus arteriosus persistens ohne Thorakotomie. 1. Mitteilung. Thoraxchirurgie 15: 199-203

Puel J, Juilliere Y, Bertrand M et al. (1988) Early and late assessment of stenosis geometry after coronary arterial stenting. Am J Cardiol 61: 546-553

Ranby M (1982) Studies on kinetics of plasminogen activation by tissue plasminogen activator. Biochim Biophys Acta 704: 461-469

Rashkind WJ, Miller WW (1966) Creation of an atrial septal defect without thoracotomy; palliative approach to complete transposition of the great arteries. JAMA 196: 991

Remley KB, Cubberley DA, Watanabe AS, Nelson JA, Colby TV (1986) Systemic absorption of gallbladder sclerosing agents in the rabbit: A preliminary study. Invest Radiol 21: 396-399

Rijken DC, Collen D (1981) Purification and characterization of the plasminogen activator secreted by human melanoma cells in culture. J Biol Chem 256: 7035-7041

Ring EJ (1984) Interventional biliary procedures. In: Moss A, Ring E, Higgins C (ed) NMR, CT and interventional radiology. Univ of California Printing Dept, San Francisco, p 159

Ring EJ, Oleaga JA, Freiman DB et al. (1978) Therapeutic applications of catheter cholangiography. Radiology 128: 333

Risius B, Graor RA, Geisinger MA et al. (1986) Recombinant human tissue-type plasminogen activator for thrombolysis in peripheral arteries and bypass grafts. Radiology 160: 183-188

Risius B, Graor RA, Geisinger MA, Zelch MG, Lucas FV, Young JR (1987) Thrombolytic therapy with recombinant human tissue-type plasminogen activator: A comparison of two doses. Radiology 164: 465-468

Roberts WC (1987) Good-bye to thoracotomy for cardiac valvulotomy. Am J Cardiol 59: 198-201

Rocchini AP, Kveselis D (1984) The use of balloon angioplasty in the pediatric patient. Pediatr Clin North Am 31: 1293-1305

Rosch J, Uchida B, Putnam JE et al. (1987) Expandable Gianturco stents in experimental intrahepatic portocaval anastomosis. Radiology 162: 481-485

Ruppin DC, Dowling RH (1982) Is recurrence inevitable after gallstone dissolution by bile-acid treatment? Lancet I: 181-185

Sackmann M, Delius M, Sauerbruch T et al. (1988) Shockwave lithotripsy of gallbladder stones. The first 175 patients. N Engl J Med 318: 393-396

Salomonowitz E, Frick MP, Simmons RL et al. (1984) Obliteration of the gallbladder without formal cholecystectomy. Arch Surg 119: 725-729

Sanborn TA, Haudenschild CC, Faxon DP, Ryan TJ (1985) Experimental angioplasty 1985: circumferential distribution of laser thermal energy with a laser probe. J Am Coll Cardiol 5: 934-938

Sasahara AA (1988) Fundamentals of fibrinolytic therapy. Cardiovasc Intervent Radiol 11: 53-55

Schatz RA, Palmaz JC, Tio FD et al. (1987) Balloon expandable intracoronary stents in the adult dog. Circulation 76 (Suppl 2): 450-457

Schoenfield LJ, Lachin JM, Baum RA et al. (1981) Chenodiol (chenodeoxycholic acid) for dissolution of gallstones: The national cooperative gallstone study. Ann Intern Med 95: 257-282

Schwarten DE, Katzen BT, Simpson JB, Cutcliff WB (1988) Simpson catheter for percutaneous transluminal removal of atheroma. AJR 150: 799-801

Shapiro WR, Green SB, Burger PC et al. (1987) A randomized comparison of intraarterial (IA) vs intravenous (IV) BCNU for patients with malignant glioma (Study 8301): INTERIM analysis demonstrating lack of efficacy for IA BCNU. Proc Am Soc Clin Oncol 6: 69

Shingleton BJ, Bienfang DC, Albert DM et al. (1982) Ocular toxicity associated with high-dose carmustine. Arch Ophthalmol 100: 1766–1772

Sigwart V, Puel J, Mirkovitch V, Joffre F, Kappenberger L (1987) Intravascular stents to prevent occlusion and restenosis after transluminal angioplasty. N Engl J Med 316: 701–706

Simon M, Kaplow R, Salzman E, Freiman D (1977) A vena cava filter using thermal shape memory alloy. Radiology 125: 89

Simpson JB, Johnson DE, Thapliyal HV et al. (1985) Transluminal atherectomy: A new approach to the treatment of atherosclerotic vascular disease. Circulation 72 (Suppl II): 146

Simpson JB, Zimmerman JJ, Selman MR et al. (1986) Transluminal atherectomy: Initial clinical results in 27 patients. Circulation 74 (Suppl II): 203

Simpson JB, Selman MR, Robertson GC et al. (1988) Transluminal atherectomy for occlusive peripheral vascular disease. Am J Cardiol 61: 966–1016

Spears JR (1986) Percutaneous laser treatment of atherosclerosis: An overview of emerging techniques. Cardiovasc Intervent Radiol 9: 303–312

Stagg RJ, Lewis RJ, Freedman MA et al. (1984) Hepatic arterial chemotherapy for colorectal cancer metastatic to the liver. Ann Intern Med 100: 736–743

Strecker EP, Berg G, Schneider B, Freudenberg N, Weber H, Wolf RD (1988) A new vascular balloon-expandable prosthesis – Experimental studies and first clinical results. J Intervent Radiol 3: 59–62

Sutton CS, Oku T, Harasaki H et al. (1988) Titanium-nickel intravascular endoprothesis: A 2-year study in dogs. AJR 151: 597–601

Tennant S, Dixon J, Venable TC et al. (1984) Intracoronary thrombolysis in patients with acute myocardial infarction: Comparison of the efficacy of urokinase with streptokinase. Circulation 69: 756–760

Teplick SK, Haskin PH (1984) Monooctanoin perfusion for in vivo dissolution of biliary stones. Radiology 153: 379–383

Thistle JL (1987) Direct contact dissolution of gallstones. Semin Liver Dis 7: 311–316

Thomsen DE (1983) A possible x-ray lasing transition. Sci News 124: 197

Thorsen S, Glas-Greenwalt P, Astrup T (1972) Differences in the binding to fibrin of urokinase and tissue plasminogen activator. Thromb Diath Haemorrh 28: 65–74

Tropp JS, Sugiura S, Derby KA et al. (1988) Characterization of MR spectroscopic imaging of the human head and limb at 2.OT. Radiology 169: 207–212

Uchida BT, Putnam JS, Rosch J (1988) Modifications of Gianturco expandable wire stents. AJR 150: 1185–1187

VandeWerf F, Bergmann SR, Fox KAA et al. (1984) Coronary thrombolysis with intravenously administered human tissue-type plasminogen activator produced by recombinant DNA technology. Circulation 69: 605–610

vanSonnenberg E, Casola G (1988) Interventional radiology 1988. Invest Radiol 23: 75–92

vanSonnenberg E, Hofmann AF (1988) Horizons in gallstone therapy – 1988. AJR 150: 43–46

vanSonnenberg E, Hofmann AF, Neoptolemus J, Wittich GR, Princenthal RA, Willson SW (1986) Gallstone dissolution with methyl-tert-butyl ether via percutaneous cholecystectomy: Success and caveats. AJR 146: 865–867

Wallace S, Charnsangavej C, Carrasco CH et al. (1984) Percutaneous transcatheter infusion and infarction in the treatment of human cancer. Current Probl Cancer 8(18): 1–76

Walls JT, Lababidi Z, Curtis JJ, Silver D (1984) Assessment of percutaneous balloon pulmonary and aortic valvuloplasty. J Thorac Cardiovasc Surg 88: 352

Wehrle JP, Glickson JD (1986) ^{31}P-NMR spectroscopy of tumors in vivo. Cancer Biochem Biophys 8: 157–166

White RI (1987) Interventional radiology: Reflections and expectations. Radiology 162: 593–600

White RI, Mitchell SE, Kan J (1986a) Interventional procedures in congenital heart disease. Cardiovasc Intervent Radiol 9: 286–298

White RI Jr, Kan JS, Anderson JH (1986b) Hemodynamics of experimental aortic balloon valvuloplasty. J Pediatr Res 20: 176A

Wholey MH, Smoot S (1988) Choledocholithiasis: Percutaneous pulverization with a high-speed rotational catheter. AJR 150: 129–130

Wierny L, Plass R, Porstmann W (1986) Transluminal closure of patent ductus arteriosus: Long term results of 208 cases treated without thoracotomy. Cardiovasc Intervent Radiol 9: 279–285

Wright KC, Wallace S, Charnsangavej C, Carrasco CH, Gianturco C (1985) Percutaneous endovascular stents: an experimental evaluation. Radiology 156: 69–72

Wright KC, Wallace S, Kim EE et al. (1986) Pulsed arterial infusion: Chemotherapeutic implications. Cancer 57: 1952–1956

Zaret MM, Ripps H, Siegel IM, Breinin GM (1963) Laser photocoagulation of the eye. Arch Ophthalmol 69: 97–104

Zigiang L, Shanxiong X, Xinian H et al. (1986) Selective bronchial arterial infusion of cisplatin for inoperable bronchiogenic carcinoma. J Intervent Radiol 1: 57–62

Zollikofer CL, Largiader I, Bruhlmann WF et al. (1988) Endovascular stenting of veins and grafts: Preliminary clinical experience. Radiology 167: 707–712

9 Ultrasound

Frank P. Leo

CONTENTS

9.1 Introduction 155
9.2 Early Scanners (Static Devices) 156
9.2.1 Bistable Systems 156
9.2.2 Analog Scan Converters 156
9.2.3 Digital Scan Converters 156
9.2.4 Processing Improvement 156
9.3 Static Scanners (Digital) 157
9.3.1 Image Improvement 157
9.3.2 Changes in Manufacturing with Respect to Power Output 157
9.4 Early Real Time Transducer Developments 157
9.4.1 Linear Array Devices 157
9.4.2 Mechanical Sector 157
9.5 Modern Real Time Transducers 158
9.5.1 Dynamic Focus and Selectable Focus 158
9.5.2 Newer Linear Array Technology 158
9.5.3 Phased Array Technology 159
9.6 What Does the Present Technology Hold? 159
9.7 Present Modes of Operation 160
9.7.1 M-mode 160
9.7.2 Doppler 160
9.7.3 Color Flow 162
9.7.4 Spectral Analysis 164
9.8 Intracavity Transducers 164
9.9 Planned Obsolescence 165
9.10 What Does the Future Hold? 166
References 167

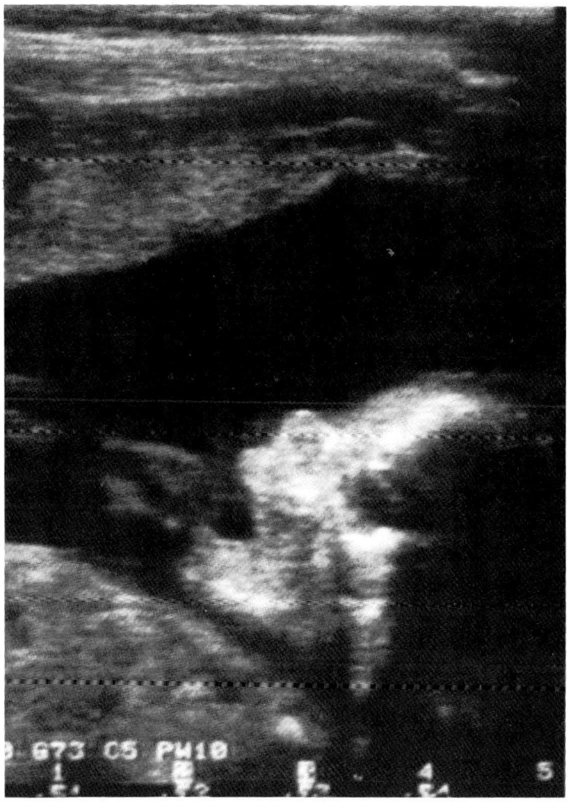

Fig. 1. 5-MHz linear array image of a fetal face. (Courtesy of Corometrics/Aloka Ultrasound)

9.1 Introduction

An early World War II development (called sonar) is presently providing images that display new life for anxious mothers prior to their normal fetal birth (Fig. 1). Ultrasound studies provide a dependable imaging modality without the utilization of ionizing radiation. Because of this, ultrasound is finding many new areas of application besides prenatal examination. Ultrasound studies of internal organs, such as liver, gallbladder, kidney, and heart, have been shown to provide information equal to and in some cases even better than other imaging modalities. Adding the ability to view moving structures in real time as well as to quantify blood flow through arteries and veins provides an extremely flexible diagnostic modality that challenges many of the other diagnostic modalities as the preferred method of examination. In addition, the introduction of smaller transducer assemblies has added a new dimension for intracavity work for prostate evaluation and for endovaginal examinations to evaluate many pelvic pathology conditions. Truly this modality offers many advantages to the physician for performing a large variety of tests using the same basic instrument but having a wide assortment of special transducers, each engineered for a specific function. The development of ultrasound in the last 5 years

Frank P. Leo, Sr. E. E., Dept. of Radiology and Radiological Science, The Johns Hopkins University, School of Medicine, 600 North Wolfe Street, Baltimore, MD 21205, USA has exploded into many facets. It has always been a prime diagnostic modality, but now it is being used for treatment (deep heating by sonic waves), for steering of other energies (kidney and gallstone lithotripsy), for cosmetic cleaning (dental teeth cleaning devices), and for determination of subsurface structures (sizmatology). It will be a very interesting modality to watch for the next few years to determine what other areas it will evolve into.

9.2 Early Scanners (Static Devices)

9.2.1 Bistable Systems

In order to appreciate the capabilities of the newer ultrasound systems, it is important to understand how this modality has developed over the years. The early systems were called "bistable static devices" because they generated one image having only two levels of contrast (black and white). If the intensity of the returned echo from an interface came up to a predefined level, it was recorded as a black dot on a white background (or in accordance with the present accepted nomenclature, as a selection of a negative image; conversely a positive image is defined as a white dot on a black background). If the amplitude of the returned echo did not reach this predefined level it was discarded and not recorded. This bistable system generated the maximum number of accepted levels from tissue interfaces separating tissues with maximum differences in acoustic impedance. In almost all cases this represented boundaries of different density tissues. Therefore this system was mainly used to outline and define the borders of different organs within the body.

9.2.2 Analog Scan Converters

Later developments of gray scale imaging proved that over 95% of the reflected imaging information from the bistable systems was being discarded. The development of the analog storage tube scan converter provided a means to accumulate and store analog intensities over a wide range of amplitudes as well as a means to "compound" scan, which enabled the sonographer to enhance low level echo areas of interest by scanning over the same area a few times and summating the information obtained. These systems provided a wide dynamic range gray scale, but the contrast resolution would tend to drift on a daily basis because of brightness/contrast changes in the analog storage tube of the scan converter. This constituted a major problem that led to the demise of this type of system because the gray level on the CRT display for a given tissue density would change from day to day. In addition, the noise content of the analog systems made it impossible to obtain low level echoes. The development of the digital scan converter corrected these problems, but introduced other problems that had to be rectified.

9.2.3 Digital Scan Converters

The digital scan converter did not have as wide a dynamic range as the analog scan converter but it did correct the brightness/contrast drift problem of the earlier analog system. This correction provided some assurance that the same area of the same body that displayed a given imaged density (gray scale) one day would appear to be the same density when imaged on other days. The limited dynamic range was corrected by changing the contrast resolution to eight bits deep. The resultant contrast quality was sufficient to produce images with enough gray tone variations to be very acceptable. The standard data format of 512×512 pixels provided adequate spatial resolution to produce diagnostic quality images.

9.2.4 Processing Improvement

With the added features of "pre-" and "post-"processing, static digital imaging systems provided the ability to tailor the digital processor to provide a better interpretation of the density values that were of interest for that particular study. If tissue values were of concern, a linear response scale was used. If bone or high echogenic areas were of concern, a response curve that provided enhancements to the upper gray/white values (with positive imaging selected) was used. If low level echo areas were of concern, a response curve that enhanced this lower segment of the darker gray/black tones was employed. In addition, selection of the response curves could be accomplished before (pre) or after (post) the scan had been completed.

9.3 Static Scanners (Digital)

9.3.1 Image Improvement

The first digital scan converter systems provided a method of acquiring an image with characteristics much different than previously available. These newer images had more contrast, were noisier (grainier), and would have missing lines (transmissions) if the operator moved the ultrasonic probe too fast. In addition, if smaller areas were magnified, the images would have a "building block" appearance similar to a mosaic image. However, this system provided an image that had a wider contrast resolution (many more gray tones were appreciated) and, as mentioned above, was reproducible when the same area of the body was imaged on different days. This last benefit was instrumental in convincing the medical community to accept digital images. The other disadvantages were partially overcome by changing the sonographers' scanning techniques and by more critical adjustment to the imaging hard copy unit (Polaroid camera or multiformat camera).

9.3.2 Changes in Manufacturing with Respect to Power Output

The early digital static scanning system had means of controlling the power output from the transducer. This was accomplished by varying the drive voltage to the crystal element that produced the transmission of intensity into the patient's body. With this method, the ultrasonic power to the patient could be controlled. A large person who required higher power for adequate transmission of sonic energy could be scanned at a higher output. A small child who needed much less power could be scanned at a very low drive voltage. The images were acceptable diagnostically, but as was mentioned in the above paragraph, they were "grainy." In order to provide a smoother and more pleasing image, the manufacturer made changes in the drive system to the crystal. These changes maximized the drive voltage to the crystal, making it constantly transmit at its maximum output, and controlled the received echo energy by varying the gain of the receiver amplifier. These changes provided "signal conditioning" (corrections and enhancements to the original signal discarding unwanted noise pulses) based on one level of transmitted power. The problem of grainy images was corrected, but fetus and small patients were being exposed to the same power output as a 250-lb. person. This approach has remained in effect for all gray scale B-scanners. With the development of more sophisticated real time computer based systems, this signal conditioning correction (based on the selected power output level) was capable of handling up to four different selections of power. These were either in a selected "db" ("0" attenuation, "- 3 db," "- 6 db," or "- 9 db") or in a coded number (0, 1, 2, or 3) that signified maximum output (100%) and lower predetermined attenuation steps to reduce the power by assigned steps.

9.4 Early Real Time Transducer Developments

9.4.1 Linear Array Devices

The first real time device was a crude but reliable linear array system. This device produced a rectangular shaped image that was presented as a longer than wider image on a CRT display (Leo 1983). This image consisted of 60 vertical lines of information generated by a transducer having 64 crystal elements. The firing sequence of this transducer was not all at one time but in sets of four crystals at a time (crystals 1 through 4 would first be fired). Echoes were accumulated to form one line of information on the display CRT and then the firing sequence would move down the transducer crystals by one crystal and fire the next four crystals (crystals 2 through 5) to acquire one more line of information. Firing the crystals in this "quad fire-step-by-one" fashion produced the 60 lines of information that made up an image.

9.4.2 Mechanical Sector

Another early type of real time transducer was the single element (19 mm diameter) crystal that was swept mechanically back and forth (using an electric motor) over a 90° angle and produced a series of images that were overlaid using a frame rate of 10 - 30 frames per second. This device produced a chevron type display that generated an increased line spreading distortion as the CRT display showed deeper areas from within the body. Spreading of the transmission lines on the display, as deeper areas of interest were presented, caused large inaccuracies in the horizontal plane. Therefore any measurement taken horizontally (i.e., femur lengths for fetal ageing) was found to be in error which was dependent on how deep within the chevron display the measurement was taken. Errors as small as 3% or 4% over a 10 cm depth and as large as 10%–12% over the same 10 cm were found to be associated with the early mechanical single element scanning devices.

9.5 Modern Real Time Transducers

9.5.1 Dynamic Focus and Selectable Focus

Real time ultrasound systems using the long linear array (with its quad fire-step-by-one fashion) or the mechanical sector device provided the diagnostician with a means to improve the speed at which images were acquired. However, the quality of the images was not greatly improved. They suffered from a lack of focus, poor spatial resolution, poor dynamic range, poor axial and lateral resolution, and poor size measurements (especially using sector transducers).

The focal zone for the early linear array system was dependent upon the physical size of the crystal elements within the transducer assembly. When four elements were fired, their combined diameter determined where the focal zone would appear, similar to the way that a single element static device transducer of a diameter of 19 mm will focus deeper than a 13 mm diameter transducer of the same frequency. Therefore, the focal zone could be controlled by the diameter of the transmitting elements. If only three crystal elements were selected from this same linear array, it would be expected that the focal zone would be closer to the transducer face. If five elements were selected, then it would be expected that the focal zone would be deeper than either the three or four element firings. If the selection of the firing sequence were controlled by the near field/far field adjustments that the sonographer has to make in order to emphasize the area of interest, then a dependable means would be found to provide both adequate penetration and best focus to the area of interest (five crystal element diameters will penetrate deeper than three crystal element diameters). This was accomplished by the early linear array systems and called "dynamic focus," because the focal area could be adjusted by the sonographer to appear at the area of interest (near field: three firing sequences; mid field: four firing sequences; far field: five firing sequences).

When a single element mechanical sector device is constructed, its focal zone is determined by the diameter and frequency of the crystal element and is made to have its best focus in the center of the chevron display. That means for a 5-MHz mechanical sector, the focal zone will be fixed (not adjustable) from about 2 to 5 cm, while for a 3.5-MHz mechanical sector, the fixed focal zone will be from about 3 to 7 cm dependent upon the fixed focus lens attached to the crystal.

Because of their multielement all-electronic construction, newer ultrasound transducers (both linear and phased array sector devices) provide three or four "selectable focal zones" that are controlled by the operator. These zones are determined by the number of crystal elements that are designed to be fired for a near, mid, or far field focal zone. In addition, dynamic focus is also available by a multifocal zone selection where the number of elements fired will cycle through and alternately fire from the smaller number (near focus) through to the larger number (far focus) to provide a long focal area display. This newer technological development has corrected the earlier system's lack of focus for the area of interest and improved axial and lateral resolution throughout the imaging field. Other developments have provided additional corrections which will be discussed below.

9.5.2 Newer Linear Array Technology

The newer linear array transducers have corrected poor spatial resolution by providing more lines of information to the image. The earlier linear array system had only 60 lines of information which produced an image with space between each transmission line. The newer devices provide 128 lines of information over the same image area as was covered by the earlier linear array systems, thereby "filling in" information into those missing line areas. This fill-in yields images that are more uniform, both spatially and contrast wise, and coupled with the dynamic focus capability provides a marked increase in both axial and lateral resolution, broadens the dynamic range of the contrast scale, and provides a more uniform focus for imaging structures deep within the body. In addition, because of the resolution and better focus capabilities of these newer linear array systems, higher frequency devices are manufactured to evaluate near field areas. "Small parts" devices have been used for carotid (Fig. 2), thyroid, and breast (Fig. 3) examinations (Dempsey 1988), and the standard 3.5-MHz linear array system has always been the system of choice for fetal examination. Many of these im-

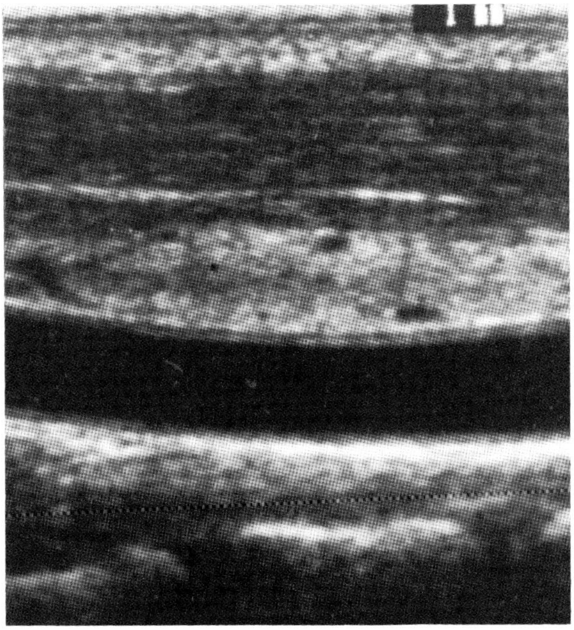

Fig. 2. 7.5-MHz high resolution linear array image of a common carotid artery, showing excellent wall detail. (Courtesy of Advances Technology Laboratories, Inc.)

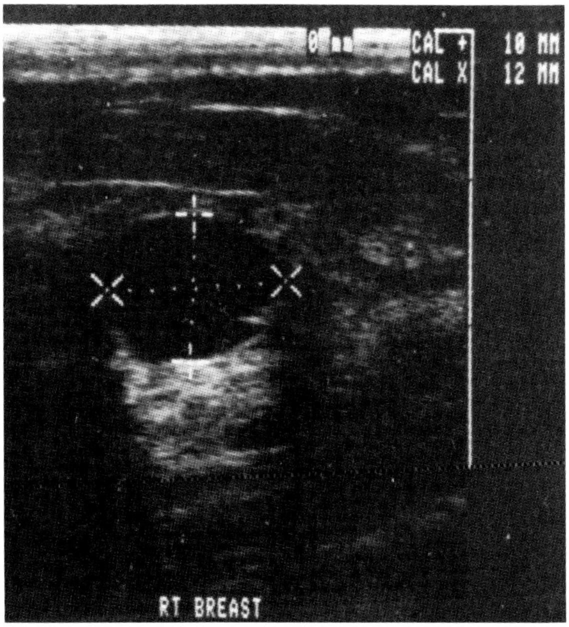

Fig. 3. 7.5-MHz high resolution linear array image of a cystic mass of the right breast, showing accurate 2D caliper measurement. (Courtesy of Advanced Technology Laboratories, Inc.)

provements are to be attributed to advances in both hardware and software: hardware because the digital scan converter has 128 parallel channels to capture information quickly and display an image made from 128 lines, and software because fast algorithms are provided to convert and enhance the data to yield a higher gain, lower noise image. The 128 parallel channels have also helped clear up problems associated with the sector device.

9.5.3 Phased Array Technology

With the development of the all-electronic phased array sector scanning device the final problems that were noted in the early development sector systems have been corrected. These problems included the horizontal distortions in measurements taken deeper in the chevron display and the "flaring-out" of the transmission lines as they moved away from the vertex of the chevron display causing noted spaces between transmission lines as one viewed deeper in the chevron display. With the generation of 128 lines of information accumulated from each frame of the scan, the line separation problem has been corrected (improved spatial resolution). The scan converter's ability to capture and store 128 parallel channels in a square format, even though it is collected in a sector format, provides the line correction necessary to produce the accurate horizontal measurements throughout the field in either direction. The displaying of sector information out of the square scan converter and presenting it on the screen as a chevron display make it possible for accurate caliper measurements to be taken to compute distance.

9.6 What Does the Present Technology Hold?

All of the above noted problems that were associated with dependable and accurate imaging have been corrected and new technology using these newer and more accurate means is emerging daily. The use of the all-electronic multielement transducer devices (linear and phased array sector) has provided the means to acquire faster imaging and controlled functions that are observed for multitasking purposes as seen in simultaneous two-dimensional (2D) and Doppler presentations (Fig. 4).

Faster and larger computer based systems have been devised to push the state of the art in acquisition and reconstruction of images at a very fast rate. At present the 128 parallel channels used to acquire data seem to be sufficient for good spatial resolution and for the update speed for image generation. Some manufacturers may increase the number of

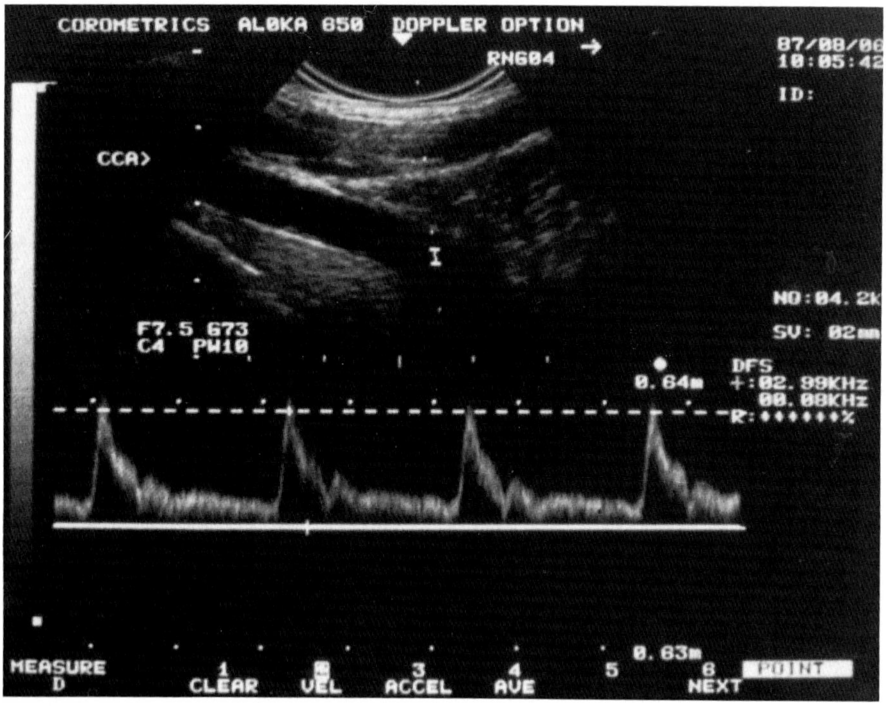

Fig. 4. 7.5-MHz duplex scan of the common carotid artery showing sample volume area *(I)* and location of sample. (Courtesy of Corometrics/Aloka Ultrasound)

channels and still provide many more multitasking capabilities because the relative speed of operation of many of the computer based systems has been increased by newer designs of transistor packs. The physical size of the computer boards has been reduced but the speed and data handling capacity have greatly increased. The physical size of sonographic equipment has been reduced but the capability of handling more data has produced small portable systems with multitasking and good imaging capabilities.

These new developed technologies have contributed greatly to the development of the multifunctional ultrasound system.

9.7 Present Modes of Operation

9.7.1 M-mode

One of the primary methods to view moving interfaces is M-mode ultrasound. With this type of study, one transmission line from an imaging transducer is selected to portray the echo interfaces that are collected for that transmission and displayed on a strip chart or on a CRT screen (Fig. 5). The data that are displayed represent the one line accumulation of all the interfaces that are stationary or have motion during that transmission period. As each transmission collects its interface data and displays the data on the strip chart with its own time reference, variations in the position of echos are recognized as motion displacements. This modality is generally used to evaluate arterial and ventricular wall or atrioventricular valve motion. This feature has also been employed to evaluate fetal heart motion prior to term.

9.7.2 Doppler

The ability to determine two very important pieces of information with respect to arterial flow is the basis for a Doppler study. The direction and flow velocity in an artery or vein can be determined from the Doppler effect (Magnin 1986; Halberg and Thiele 1986). An ultrasound beam of a given frequency is transmitted into the body at a known angle and is then reflected from a moving interface such as the red cells flowing in the blood of an artery or vein. The reflected sound wave will differ in frequency from the transmitted wave in accordance to whether the flow is toward the transducer or away from the transducer. If the flow is toward the transducer, the reflected frequency will be higher than the transmitted frequency. If the flow is away from the transducer, the reflected frequency will be

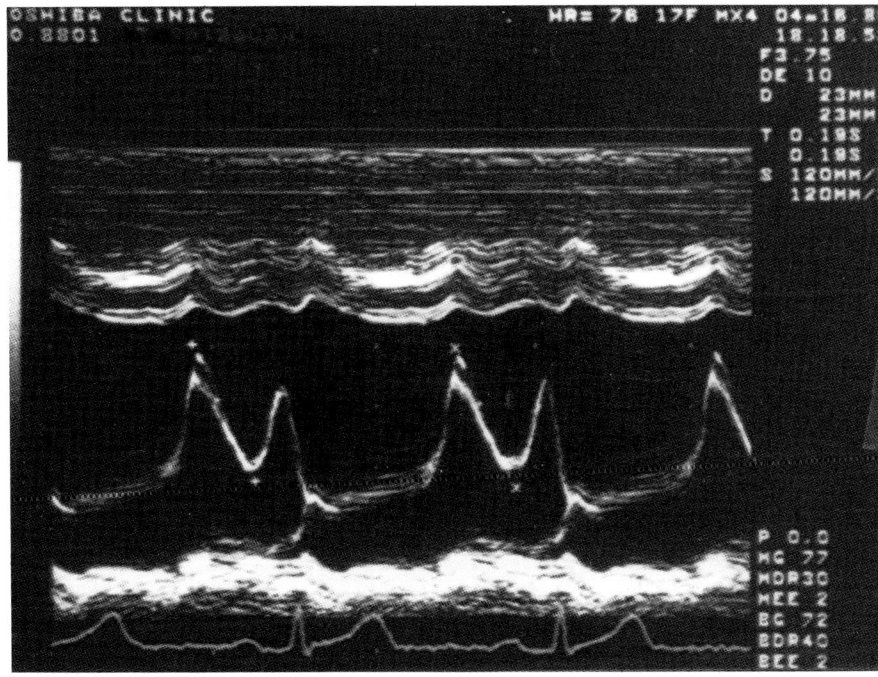

5

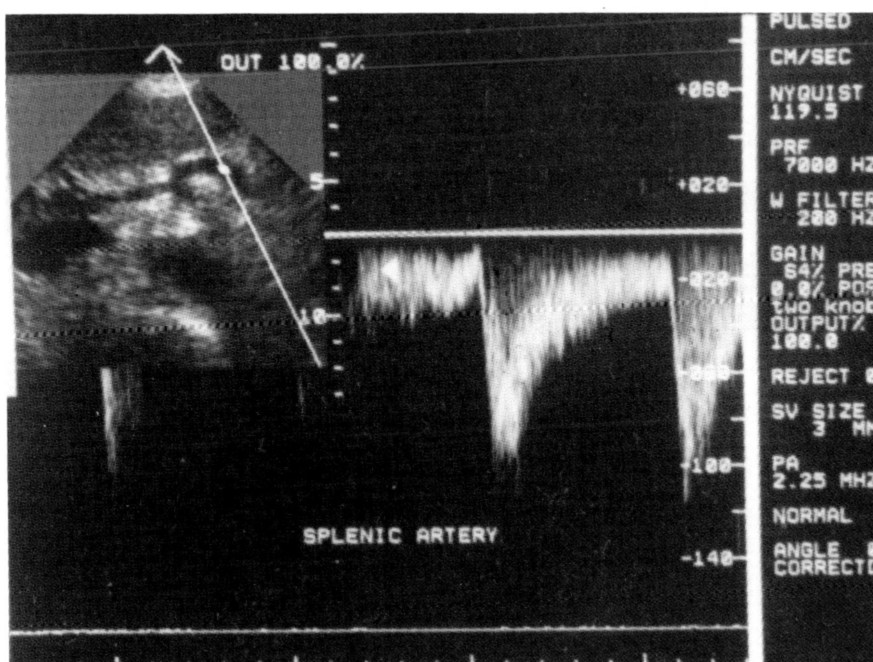

6

Fig. 5. CRT displayed M-mode study of a circulatory investigation. In the "frozen" mode, the distance between two points, the time and slope, can be determined. (Courtesy of Toshiba America, Inc.)

Fig. 6. Simultaneous duplex display of splenic artery by pulsed Doppler showing 3 mm sample volume location, size, and angle. (Courtesy of Advanced Technology Laboratories, Inc.)

lower than the transmitted frequency. The difference in the offset frequency from the original frequency is a function of the velocity of the flow. A small proportional offset is the result of a slow velocity flow; a large proportional offset is the result of a fast velocity flow. These data determine the blood flow direction (+ or − the original frequency) and velocity (the difference in the frequency of offset) (Fig. 6).

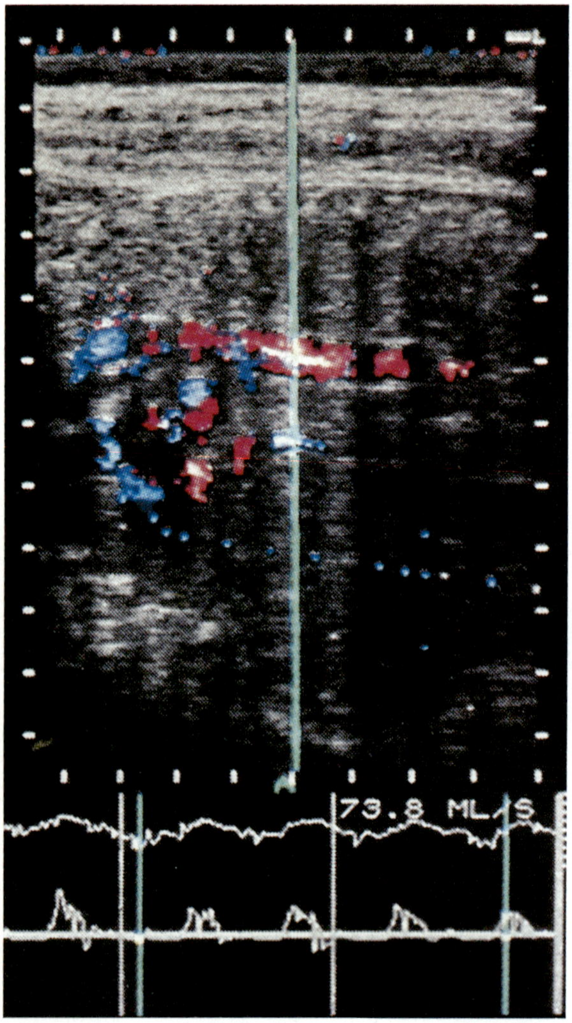

Fig. 7. Volume color flow measurements on a fetal dorsal aorta showing sample area and location as well as reverse flow indications. (Courtesy of Quantum Medical Systems, Inc.)

Earlier Doppler systems using a single element sector scanning device could not provide simultaneous 2D imaging and Doppler information. The 2D image was displayed with the Doppler sampling volume and angle of projection line over the sample area. At a switch command, the 2D image froze on the screen and the Doppler accumulation function would be active. An audio output device would alert the operator to the accuracy of placement of the sampling volume indicator. Modern real time electronic multielement transducers can provide simultaneous 2D imaging and Doppler information at a constant frame rate. This is due to the ability of utilizing a few lines of information from the 128 lines that are generated from the many transducer elements within the transducer to accumulate

Fig. 8. Complex, stable, poststenotic color flow pattern in an internal carotid artery with associated spectrum at the loction of the indicated line position. (Courtesy of Quantum Medical Systems, Inc.) ▷

the Doppler information while all the other elements are providing image information. Some single element mechanical sector devices "time-share" the 2D image information with the Doppler information to provide a very slow updated imaging capability as well as a slow updated Doppler single. This type of system tends to degrade both flow and image presentation, and it is more difficult to obtain acceptable patient studies.

9.7.3 Color Flow

When added features were incorporated into the Doppler information, a more definitive interpretation of patient diagnostic problems became possible. Color flow imaging is the incorporation of both high resolution ultrasound and Doppler information to display blood flow in color. This simple explanation really does not completely define color flow technology but is a useful starting point for understanding this powerful modality. Earlier it was stated that there are two types of data that are acquired with a Doppler study, i.e., flow direction and velocity. When a separate color scale is assigned to the direction of flow, where one color designates flow toward the transducer (red) and another designates flow away from the transducer (blue), quick visual means are established to show flow direction. In addition, hues of these colors (up to white in some systems; in others red moves toward yellow and blue moves toward green) are assigned to define the speed of flow (velocities) through the artery or vein under test. Therefore a color flow imaging system utilizes a high resolution ultrasound imaging device performing simultaneously with real time imaging of blood flow and tissue (Fig. 7).

The quality of the color flow images (Gooding 1988) is dependent upon many factors, including the ability to distinguish accurate flow information

Fig. 9. 7.5-MHz medial scan of a renal transplant showing cortical color flow with corresponding spectrum. Flow direction from sample along the indicated line shows a bidirectional flow spectrum. (Courtesy of Quantum Medical Systems, Inc.) ▷

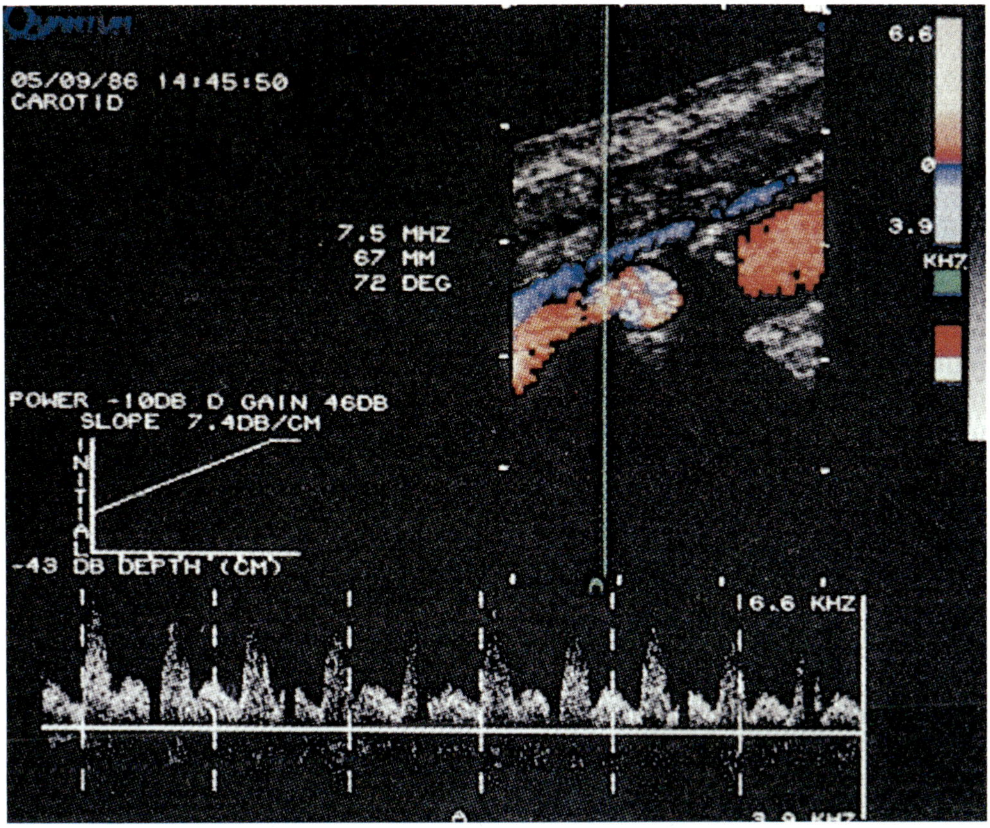
05/09/86 14:45:50
CAROTID
7.5 MHZ
67 MM
72 DEG
POWER -10DB D GAIN 46DB
SLOPE 7.4DB/CM
INITIAL
-43 DB DEPTH (CM)
16.6 KHZ
6.6
0
3.9
KHZ

Fig. 8

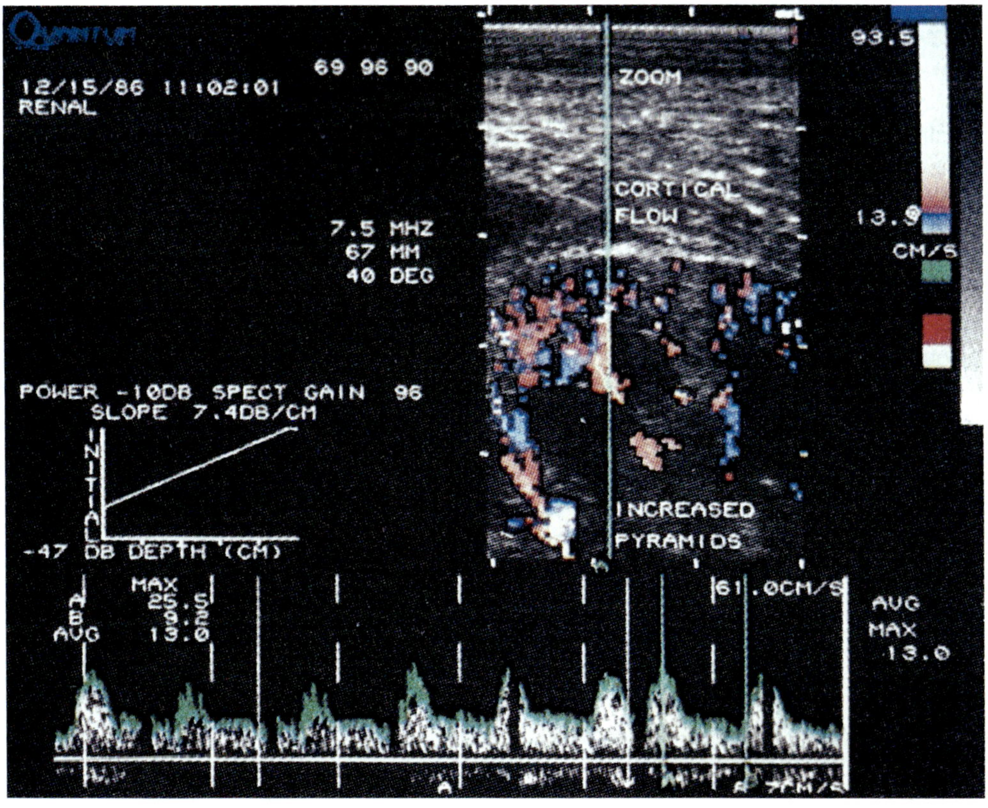
12/15/86 11:02:01
RENAL
69 96 90
7.5 MHZ
67 MM
40 DEG
ZOOM
CORTICAL
FLOW
INCREASED
PYRAMIDS
POWER -10DB SPECT GAIN 96
SLOPE 7.4DB/CM
INITIAL
-47 DB DEPTH (CM)
MAX
A 25.5
B 9.2
AVG 13.0
61.0CM/S
AVG
MAX
13.0
93.5
13.9
CM/S

Fig. 9

from wall to wall across the diameter of the vessel. In addition, flow information should not be "smeared" out of the vessel walls and should not interfere with the ability to visualize these walls accurately with the gray scale portion of the system. In order to accomplish these two functions, high flow sensitivities are needed so that low flow velocities can be detected and small sample volumes can be used to accurately define true flow at the true vessel wall. This provides the ability to view vessel walls that exhibit roughening and irregularities, and to visualize the small eddy currents (reverse flow) that these rough walls will cause in the blood flow. It will suffice to say that blood flow through arteries and veins is not at the same speed from wall to wall because of the condition (roughness) of the walls. Therefore the color of the flow at the walls may appear slightly darker for a smooth walled than for a rough walled artery or vein due to the low restriction in flow (Fig. 8).

The accuracy of flow measurements is highly dependent upon the correction angle of the probe to the flow angle. Some systems provide a fixed angle transducer so that the correction angle is constant. Others provide a variety of correction angles that require assumptions for data reduction, the major assumption being that the major flow streamline is down the center axis of the vessel lumen or parallel to the vessel wall. These assumptions have been proven to be wrong and therefore the data reduction is not correct. A fixed angle transducer device has been shown to yield more accurate measurements of flow velocities.

9.7.4 Spectral Analysis

The major contribution of the spectral analysis portion of Doppler systems is to provide a means to accurately quantify the Doppler or color flow results seen on the imaging device. In most cases sophisticated electronics are used to convert flow events into a precise quantified frequency display that reinforces the presented image data (Fig. 9). Automatic calculations have been incorporated into the systems' software to provide spectral display information on real velocity, velocity profile accelerations, percent stenosis, percent window, pulsatility index, and much more. The electronics that provide these results are so designed as to simultaneously provide image data, Doppler flow data, flow direction data, color conversion data, frequency conversion data based on the Doppler offset, and frequency conversion data based on the Doppler flow direction information. To perform these functions correctly, these systems are required to have a very large dynamic range (about 100 db) in order to have the capability to discriminate low level signals in the presence of other signals with magnitudes 100000 times larger. To put this into proper perspective, the Doppler signal acquired from blood flow in an artery is about 100 times smaller than the signal that is acquired from the wall of that artery. The electronics must be able to recognize this small signal and provide accurate information from it. Problems that are associated with these spectral displays in general are few; but the predominant problems are generally limited to the jitter in the image and/or in the spectral display and also a mirrored spectral display (simultaneously seeing flow in both directions) caused by phase errors in the reduced data even though there is no audible change on the audio output signal from the stereo discriminator.

Recent evaluations of these spectral analyzer systems have shown promise for defining problems in placental circulation (Woo et al. 1987). The results of a measurement based on the ratio of systolic velocity to diastolic velocity (S/O) determine a "resistance" value which is compared to an established table of normal ratio values for a given fetal age. There are also other conditions that may prove useful for this spectrum analyzer system, such as umbilical artery velocity for twin pregnancies, hypertension, diabetes mellitus, and unexplained fetal death. More investigations are being pursued to further expand this modality's usage.

9.8 Intracavity Transducers

New uses for ultrasound have been found with the development of small physical sized all-electronic transducers. Small rectal probes for prostate evaluation (Sanders et al. 1987) have been developed recently that assist the physician to investigate an area of the body where only a blind type of investigation could previously be performed (Fig. 10). With the use of another type of small transducer assembly, intravaginal investigations (Timor-Tritsch et al. 1988; Sacks et al. 1988) have proved to be more conclusive for pelvic studies and fetal evaluation than the previous standard outer abdomen skin line approach. Unlike the previous method, this intravaginal examination does not require a full bladder to provide an adequate imaging window, and has thus been achieving a large degree of acceptance by eliminating patient discomfort.

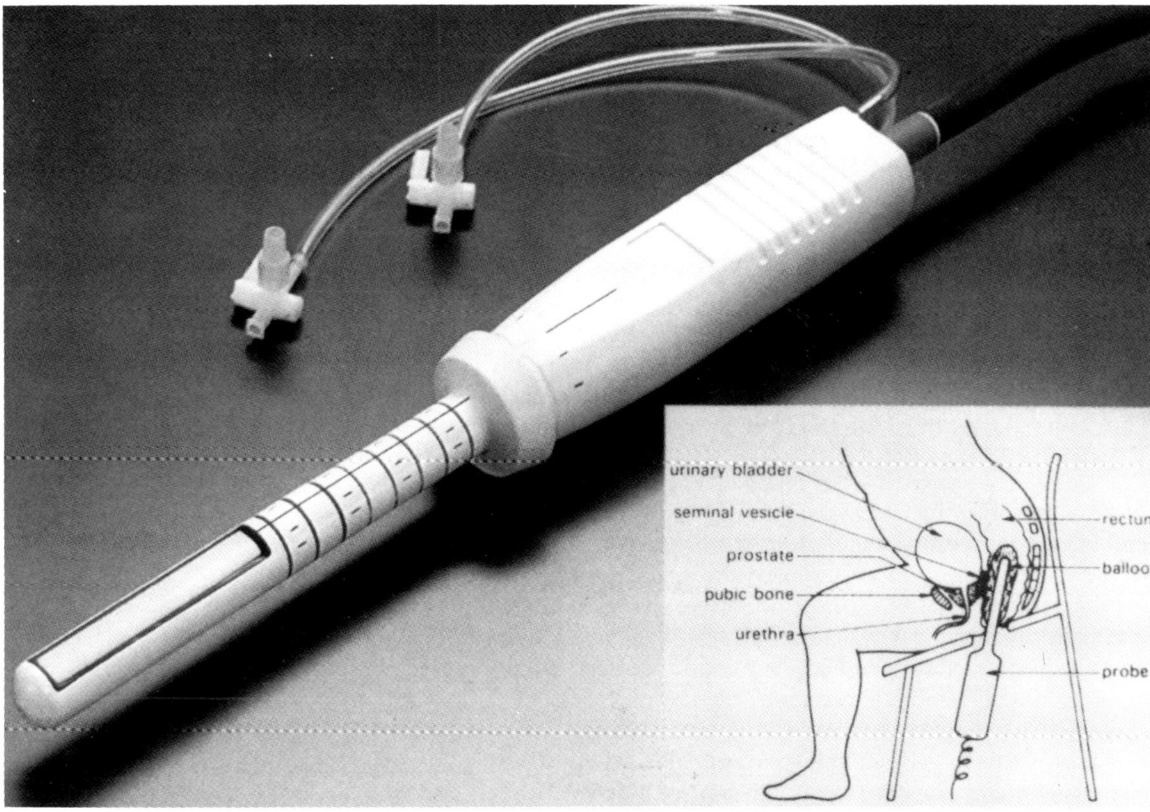

Fig. 10. Prostate intracorporeal evaluation probe and manufacturer-suggested positioning for use. (Courtesy of Toshiba America, Inc.)

Another benefit derived from these intracavity type transducers is the ability to acquire biopsy specimens from areas of interest with the use a biopsy attachment mounted on these probes. The sensitivity of the newer systems allows viewing the passage of the biopsy needle under ultrasound control. These studies can be performed on an outpatient basis, thus providing a quick and simple method to evaluate a previously difficult situation.

9.9 Planned Obsolescence

The ability to update a system for new technology without having to discard half the system's hardware is a good indication of whether the manufacturer has produced a "planned obsolescence" system. Users who have been told that their 2-year-old system cannot be updated for Doppler technology find themselves with a "dead technology system" that has reached the end of its useful life very quickly. The same situation applies to the user who has a mechanical sector system and wants the capabilities for an all-electronic linear or phased array sector device to be incorporated into the basic system. If this change cannot be made for a nominal cost, then the manufacturer has again produced a "planned obsolescence" system. What does a user look for to offset this planned obsolescence? In general, "equipment that utilizes the building block designs and plug-in modular units with nonobsolescent features, should be preferred, so that as new advances occur, these can be incorporated without having to replace the entire system." This statement was first made by this author in an earlier paper (Leo and Rao 1975). It was an extremely pertinent statement at that time and is just as pertinent and important at this time. Good ultrasound systems are very costly and to replace a whole system in order to acquire an added technology is very wasteful. It is advisable for the potential purchaser to be aware of what new technology is being developed and to obtain from the manufacturer an assurance that it could be incorporated into his system at a later date (at a nominal charge). In general we have found that the systems that are large computer based software driven devices have the best track record in providing nominal cost updates to technology.

These are all modular design, where individual plug-in boards control each different function of the system, which are tied together for operation by software commands and controls. These types of system also provide the user with the added features to update software functions in order to improve the overall performance of the system at a very moderate cost. It is still the responsibility of the purchaser to safeguard his or her investment in equipment to assure its use and application as technology expands.

9.10 What Does the Future Hold?

Intracavity work (prostate and intravaginal) is currently developing into a major modality. There will be further developments to improve the size, frequency, and image plane of these probes as well as to provide them with a new design of biopsy attachments for more accurate placement and needle viewing. In addition the intravaginal probe will be equipped with Doppler and color flow capabilities in order to provide more definitive information relative to fetal and placental condition and well-being.

General transducer improvements will be expected for imaging quality, resolution, and penetration. There will also be improvements to the efficient usage of the power output of these all electronic transducers to provide greater penetration with lower power output. This particular improvement will be stimulated by the requirement of the FDA to provide a warning label (FDA 1985) on the ultrasound system when it is to be used for some fetal studies. Recent investigations (DUCK et al. 1985) have shown that the newer all-electronic real time ultrasound system have a marked increase in power output, which has caused concern to the Center for Devices and Radiological Health. Therefore this labeling concern has also been of importance to the American Institute of Ultrasound in Medicine and the National Electrical Manufacturers Association, who have combined talents to devise a new method to acquire accurate measurements of acoustic output from ultrasound equipment (AIUM-NEMA STANDARD 1988).

Another improvement that might be available shortly is the capability to provide many varieties of transducer (mechanical as well as all electronic) all interfacing with the same basic system and all specifically designed for a particular study. One manufacturer currently provides mechanical and electronic transducers of all varieties to operate on one basic system (Fig. 11). In addition the systems themselves will also have the ability to highlight the keyboard functions that would be used for that transducer and that study. The ability to store particular studies and images as a means for comparison with future studies on that patient will also be provided by network interfacing capabilities.

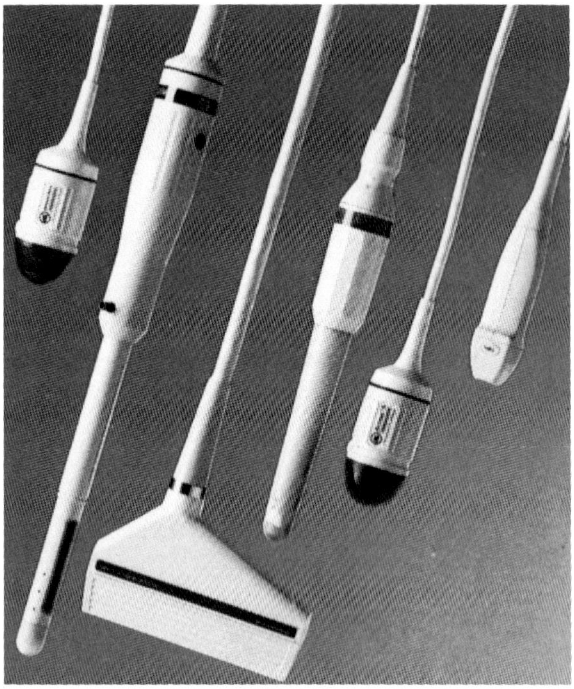

Fig. 11. One manufacturer's complement of ultrasound probes for a system used for many varieties of study. (Courtesy of Advanced Technology Laboratories, Inc.)

It would also be within the realm of reason to hope for a needleless biopsy based on the frequency spectrum that is available from the results of spectral analyzers. If one could define the appearance of a "normal" tissue spectrum profile, it could be stored in the software for comparison with other pathological tissue specimen profiles. If this reasoning could be expanded to where spectrum profiles for other tumor and cystic areas could be resident in the software, a means could be established of identifying these areas using only a well defined sonic beam echo frequency spectrum.

Another area where ultrasound may find application involves cancer treatment. If a special transducer head were designed to have a concave array face (the concave head is already in use for general sector imaging on present systems) and high power output from any segment of the crystals were achieved at any given time, then the concentration

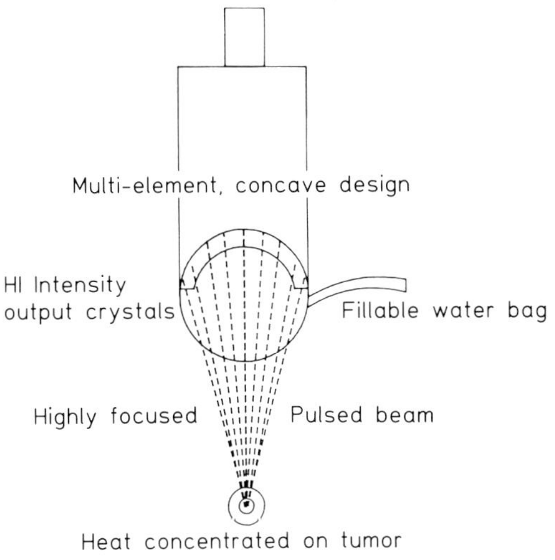

Fig. 12. Artist's conception of a concave, multielement high intensity output probe that futuristically may be used for tumor treatment

of the intensities from many directions could be focused on the tumor (Fig. 12) and produce a concentrated heating of the tumor tissue. The focus area could be controlled by the filling or emptying of the water bag on the face of the transducer to assure the concentration of heat at the proper depth. This may well be a new approach for ultrasound because in the past it was a diagnostic tool to define and locate problems. With this new approach it could become a treatment device.

Ultrasound has already found its way into a new treatment system as a steering device for breaking up kidney stones and gallstones. This sonic generation system, called the lithotriptor, concentrates sonic energy produced from a spark gap (via a parabolic reflecting device) on the stone to cause it to "spall" (outer edges of the stone break up into a fine sand rather than cracking apart in large pieces) and break up. This system is finding use as a noninvasive stone removal device. The viewing of the stone and the steering of the high intensity sonic energy are provided by an ultrasound probe that is an integral part of this system. The ultrasound probe can detect the stones very easily because of their high echogenity to the transmitted ultrasound wave, and thereby provides a location for concentrating the high intensity wave. It is anticipated that eventually this device will be completely automated, so that once the stone is found by the ultrasound system, servo drives will orient the patient to produce the correct angle and focal depth to the center of the stone for best energy transfer.

The future looks very challenging for ultrasound. Many problem areas have been defined and corrected. Improvements in equipment are the results of correction to problems, including those resulting from the need to provide additional capabilities. As long as such problems are solved, ultrasound capabilities will continue to expand, and the medical community will be provided with a valuable modality for diagnosis and eventually for treatment.

References

AIUM/NEMA Acoustical Output Measurement and Labeling Standard (1988)

Dempsey PJ (1988) Breast sonography: historical perspective, clinical application, and image interpretation. Ultrasound Quarterly 6 (1): 69–90

Duck FA, Starritt HC, Aindow JD et al. (1985) The output of pulse-echo ultrasound equipment: a survey of powers, pressures and intensities. Br J Radiol 58: 989–1001

FDA (1985) 510 (K) Guide for measuring and reporting acoustic output of diagnostic ultrasound medical devices. Center for Devices and Radiological Health, final draft

Gooding GAW (1988) Color-flow doppler imaging. Appl Radiol, January, p 11

Halberg LI, Thiele KE (1986) Extraction of blood flow information using Doppler-shifted ultrasound. Hewlett-Packard Journal, June, pp 35–40

Leo FP (1983) Real time ultrasound technology. In: Sanders RC, Hill M (eds) Ultrasound annual. Raven, New York, pp 47–68

Leo FP Rao GUV (1975) The technology of diagnostic ultrasound. Radiol Clin North Am 13: 403–415

Magnin PA (1986) Doppler effect: history and theory. Hewlett-Packard Journal, June, pp 26–31

Sacks GA, Fleischer AC, Kepple DM (1988) Clinical applications of transvaginal sonography in obstetrics and gynecology. Vanderbilt University Medical Center. Reprinted from Toshiba Medical Review

Sanders RC, Hamper UM, Dahnert WF (1987) Update on prostatic ultrasound. Urol Radiol 9: 110–118

Timor-Tritsch IE, Rottem S, Thaler I (1988) Review of transvaginal ultrasonography: a description with clinical application. Ultrasound Quarterly 6 (1): 1–34

Woo J, Liang S, Lo R et al. (1987) Doppler blood flow velocity waveforms in alpha-thalassemia hydrops fetalis. J Ultrasound Med 6: 679–684

10 Imaging Distinct Points in Left Ventricular Myocardium to Study Regional Wall Deformation

WILLIAM C. HUNTER and ELIAS A. ZERHOUNI

CONTENTS

10.1 Overview of Cardiac Imaging 169
10.2 Significance of Studying Regional Cardiac Motion 170
10.3 Conventional Imaging of Regional Wall Motion 170
10.3.1 Comparison of Systolic vs Diastolic Chamber Outlines 170
10.3.2 Limitations of Chamber Outlines for Studying Regional Wall Motion 171
10.3.3 Potential Use and Limitations of Regional Wall Thickness 172
10.4 Advantages of Identifying Specific Myocardial Points 173
10.5 Techniques Based on Implanted Myocardial Markers 174
10.5.1 Global Sets of Markers 174
10.5.2 Local Pairs of Markers 175
10.5.3 Local Triplets of Markers 175
10.5.4 Local Tetrahedra and Prisms 175
10.5.5 Computer Automated Tracking and Three-dimensional Reconstruction 176
10.5.5.1 Calibration of Divergent X-ray Field 176
10.5.5.2 Three-dimensional Reconstruction 177
10.5.5.3 Avoiding Artifacts in Position Measurements . 179
10.5.5.4 Locating Centers of Spherical Markers 180
10.5.5.5 Computer Automation 181
10.6 Identifying Myocardial Points Without Implanting Markers 181
10.6.1 Epicardial Bifurcations of Coronary Arteries . 181
10.6.2 Magnetic Resonance Tagging of Specific Myocardial Points 183
10.6.3 Range-Gated Doppler Ultrasound to Determine Strain 186
10.7 Applications of Marker Motion Analysis to Other Organs 187
10.8 Future Directions of Motion Analysis Systems in Research and Clinic 187
References 188

10.1 Overview of Cardiac Imaging

Generating motion is the essence of cardiac function, and imaging that motion has played an increasingly important role in modern developments in cardiology and cardiac research. In fact, one could say that evaluation of almost every aspect of cardiac function has benefitted from the availability of special imaging techniques: (1) global and regional motion of the myocardial walls, (2) motions of the valvular apparatus, (3) blood flow within and between cardiac chambers, (4) coronary artery patency and ability to deliver myocardial blood flow, (5) metabolic state of the myocardium, (6) localization and visualization of infarcted zones within the myocardium. Especially in clinical situations, where the most prevalent problem involves *local regions* with differential behavior (caused by local blockages of coronary arterial blood flow), some form of cardiac imaging is now almost considered mandatory.

The techniques applied to cardiac imaging problems have covered the full spectrum of radiological approaches:

1. Classical contrast angiography in single or biplane views (DODGE and SHEEHAN 1986).
2. Rapid X-ray tomographic imaging at cine rates (BRUNDAGE 1987; REITER et al. 1986), which has even been extended to three-dimensional reconstructions (RITTMAN et al. 1980; ROBB et al. 1980).
3. Radionuclide imaging of both mechanical performance and myocardial state (metabolic or pathological) (HOLMAN 1980; POHOST et al. 1986).
4. Nuclear magnetic resonance (CANBY et al. 1986) for both imaging of moving cardiac structures and spectroscopic evaluation of the chemical state of the myocardium. Potentially, the combination of spectroscopic information with its spatial localization should offer an extremely powerful tool to observe regionally both the metabolic and mechanical behavior of the myocardium.

WILLIAM C. HUNTER, Ph.D., Dept. of Biomedical Engineering, The Johns Hopkins University, School of Medicine, 720 Rutland Ave, Baltimore, MD 21205, USA
ELIAS A. ZERHOUNI, M.D., Dept. of Radiology and Radiological Science, The Johns Hopkins University, School of Medicine, 600 North Wolfe Street, Baltimore, MD 21205, USA

5. Ultrasonic imaging (LEVINE et al. 1986) using both the discrete echoes reflected from interfaces and the Doppler shifted echoes reflected from moving structures.

In many cases, application of these imaging modalities to the heart has occurred only after initial success in imaging other organ systems. The major complicating factor making the heart difficult to study has been its rapid motion, but that rapid motion is also the essence of the information that needs to be retrieved. Whereas images often provide primarily *structural* information about many other organs, images of cardiac motion are critical for *functional* evaluation of the heart – particularly for studying differences in myocardial function between local regions of the heart wall. In fact, many of the quantitative techniques described in this chapter that were developed for functional evaluation of cardiac wall motion can also be applied to other organs for which displacement, deformation, or motility are functionally important. Several examples of studies in the lungs and digestive tract are cited in Sect. 10.7.

10.2 Significance of Studying Regional Cardiac Motion

With the multiplicity of techniques and the variety of functional questions for which cardiac imaging has served, it is clear that the scope of cardiac imaging is immense. It is also growing rapidly as improvements in imaging technology provide more opportunities to evaluate cardiac function. Other than just sketching out the terrain, as done above, this chapter is not intended to survey in detail the vast range of imaging applications in cardiology. Instead, the focus will be on one particular aspect of cardiac functional measurements – regional cardiac motion – and on particular problems with such measurements that come into play regardless of the imaging modality. In general, to extract functional information from these images requires more attention to calibration and distortion of the images than may be necessary just to display the structures.

The function of cardiac muscle is both to develop tension and to shorten, thus ejecting blood into the high pressure arterial system. Global measures of how well the left ventricle accomplishes this task are routinely obtained during cardiac catheterization by measuring left ventricular pressure via a catheter and chamber volume via quantitative contrast ventriculography (DODGE and SHEEHAN 1986). However, myocardial ischemic disease (the most prevalent cardiac problem) is a *regional* disease that attacks only the localized segments of myocardium which are underperfused. Given this regional nature, measurements have been sought to evaluate the specific contractile performance of such an underperfused region of myocardium. For this case, the tension and shortening generated by that local segment of myocardium would be the appropriate measurements. However, local tensions cannot yet be accurately measured (YIN 1981), although indices that may relate to local wall stress are being developed (HALPERIN et al. 1987). Consequently, local shortening by itself has often served as an incomplete, but still useful measure of local myocardial performance.

In addition to improving clinical diagnosis, there are significant basic research questions that have also recently motivated several groups of investigators to study measurements of the local motions undergone by small myocardial regions (HUNTER et al. 1986; WALDMAN et al. 1985). The long-range goal of such measurements is to unravel the interactions among cardiac muscle fibers in the walls of the heart, and to discover how the muscle fibers accommodate the global volume changes both in healthy myocardium and in pathological situations, such as regional ischemia.

10.3 Conventional Imaging of Regional Wall Motion

10.3.1 Comparison of Systolic vs Diastolic Chamber Outlines

In the most common clinical diagnostic situation, silhouettes of the left ventricular chamber (viewed from the 30° right-anterior-oblique orientation after opacifying with contrast) are recorded on cine film during catheterization. The outlines of the chamber are then compared for the end-diastolic frame versus the end-systolic frame. Since qualitative assessment of "hypokinetic," "akinetic," or "diskinetic" motion of a local wall segment has been found to lead to significant errors (CHAITMAN et al. 1975), numerous techniques have been proposed that attempt to quantify regional differences in shortening at locations around the perimeter of the silhouette. In order to devise a regional shortening measure from just the outline of the chamber, all these techniques have resorted to defining some reference point or points, the distance to which can be defined for each point on the chamber outline. Some proposed a unique center of contraction (RICKARDS et al. 1977), but others challenged the notion that there would be just one center towards which all contraction would be oriented (GOODYER and LANGOU 1982). Sometimes a long axis (from ventricular apex to the middle of the aortic valve) was defined (GELBERG et al. 1979), and the contraction of the ventricular endocardial outline was assumed to occur only along radial lines directed perpendicular to this axis. In the most sophisticated technique (SHEEHAN et al. 1983), endocardial surfaces from end-diastole and end-systole were combined to form a "centerline." Normal to this, and distributed equally around its perimeter, a set of 100 locally varying orientations (vectors) was defined, as shown in Fig. 1. Shortening between the diastolic and systolic chamber silhouettes was then measured along each of the 100 local vectors.

Not only contrast ventriculography, but also the noninvasive technique of two-dimensional echocardiography has been used to visualize the motion of the endocardial border (KISSLO et al. 1977). Ultrasonic imaging offers the advantage of obtaining several different projections of the chamber border; in particular, a short-axis cross-section can be observed, which is not obtainable with ventriculography. Since the ultrasonic image often does not produce as sharp an endocardial border as seen with ventriculography, computer aided techniques have been used to refine the contour of the endocardial border (WEISS et al. 1981). Analyses to quantitate the amount and sites of wall motion abnormalities can be done with two-dimensional echocardiographic images using techniques that are very similar to those used for images from contrast ventriculography (FORCE et al. 1984).

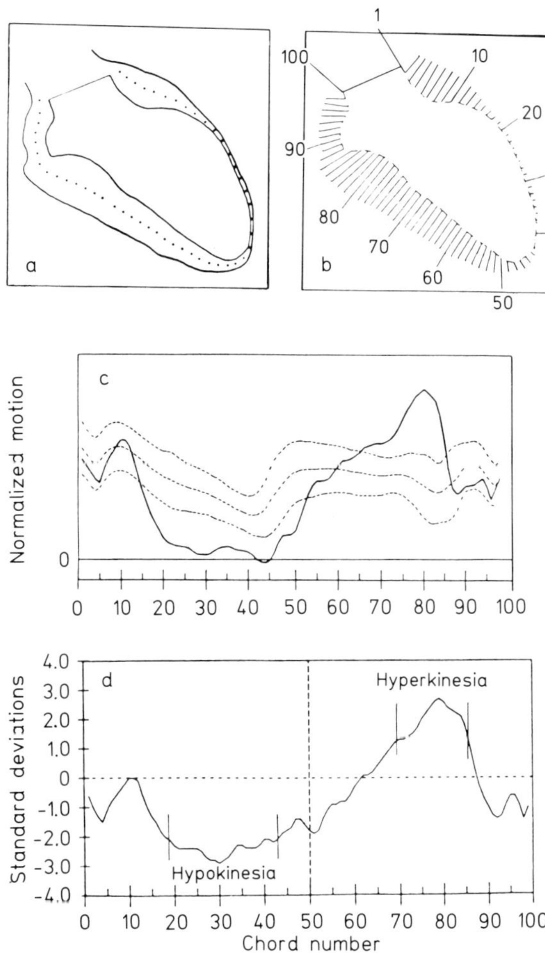

Fig. 1a–d. Sample of the centerline method for estimating left ventricular local wall motion from outlines of cavity silhouettes at end-diastole and end-systole. **a** *Solid lines:* contours of cavity silhouette from cine frames closest to end-diastole and end-systole. *Dotted line:* centerline constructed by computer algorithm to fall midway between diastolic and systolic contours. **b** Local wall motion is measured as displacement along 100 evenly spaced chords, each perpendicular to the centerline. **c** *Solid line:* displacement at each chord normalized by the end-diastolic perimeter. *Dotted lines:* mean motion (±standard deviation) from a group of normal patients. **d** Standardized motion: i.e., normalized wall motion for the individual case being studied has been plotted as the deviation from the mean (of normal patients) in units of standard deviation. (DODGE and SHEEHAN 1986)

10.3.2 Limitations of Chamber Outlines for Studying Regional Wall Motion

For measurements of local wall motion, however, the majority of cardiac imaging schemes appear to be less than ideal. Quantitative contrast angiography, echocardiography, and magnetic resonance imaging all attempt to define the surface boundary between myocardium and blood within the cardiac chambers (i.e., the endocardial surface) or the boundary between myocardium and surrounding pericardial or pulmonary tissues (i.e., the epicardial surface). Information is therefore absent concerning the motion of any myocardial points in the middle of the heart wall – away from the identifiable surfaces. Furthermore, echocardiography and magnetic resonance imaging, as usually applied, present two-dimensional images from a plane located at a fixed position in space; the resulting images of the endocardial border may thus portray somewhat varying anatomical portions of the ventricular wall as the heart translates through the fixed imaging plane during the cardiac cycle. Thus, these techniques, as usually applied, offer no way of defining specific, unique *points* within a local region of myocardium, from which the shortening within that region could be discerned. Accurate analysis of regional motion requires a way to *identify* many specific points within the ventricular wall, as well as a way to track the motion of their movements in three dimensions over several cardiac cycles. The key information is most often not just the individual motion of a single point but its *relative* motion with respect to other neighboring points.

All of the above methods to analyze local ventricular wall motion actually *model* ventricular wall motion rather than measure it (SHEEHAN et al. 1986). Each analysis relies strongly on one or another type of assumption about the pattern of local contractions. In fact, there may actually be no one-to-one correspondence between points on the radiographically determined endocardial contour at end-diastole and end-systole, because of the infoldings of trabeculae during systole and papillary muscle exclusion of dye (SHEEHAN et al. 1986; INGELS et al. 1980). These two phenomena may effectively uncouple the motion of the observed contrast border from the motion of the majority of the ventricular wall in that region.

In an attempt to test whether the patterns of local contraction assumed by the analytical models of regional wall motion are realistic, INGELS et al. (1980) compared the actual motion of markers implanted at midwall to the motion predicted by each of several analytical models of local wall motion. They found that the error in predicted marker position was often greater than 40% of the actual motion of the marker during its systolic excursion. Particularly late in systole, they often observed abrupt, discontinuous motion of the contrast border (presumably as dye was squeezed out of enfolding regions) when simultaneously such abrupt motions were absent from adjacent markers implanted in the midwall. While important clinical information can and has been derived from observing the motion of contrast borders, such motion is not necessarily well correlated with the motion of the adjacent myocardium.

Finally, the motion of any one point in the myocardium – even if it can be unambiguously identified by the use of a marker – is not only the result of *local* contractile forces, but also the result of more *global* influences. The heart may translate as a unit (e.g., due to the recoil force of blood acceleration into and out of the chambers) or it may rotate as a unit (e.g., due to forces exerted by the great vessels) (PANDIAN et al. 1983). For example, suppose that in panel a of Fig. 1 the end-systolic contour were shifted slightly to the left; the distribution of vectorial segments between diastolic and systolic contours (as in panel b) would then be significantly altered. There has been considerable debate about whether to attempt to remove some of the potential translational or rotational effects by expressing all local segmental motions relative to some axis and some centroid that is defined by landmarks observable in each frame (CLAYTON et al. 1982; INGELS et al. 1980). In principle, such corrections would seem useful, but in practice their use may sometimes lead to increased errors because of the inability to accurately locate the specific landmarks (SHEEHAN et al. 1986). Moreover, some methods of removing bulk translation (e.g., setting the origin of the coordinates to the centroid of the cavity silhouette) may lead one to either underestimate (SHEEHAN et al. 1983) or overestimate (FORCE et al. 1986) the degree of abnormality, depending upon the method of analysis.

10.3.3 Potential Use and Limitations of Regional Wall Thickness

Shortening of myocardial muscle fibers, which lie predominantly in planes parallel to the epicardium, is accompanied by transverse thickening required to maintain myocardial volume constant. Thus, there is a tight correlation between local shortening in the direction of muscle fibers and local wall thickening. Ventricular wall thickness can be readily quantitated by echocardiography, since ultrasonic echoes clearly identify *both* the endocardial and epicardial surfaces of the heart. Thus, several studies have tested the utility of two-dimensional echocardiography for mapping regional disorders of contraction around the circumference of the left ventricle.

Perhaps because wall thickening is inherently a more "local" measurement than the motion of the endocardial outline (which can also be influenced by the global factors outlined above), thickening has been found to discriminate more precisely between infarcted and normal zones of myocardium (LIEBERMAN et al. 1981). Using two-dimensional echocardiography, maps of systolic wall thickening have been generated at a resolution of 16 sectors per complete circumference (BUDA et al. 1986, LIEBERMAN et al. 1981; LIMA et al. 1985). This resolution was sufficient to demonstrate clearly that impairment of fiber shortening (and thus wall thickening) occurs in zones of normal tissue adjacent to infarcted myocardium (BUDA et al. 1986; LIMA et al. 1985). Thus, more highly refined information about local contraction of the myocardium appears to be derivable from measurements of thickening rather than the motion of the endocardial border alone.

Measurements of wall thickening by two-dimensional echocardiography also have potential limitations (FALSETTI et al. 1981; PANDIAN et al. 1983). For one, the identification of the endo- and epicardial borders is more difficult than with M-mode echocardiography, so that computer assisted techniques have been almost always used to determine these surface contours. Also, unless special precautions are taken, there is no guarantee that the images from end-diastolic and end-systolic frames correspond to the same cross-section of the left ventricle, because during contraction the heart may have translated through the fixed plane in space that is being imaged. To overcome this problem in animal experiments, LIMA et al. (1985) attached three surface markers to the canine hearts they studied to define uniquely the particular anatomical cross-section that they wanted to observe. By requiring the echocardiographic image to contain those three markers, it could be assured that the same *anatomical* section was being imaged in both diastole and systole.

Finally, even measures of wall thickness may not be immune from the problem of defining the reference point to which such measurements will be referred. Because of the nonuniformities of circumferential motion during regional ischemia, FORCE et al. (1986) showed that a particular radial geometric line (along which thickening is measured) may correspond physically to different myocardial segments in the systolic vis-à-vis the diastolic image. By their analysis, this could lead to significant overestimation of the region of apparently reduced thickening. Furthermore, the results also depended on what point was chosen as the center from which the "radial" lines emanated along which wall thickness was measured. The overestimation of the region of reduced thickening was exacerbated if the radial lines were drawn to the centroid of each respective image, rather than consistently using the same central focus point (which was chosen reasonably as the end-diastolic centroid).

10.4 Advantages of Identifying Specific Myocardial Points

The motion of any single point in a biological material (such as the myocardium) is governed by the bulk translation and bulk rotation of the organ it is part of (such as the heart) as well as the local deformation of the tissue in the neighborhood of the point. For insight into the contractile shortening of cardiac muscle fibers in vivo, only the deformational component of motion is meaningful. Translation or rotation of the heart as a unit would not alter the length of any cardiac muscle fibers.

To measure myocardial deformation (e.g., systolic shortening), the motion of at least *two* uniquely identifiable points must be known. That is, shortening presupposes the existence of a line segment, which is defined by the location of its end-points. Lack of such uniquely identifiable points is the crux of almost all the theoretical difficulties experienced by the methods to study left ventricular regional wall motion that were outlined above. For instance, there are few useful landmarks along the outline of the endocardial silhouette obtained from contrast ventriculography. Even if there were unique landmarks along the contour, the analysis schemes described previously would still have trouble because they *assumed* line segments drawn to imaginary points in the center of the ventricular cavity.

Most of the imaging techniques used to observe cardiac motion only identify surfaces (e.g., endocardial boundary) and not discrete, individual points. Even then, these "surfaces" are usually only observed as the boundary obtained by projecting the surface of the three-dimensional reality onto a two-dimensional image. Recent tomographic extensions of contrast ventriculography (REITER et al. 1986, 1987; RITTMAN et al. 1980; ROBB et al. 1980) will allow one to reconstruct the complete three-dimensional surface, but they do not overcome the fundamental limitation that only surfaces are being imaged and not individual points.

The advantages that would be offered by imaging anatomically specific points have been clearly recognized by the investigators studying regional wall motion of the left ventricle. In the rare clinical cases when patients have had radiopaque markers implanted at the time of cardiac surgery or transplant, such data have been treated as the "gold standard" with which to evaluate the assumptions inherent in the more indirect approaches to quantifying regional wall motions (INGELS et al. 1980). Similarly, direct measurement of myocardial segment lengths by transit-time sonomicrometry has been the standard for basic studies of regional wall motion in experimental animals.

However, in clinical situations it has proven difficult to define sufficient numbers of suitable, anatomically specific points with small enough spacing between the points to be adequate for studies of regional wall motion. This limitation has all but precluded the general clinical use of methods based on specifically marked local myocardial points. It has remained a tool almost exclusively for the research scientist - whether clinically or basically oriented. Only in the cardiac transplantation program at Stanford has the use of myocardial markers become part of standard clinical practice, and this can hardly be considered typical. However, in the foreseeable future, the possibility of tagging specific myocardial anatomical sites *without having to physically implant markers* (see Sect. 10.6) offers the exciting potential of moving this powerful technique off of the research bench and into the clinic.

10.5 Techniques Based on Implanted Myocardial Markers

10.5.1 Global Sets of Markers

The first applications of implanted myocardial markers in humans were not motivated by the desire to image *regional* wall motion, but by other advantages of markers for studies of global ventricular function. For example, in the earliest human study with implanted markers, HARRISON et al. (1963) chose to use the marker method because they needed to measure global cardiac dimensions throughout each individual cardiac cycle and over the course of many cycles in intact, unanesthetized human subjects during various states of voluntary respiration and muscular exercise. Similar considerations motivated the use of markers to monitor cardiac function in transplanted hearts (INGELS et al. 1975) and for long-term longitudinal monitoring following valvular surgery (MCDONALD 1970, 1972). In most present clinical situations, however, the use of echocardiography or magnetic resonance imaging should be able to provide the required global information on cardiac volumes, ejection fraction, diameters, etc., without the need for implanted marker methodology.

There are other important aspects of global left ventricular deformation that *do* require knowledge of how specific anatomical sites move, however. In particular, the torsion of the left ventricle around its apex-base axis has recently been advanced as an important mode of cardiac deformation (ARTS et al. 1984; HANSEN et al. 1987). Torsion is thought to be related to the balance of myocardial fiber forces exerted between subepi- and subendocardial fibers, which tend to twist the ventricle in opposite directions because of their fiber orientations. Although there are not yet any experimental data, theoretically, deviations in torsion from the normal pattern of changes during systole may be a sensitive indicator of transmural imbalance in contractile state - perhaps related to subendocardial ischemia. Torsion cannot be sensed from the usual long-axis projection of the endo- or epicardial surfaces, because the relevant rotations around the long axis are not evident in these views. A crude measure can be derived from two-dimensional echocardiographic cross-sections taken at two widely spaced levels along the apex-base axis (ARTS et al. 1984). However, the most accurate measures of torsion to date have come from analyses of the motion of implanted myocardial markers (HANSEN et al. 1987; INGELS et al. 1987).

Analysis of the global motion of implanted markers has also been utilized to give a sense of the overall pattern of shape changes occurring in the left ventricle (WALLEY et al. 1982). Assuming that the whole left ventricular cavity deforms as a relatively homogeneous unit, such a deformation would have three principal directions in which the amount of change in chamber diameters would take on its extreme values. Determining the orientations of these characteristic directions may be a new way to study shape changes in the left ventricle. Furthermore, the product of the fractional stretch ratios in these three (mutually perpendicular) principal directions may provide a reliable index of ventricular volume changes (WALLEY et al. 1982). Such a method to determine ventricular volume, while interesting for the left ventricle, may not necessarily be of major utility in clinical determinations because there appear to be several acceptable clinical alternatives for determining left ventricular volume. However, this method of volume determination may offer advantages for the right ventricle (SCHWIEP et al. 1986), because its complex, asymmetrical geometry invalidates many of the formulae used to calculate left ventricular volume from two-dimensional projections.

10.5.2 Local Pairs of Markers

The simplest possible study of local wall motion is to monitor changes in the lengths of several separate line segments, each one determined by the distance between a pair of implanted markers. Some of the earliest animal experiments (HEIKKILA et al. 1972) and clinical studies (BROWER et al. 1978, 1979) of regional wall motion by implanted markers used this approach. In animal experiments, this method has been supplanted by sonomicrometry, because of its greater ease of use. In man, the opportunity to "apply" noninvasive tags at specific myocardial points (Sect. 10.6) may rekindle interest in this approach. However, by incorporating just one more marker into the local group, thus forming a triplet, two additional and independent measures of local wall deformation can be obtained (see Sect. 10.5.3). Since so much can be gained with so little investment, the appeal of just studying pairs of implanted markers is diminished.

10.5.3 Local Triplets of Markers

In several studies of local deformation of the epicardium of the right ventricle in dogs, MEIER (1980 a, b) pioneered the development of the technique for determining the components of planar mechanical strain by observing the relative motion of a triplet of implanted markers. By implanting the markers in the subepicardium, he could be fairly certain that the plane of markers that he studied would closely parallel the local plane of cardiac muscle fibers. The same idea can also be used for deeper muscle layers in the heart wall, but implanting the three markers at equal depths so that their plane will be approximately parallel to the local fiber plane can be more problematical than for the epicardium.

From the relative motion of the three markers, the three independent components of the local deformation in that plane can be determined. Suppose for the purpose of explanation that the three markers form a right triangle when they are implanted. The three components of deformation are: (1) stretch along one leg of the right triangle, (2) stretch along the orthogonal leg, (3) change in the angle between the two legs (shearing deformation). While the first two of these components are just simple extensions of the idea of segment lengths determined by marker pairs, the shearing deformation adds a qualitatively new type of information to the deformation picture. Such shears may well be very important because they may be directly relatable to the global torsional deformation that was discussed above (Sect. 10.5.1).

As MEIER's (1980 a, b) articles showed, the triplet of beads does not in practice have to be implanted as a right triangle. Any shape of triangle will do; however, the more the shape deviates from an equilateral triangle, the more susceptible the derived deformation components will be to random noise in the determination of marker positions. Triangles with long, narrow shapes should be avoided. The mathematical transformations required are combinations of standard matrix operations [see MEIER (1980 a, b) for details], and thus can be programmed readily for computer solution. The validity of these computations rests on the assumption that the local region of the myocardium lying within the marker triangle deforms in a homogeneous way (i.e., that one subregion of the triangle does not deform differently than any other). With a sufficiently small triangle, this appears to be a reasonable assumption. A commonly used size that has produced reasonable results in canine experiments is a triangle of approximately 1.0 cm per side (for canine left ventricles weighing approx. 100 g).

This technique has so far only been applied in animal experiments. It appears to be well suited for eventual clinical application, particularly if suitable noninvasive markers can be used (see Sect. 10.6). Since rather arbitrarily shaped and sized marker triangles can be used (within the limits set out above), there is considerable potential for using already existing cardiac landmarks (e.g., epicardial bifurcations of coronary arteries, Sect. 10.6.1), if the spacing of such landmarks is such that suitable triangles can be formed. Usually, the triplet of markers will lie in a plane either at the epicardial surface or parallel to it but deeper in the ventricular wall, because myocardial fibers run approximately in such planes. However, for experimental work, implanting three markers at precisely the same desired depth below the epicardium can be a difficult experimental task. If such problems are of concern, then three-dimensional imaging (next section) may provide a solution

10.5.4 Local Tetrahedra and Prisms

The concepts described in the preceding section can be easily extended from the planar case to three dimensions (FENTON et al. 1978; WALDMAN et al. 1985). Now, there will be six independent components describing the deformation: three stretches in mutually perpendicular directions, and three shearing deformations – each one in a plane mutually perpendicular to the others. The minimum number of markers required to generate this complete three-dimensional set of strains is four noncoplanar markers, which form a tetrahedron. Once again, an equilateral tetrahedron would probably be ideal.

Just as in the case of a triangle of markers, the strain calculation in three dimensions from a marker tetrahedron requires that the myocardium lying within the tetrahedron deforms in a homogeneous way. Homogeneity does not mean that the deformation must be the same in all directions; rather, it requires that the deformation be equivalent over all subregions within the tetrahedron. Within the thick walls of the left ventricle, however, the fact that the myocardium cannot change its tissue volume significantly during one contraction requires there to be nonuniformity in the amount of thickening for layers at different depths within the wall: deeper layers must thicken considerably more. For example direct measurements (GALLAGHER et al. 1985) show that the inner half of the left ventricular wall thickens approximately 50% more than the outer half during each contraction. Thus, the assumption of homogeneous deformation is violated in the radial direction, and any component of strain that involves the radial direction (e.g., radial thickening, radial-circumferential shears, tissue volumetric strain) becomes questionable for the left ventricle when calculated from a tetrahedron of markers. In nonradial directions (i.e., in planes parallel to the epicardial surface, as in the triangle of markers discussed in Sect. 10.5.3), homogeneity still appears to be a workable assumption for points separated by approximately 1 cm.

For the left ventricle, it appears that more accurate deformations can be calculated from a prism with vertices defined by six implanted markers rather than from a tetrahedron (WISEMAN et al. 1987). The six markers compose two triangles in planes parallel to the epicardium; the calculated strain should approximately correspond to the actual strain at the centroid of the six markers. The error that still remains (due to the inherent nonuniformity of the deformation) is reduced when using a six-marker prism by approximately an order of magnitude compared to the error in calculating strain for a tetrahedron of markers. Much of the improvement using the prism approach is due to a better radial balance of markers: In the prism, there are equal numbers of markers in two layers that approximately symmetrically bracket the location (centroid) for which the strain is being calculated. In the tetrahedron, such symmetry is lost, and one triangle of markers (which is the primary basis for all the tangential components of strain) is derived from a layer at one extreme of the tetrahedron, while strain components involving the radial direction are based on the motion of just a single point from another layer.

10.5.5 Computer Automated Tracking and Three-dimensional Reconstruction

To reconstruct the three-dimensional position of a marker, projected images of the marker must be recorded in two approximately orthogonal planes. Both cineradiography and fluoroscopy (with video recording) have been used to capture the images (GARRISON et al. 1982; INGELS et al. 1975), with film speeds from 50 to 90 frames/second required to capture information from the moving heart. For example, Fig. 2 shows one frame from a cineradiograph of an in situ canine heart that had previously been implanted with 18 marker beads. This image is from the lateral X-ray system; an orthogonal view (anterior-posterior) was also recorded simultaneously. In an idealized situation, the image in one plane could be considered to give the (x, y) coordinates of the marker, and the orthogonal image would give the (y, z) coordinates. The common y information is used when there are multiple markers to match the images of the same marker in the two planes. In practice, however, there are many technical factors that must be overcome to allow this scheme to work. These factors will be explained in the next sections.

10.5.5.1 Calibration of Divergent X-ray Field

A common problem when measuring dimensional information from radiographic images is the divergence of the X-ray beam. This causes the distance between two markers in the recorded image to be magnified by a variable amount, depending on the locations of the X-ray source and image plane relative to the markers. Often, magnification has been quantified by imaging a grid of known spacing which is placed as close as possible to the position where the heart had been located during its imaging. However, GARRISON et al. (1982) suggested a better procedure, that overcomes errors due to inaccurate placement of the reference grid and also due to variations in magnification for parts of the heart located closer to or farther from the X-ray source

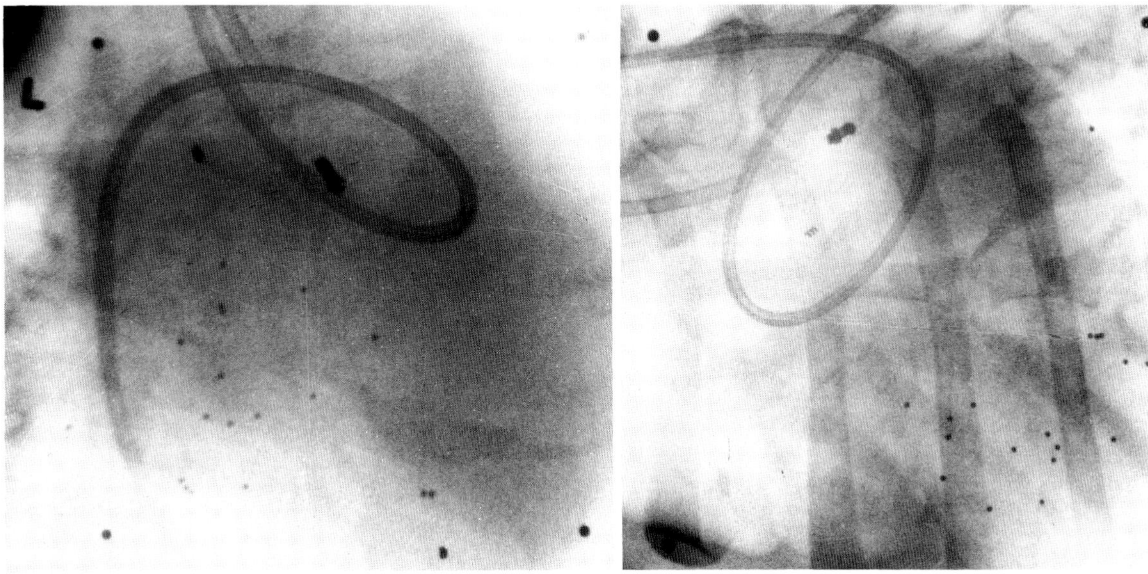

a b

Fig. 2a, b. One frame of a cineradiograph of an in situ canine heart marked with implanted stainless steel markers. At each of the corners of the frame are reference markers used for frame alignment. **a** Lateral view; **b** simultaneous anterior-posterior view

than where the reference grid was placed. They devised a calibration fixture (Fig. 3 a) that contains a dozen markers whose locations are precisely known. From the biplane images of this fixture (Fig. 3 b), the locations of the two X-ray sources and the locations and orientations of the two imaging planes can be calculated. As shown in the next section, this is all the information that is required to calibrate the images and allow reconstruction of the marker positions in space from their film images.

The calibrated locations of the X-ray sources and imaging planes are all specified in terms of a coordinate system that is defined by the placement of the calibration fixture. If it is important to have a less arbitrary coordinate system, then the location and orientation of the calibration fixture with respect to the desired coordinates would also have to be determined.

One drawback of the calibration fixture designed by GARRISON et al. is that the markers have been placed so that images of pairs of them often overlap (Fig. 3 b). This disadvantage may be overcome by a calibration fixture designed by DAUGHTERS (personal communication), that uses calibration markers placed at nonuniform intervals along a helical line on a Plexiglas cylinder.

10.5.5.2 Three-dimensional Reconstruction

Knowing the locations of the two X-ray sources and imaging planes, it is possible to reconstruct the three-dimensional placement of a marker from its images in the two films. Figure 4 shows how the reconstruction works. After constructing a line connecting the lateral X-ray source to the image of the marker in the lateral image plane, one knows that the physical marker should lie somewhere along this line. A similar line can be constructed between the anterior-posterior X-ray source and its imaging plane; the marker should then have been located where these two lines cross. As the inset in the figure shows, however, the two lines will rarely intersect precisely, because of measurement errors. The best estimate of marker location is then the point halfway between the two source-to-image lines at the place where they come closest to each other.

The distance between this point and either line is called the "miss distance," which serves to evaluate how accurately the location of the marker has been reconstructed. Random variations in the miss distance usually reflect small inaccuracies in locating the marker image in each film. A miss distance that has a constant component from frame to frame suggests inaccuracy in calibration (i.e., the determination of source and image locations from films of the calibration fixture). Such calibration errors can occur if the X-ray equipment moves slightly between the time of imaging markers in a heart and imaging the calibration fixture.

When there are many markers in each view, there is an additional problem to be overcome: how to

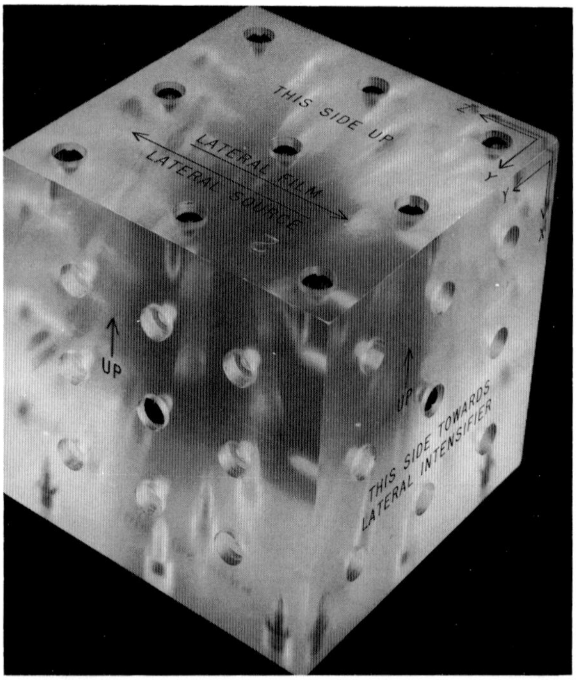

a

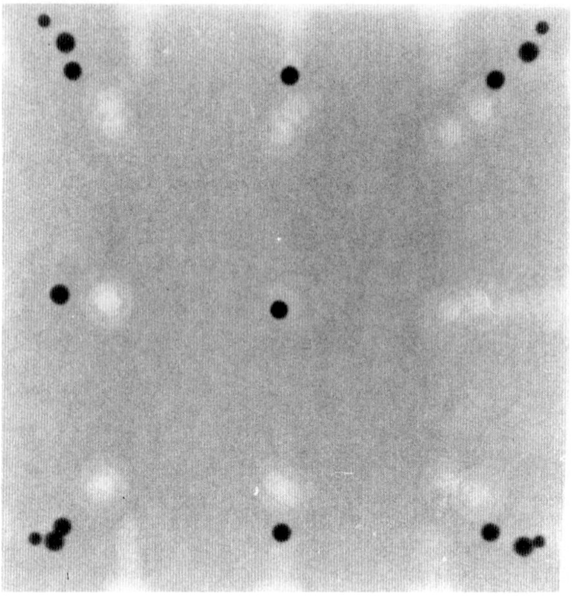

b

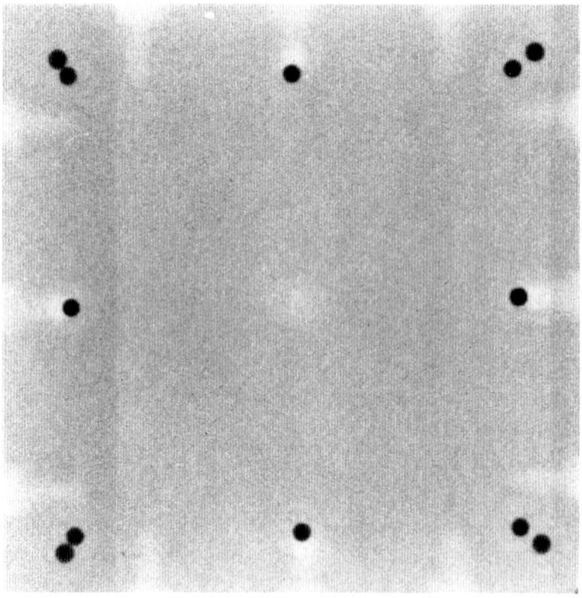

c

Fig. 3a–c. Calibration fixture used by GARRISON et al. **a** Fixture is a Plexiglas cube with precisely located holes drilled on each face and radiopaque beads placed in 12 of the holes. Top right corner of the cube shows the origin of the coordinate axes derived from calibration. **b** Lateral image of the calibration cube. Note *(at bottom left)* that two images of individual beads in the cube sometimes overlap. Smaller diameter dots are images of reference markers placed on face of image intensifier. **c** Image of calibration cube in the orthogonal (vertical) view

match the image of a bead in one view with its corresponding image in the orthogonal view. To solve this, one can use the redundant information provided by having a common coordinate. For example, having (x, y) coordinates in one view and (y, z) coordinates in the other, one would use the common y coordinate to match images. Those two images with identical y coordinates would be paired together. As Fig. 5 shows, because of the divergence of the X-ray beams, what actually needs to be paired is not a common y coordinate but a common angular orientation.

In practice, pairing becomes more complicated when there are many beads in each image, because there is a rather likely chance that two markers will have the same y coordinate – "same" that is within the resolution determined by system errors. GARRISON et al. (1982) estimated that for markers distributed randomly on an 8 cm square surface (angled at 45° to each image plane) and for a system resolution of 0.1 mm, there would be a 50% chance of two markers having the "same" y coordinate if there were only 20 markers on the square surface. In practice, this many markers are often

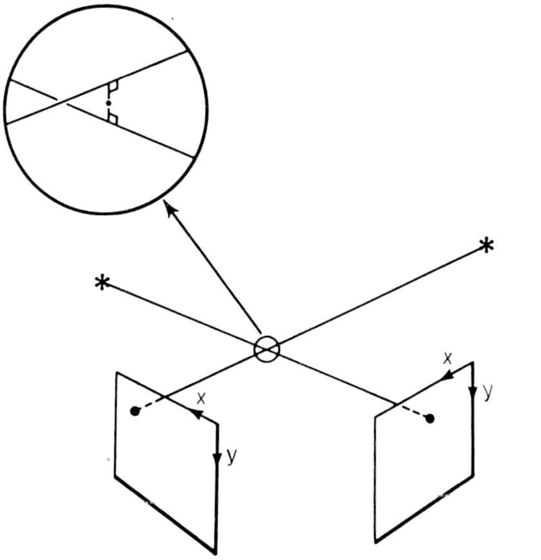

Fig. 4. Sketch of method to determine the three-dimensional position of a marker from its images in biplane films. *Asterisks* denote the locations of X-ray sources. The (x, y) and (z, y) image planes are also shown. Lines are drawn from each X-ray source to the projected image of the marker. The *inset* shows that the lines from X-ray source to image will not necessarily intersect precisely, so the midpoint is chosen as the best estimate of marker location. The miss distance is the distance from estimated marker location to either line. (MAUGHAN et al. 1984)

placed in a heart, and experience has generally borne out GARRISON et al.'s prediction that having a pair of markers with equivalent y coordinates is a fairly common occurrence. Fortunately, there is more redundant information that can be utilized to pair beads that happen to have a common y coordinate in one frame. This approach employs the fact that each bead image is tracked and identified from frame to frame in each of the two planar views. Although two markers may have equivalent y coordinates in one frame, they are much less likely to have equivalent y coordinates in *all* frames. If just one frame can be found where their y coordinates are sufficiently separate, then the marker images can be paired for that frame; subsequently, the pairing can then be extended separately in each view to all other frames. As an alternative approach, the pattern of changes in y coordinates over the whole set of frames can be compared between the two views. Correlating these patterns can also provide the information sufficient to pair a bead image in one view with its mate in the other view.

10.5.5.3 Avoiding Artifacts in Position Measurements

Two other special fixtures were also designed by GARRISON et al. (1982) to overcome other imaging artifacts (SMITH and STARMER 1978) so that position accuracy could be improved. When cine film is being exposed (at 90 frames/s) or when it is being projected, there may be a small jitter in the location of the film frame with respect to the body of the camera or projector. By imaging markers in each frame that are permanently fixed on the image intensifier, errors in film positioning can be removed. A second common artifact of image intensifier systems is pin-cushion or other similar distortions of the image. By imaging a grid of markers (Fig. 6) placed in a rectangular array (1 cm spacing) the amount of image warping can be measured and a suitable dewarping correction can then be applied to the images containing cardiac data. A third source of inaccuracy arises from the fact that the two X-ray sources do not fire simultaneously, so

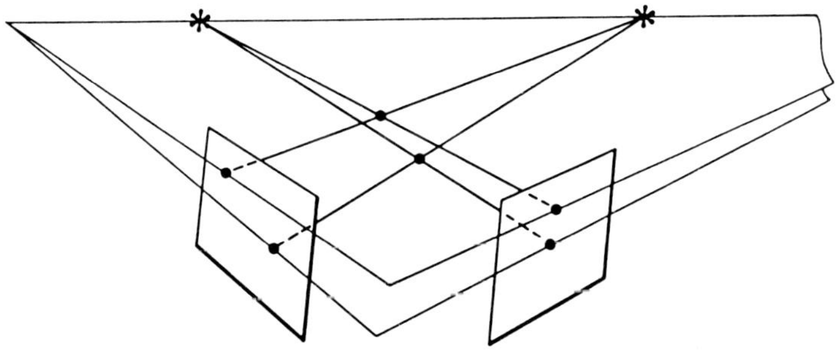

Fig. 5. Sketch of the method to pair the image of a marker in one view with its image in the orthogonal view. *Asterisks* denote X-ray sources, and image planes are also shown, as in Fig. 4. Note that for any one marker, the actual marker, its images in either image plane, and the X-ray sources are all coplanar (within the miss distance). A different marker will lie on a different plane. The angulation of each plane is the criterion by which images of the same bead are paired between views. (MAUGHAN et al. 1984)

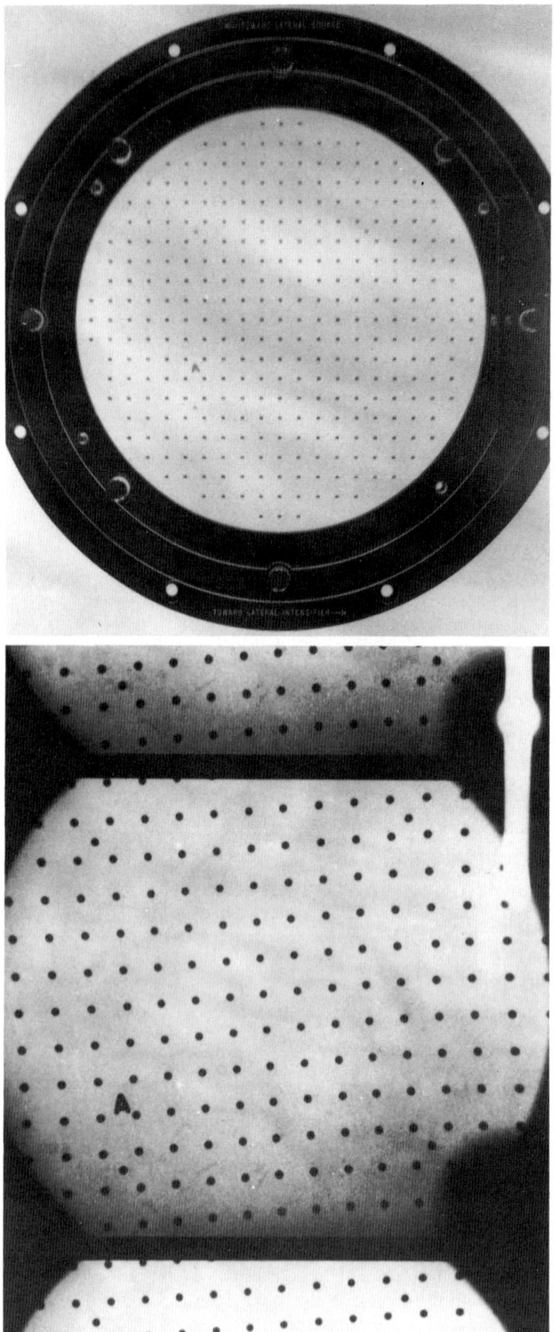

Fig. 6. The dewarping fixture *(top)*, which is attached to the face of the image intensifier, contains a precisely rectangular array of markers at 1 cm spacing. Its image *(bottom)* is used to determine the magnitude of any distortion. As determined from this image, the compensation to remove the indicated distortion is part of the processing of each film frame. (MAUGHAN et al. 1984)

that a marker will have moved slightly between its image in one view and the other. This problem can be overcome by interpolating the coordinates between two successive frames in one view to match the time of exposure of the cine film in the other view. With these corrections and using the calibration described above, three-dimensional locations of markers spaced over a range the size of a canine heart can be determined within a standard deviation of approximately 0.1 mm. (That is, the standard deviation of the miss distance is on the order of 0.1 mm)

10.5.5.4 Locating Centers of Spherical Markers

To achieve an accuracy of 0.1 mm when using physical markers that are ten times greater in diameter (1.0-mm stainless steel beads) also requires a very precise method for locating the center of the bead image in each plane. GARRISON et al. also developed an automated procedure that can achieve this degree of precision. Their algorithm is based on comparing the two-dimensional distribution of image intensities in the neighborhood of a bead image to the distribution of intensities for an "ideal" image of a bead. Numerical values for the intensity at each point (pixel) in the image are obtained by projecting a frame of cine film into a video camera whose output is digitized and stored in a computer memory. Next, a trial position for the bead center is assumed, and the distribution of intensities for the "ideal" bead is shifted so that its center is at that trial point. A mathematical correlation between the two distributions of image intensity ("ideal" bead vs data bead) is then performed. After many trial positions for the bead center have been selected, and the correlation process repeated for each, the trial position having the highest correlation between the image intensities of "ideal" and data beads becomes the best estimate of the center of the bead image.

When there are many beads (15–20) implanted in a heart, it is also not uncommon for the images of two of them to overlap slightly in one plane. To handle such occurrences, the correlation method described above must be altered slightly. Basically, the "ideal" pattern of image intensities is changed to a dumbbell shape with variable orientation and spacing between the two centers of peak intensity. This mask is moved around (as before) searching for the largest correlation, and the parameters of dumbbell are varied as well. The pattern with highest overall correlation is chosen to represent the positions of the two overlapping marker images.

So that the correlation method can reliably locate the precise centers of each marker, it is important that the markers have spherical symmetry. When the correlation method was used on images of small wire helices, which have also been used as myocardial markers (INGELS et al. 1975; WALLEY et al. 1982), the variance in miss distance was several times larger than with spherical bead markers. Evidently, as the helical marker rotated slightly from frame to frame, the intensity pattern of its image changed sufficiently that the correlation algorithm would not consistently choose the same place in the image as the "center." Perhaps this difficulty could be overcome by having the correlation method try to identify both the location and also the orientation of an asymmetrical marker (similar to what was done for the dumbbell shaped image of two beads as described above). The speed of marker tracking would suffer with this approach, however.

10.5.5.5 Computer Automation

For images acquired on 35-mm cine film, the equipment required to automate the calculations outlined in the preceding sections is sketched in Fig. 7. This figure specifies the original equipment as used by GARRISON et al. (1982). More recently, the entire system has been adapted to run on an IBM AT-class personal computer. In this configuration the required computer equipment (i.e., everything excluding the 35-mm projector and video camera)

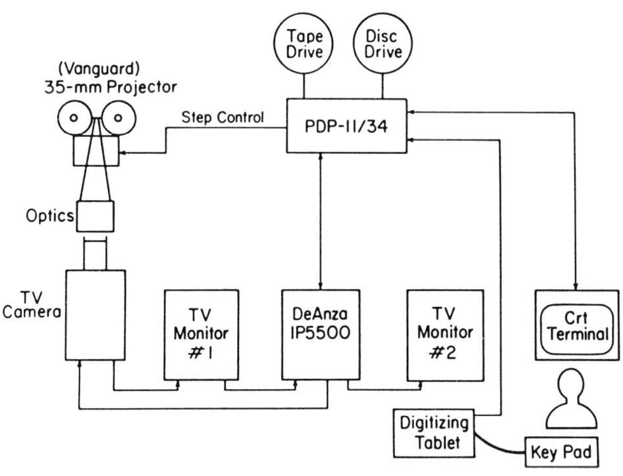

Fig. 7. The equipment utilized by GARRISON et al. to implement their computer automated marker tracking system. The PDP-11/34 is a minicomputer; the DeAnza unit is an array processor and array memory (used for digitized images). The user can view a TV monitor and terminal, and he interacts with the program via a digitizing tablet and key pad. (MAUGHAN et al. 1984)

would cost on the order of $ 13000. Thus, cost no longer appears to be a barrier to automated quantitative studies of marker motion.

The computer operations are divided into two phases: (1) semiautomatic tracking of the marker images as projected individually by both of the biplane films (two-dimensional tracking), and (2) three-dimensional reconstruction of the location of markers in space. The first phase requires an operator: (a) to select the proper sequence of film frames, (b) to focus the projection optics and set lighting levels, and (c) to locate for the computer the initial neighborhood within which each marker is located in the first frame of the sequence being tracked. The computer then automatically finds the precise center of each marker image (using the correlation scheme outlined above), advances the film to the next frame, and uses the preceding history of the motion of the image of each marker to predict for itself the neighborhoods in which it will search for each marker in the next frame. Thus, once started, the two-dimensional tracking operation could proceed entirely automatically (although in the initial prototype system, operator interaction was still required at each frame to "approve" the automatically generated locations for the purpose of quality control).

10.6 Identifying Myocardial Points Without Implanting Markers

10.6.1 Epicardial Bifurcations of Coronary Arteries

While implanted markers have been used in a few, research oriented clinical studies following cardiac surgery, their primary use has been for basic research in animal models. If naturally occurring markers could be developed for clinical use, a much broader spectrum of clinical applications for wall motion studies would become possible. The first type of natural markers to be used in patients were the branching points of epicardial coronary arteries, which were visualized by routine coronary angiography (KONG et al. 1971). With normal coronary arteries, 15–30 bifurcation points are readily identifiable, and this density of "markers" on the epicardial surface is more than sufficient for most local motion studies. Figure 8 shows a typical pair of biplane coronary angiograms and also a typical set of branch points identified for use as markers for analysis of local wall motion.

While the initial paper describing the use of coronary bifurcations as markers for wall motion analy-

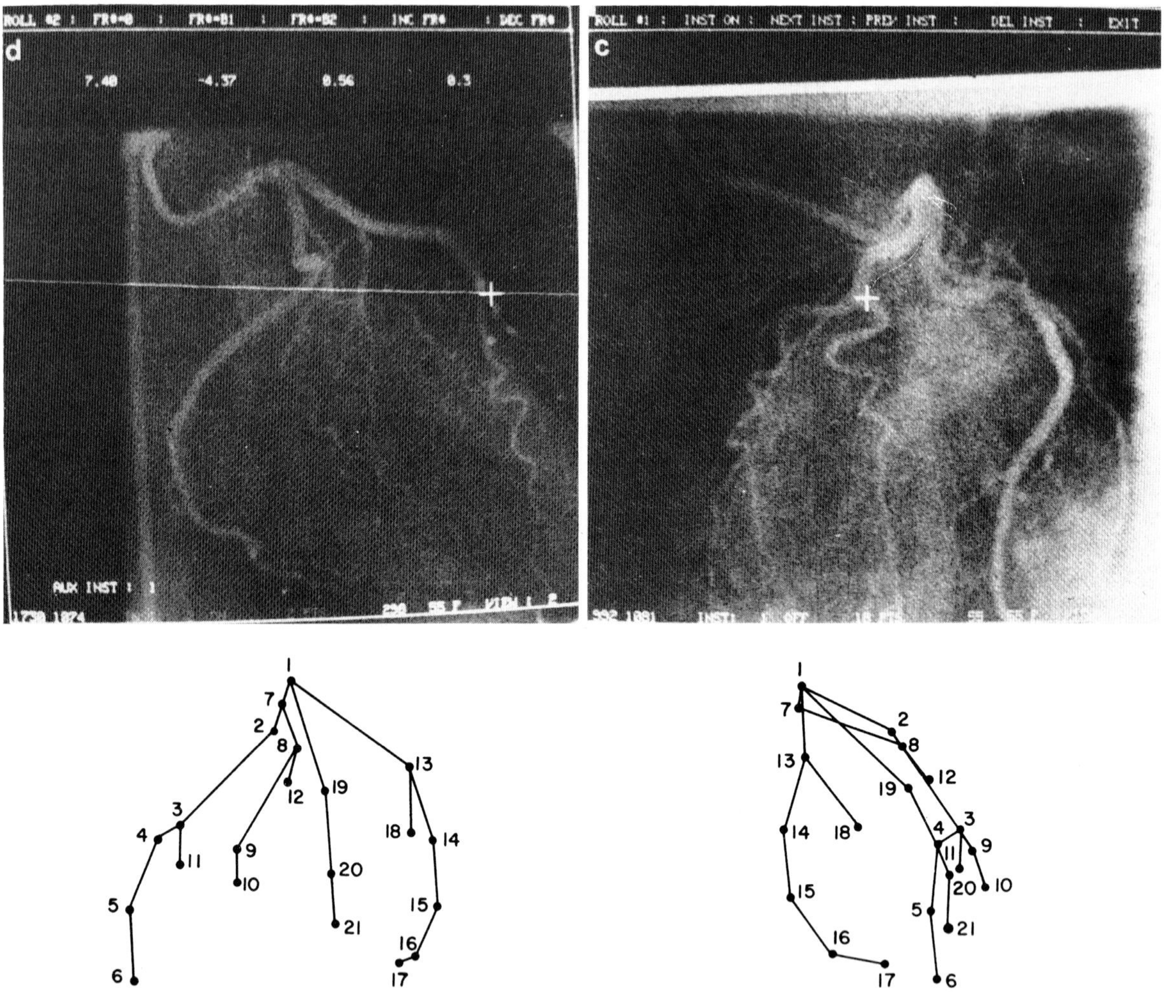

Fig. 8. Identifying epicardial "markers" from the bifurcation points of the coronary arterial tree visualized by biplane angiography. *Top:* Images of the coronary system in the two orthogonal views. Note the arterial bifurcation point (+) identified in the right-hand view, and its "back projection" (see text) shown by the superimposed line in the orthogonal view. *Bottom:* The set of indentified epicardial arterial bifurcation points are numbered and interconnected with lines that follow the arterial tree. Two orthogonal views are shown that correspond approximately to the X-ray images shown in the top panels. (MacKay et al. 1982)

sis was enthusiastically received (earning a Young Investigator's Award), practical application of the concept has proved difficult. The first impediment was the overwhelming work load and difficulty of identifying the branch points by hand and correlating a branch point in one view with its mate in the orthogonal view. This roadblock has been removed by a computer assisted system having specially designed graphical overlays (MacKay et al. 1982; Potel et al. 1983). Key to this system is the display of "back projections" of positions from one view onto the display of the other view (see Fig. 8). That is, having identified a bifurcation point in one view, and knowing the location of the X-ray source from calibrations similar to that described in Sect. 10.5.5.1, one can draw a line in space (connecting the X-ray source and image point) along which the bifurcation point must lie. Projecting this line onto the orthogonal view aids greatly in identifying the corresponding image of the same branch point in this second view.

Despite the successful automation of part of the process of tracking epicardial coronary bifurcations, many problems remain to be resolved. Foremost is precise localization of the bifurcation point in either view. Since the large epicardial arteries have significant width, how to pinpoint what will be called the precise *point* of bifurcation has not yet been objectively determined. One cannot just pick the point at the base of the internal V at a branch, because any rotation of that region of the heart will make the V-point *appear* to move as a result of viewing different amounts of overlap between the two branches. In the computer assisted system developed so far (MACKAY et al. 1982), a trained "analyst" was required to determine (ultimately, somewhat subjectively) the precise positions of the bifurcation points. A computer assisted method that takes into account the three-dimensional nature of the arteries should provide a more objective and precise localization (YOUNG et al. 1989). Using digital subtraction angiography to more clearly define the opacified arteries may also be advantageous in this process.

Should all technical problems be overcome, there may still be a critical limitation in the coronary bifurcation approach, however. Many clinical applications of local cardiac wall motion arise as a result of narrowings or blockages of coronary arteries. The important question is whether it would be possible to opacify sufficiently the poststenotic coronary arteries, which would be located in the regions where one would most require regional wall motion measurements to evaluate myocardial performance in the ischemic zone.

10.6.2 Magnetic Resonance Tagging of Specific Myocardial Points

Magnetic resonance imaging (MRI) is the newest imaging modality. Its potential for cardiac imaging was recognized very early (POHOST and CANBY 1987). The fundamental reason for the early application of MRI to cardiovascular imaging is the sensitivity of the method to flow and motion. The image signal in MRI is generated by hydrogen nuclei that have been preexcited by a resonant radiofrequency (RF) pulse. The reader is referred to more basic texts for a fuller understanding of this mechanism (SINGER 1959; AXEL 1984). For the purpose of this chapter, the reader only needs to know that the ultimate signal intensity of any tissue is determined by: (1) the relaxation times of the tissues, (2) the degree of RF excitation imparted to the tissues, and (3) the degree of motion occurring during image acquisition. To allow for recovery, RF excitation of tissues is generally performed at intervals greater than the relaxation time. For the heart this implies repetition rates of several hundred milliseconds. As the velocity of flowing blood and that of moving myocardial walls are greatly different, it is possible to create MR images where the blood pool will have a different signal intensity than the myocardium. As the time to acquire a single data point for an image is in the order of 20 ms, adequate images of the heart, without much motion blurring, can be obtained if cardiac gating is used. Newer methods permit the acquisition of cinematic sequences comprising 16–32 frames per cardiac cycle (SECHTEN et al. 1987). However, to date all of these MRI techniques suffer from the same limitation as all conventional tomographic imaging modalities, i.e., there is no way of following the displacements of a specific point in the myocardium throughout the cardiac cycle. To overcome such limitations, a novel imaging approach was developed which permits noninvasive "labeling" or "tagging" of defined regions of the myocardium.

This new method of cardiac tagging is based on the concept of generating a difference in MR signal intensities between tagged and nontagged regions of the myocardium that can persist for several hundred milliseconds. This allows images taken at different points in the cardiac cycle to reflect intervening rearrangement of myocardial fibers demonstrating the relative deformation of the tagged regions (Figs. 9–11).

To understand this technique it is important to realize that the signal intensity of tissues imaged by MRI depends upon the T_1 and T_2 relaxation times and proton density of the tissues, the degree of RF excitation imparted to these tissues, and the repetition time and echo time used in the particular imaging sequence. Obviously, relaxation times, proton density, and the imaging sequence are parameters that cannot be modified for selected regions of the myocardium. However, the degree of RF excitation of specific regions can be modulated so as to generate differences in signal intensity. This is the fundamental idea behind tissue labeling with MRI. In fact, our method works in the following manner:

An RF pulse is first imparted to thin bands of myocardial tissue at or near diastole. This is done by the use of narrow and very selective RF pulses in the presence of linear magnetic field gradients. By modulating the gradients and the RF pulse we can create various patterns of tissue labeling such as a grid-like pattern or a series of parallel lines throughout the heart and even a radial pattern centered on the long axis of the left ventricle (see Figs. 9–11). This is generally done by using 180° RF pulses or so-called inversion pulses that are capable of inverting the magnetic vector in the particular band of excited tissue. Therefore, the magnetic vector of the tagged region is now in direct opposition to the magnetic vector of the nontagged regions.

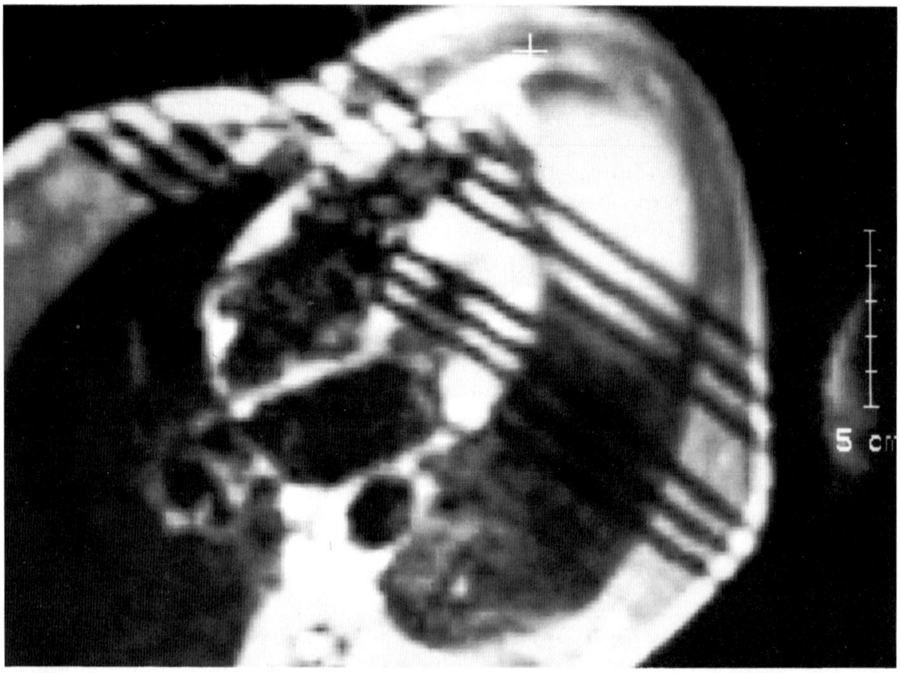

9

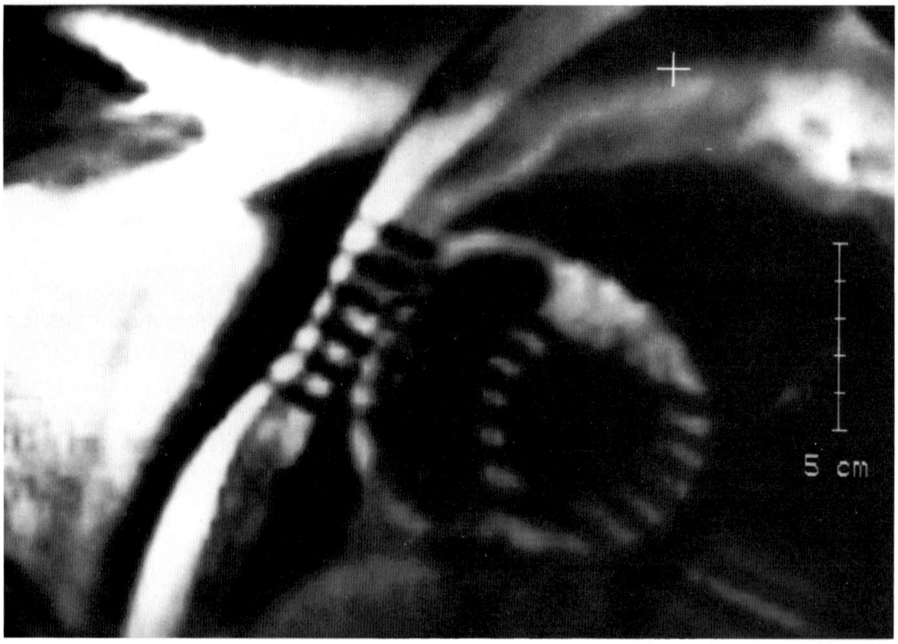

10

Fig. 9. Example of tagging for analysis of base to apex motion. Two sets of three parallel linear tags were generated at end-diastole and localized by proper matching of the radiofrequency and gradient strength of the system to the base and apex of the heart. RF tagging required a total time of 12 ms. The image presented here was obtained 150 ms after completion of tagging in a plane orthogonal to the plane of imaging which is parallel to the long axis of the left ventricle. Displacement of the cardiac tags relative to the tags seen in the chest wall reflects base to apex motion. Note the basal tags which have translated towards the apex to a greater degree than the tags located in the apical region of the heart

Fig. 10. A set of six parallel tags were generated at end-diastole. This image was obtained 90 ms after generation of the tags. Reorientation of the tag lines relative to their original position as marked in the anterior chest wall reflects reorientation of fibers within the myocardium. (ZERHOUNI et al. 1988)

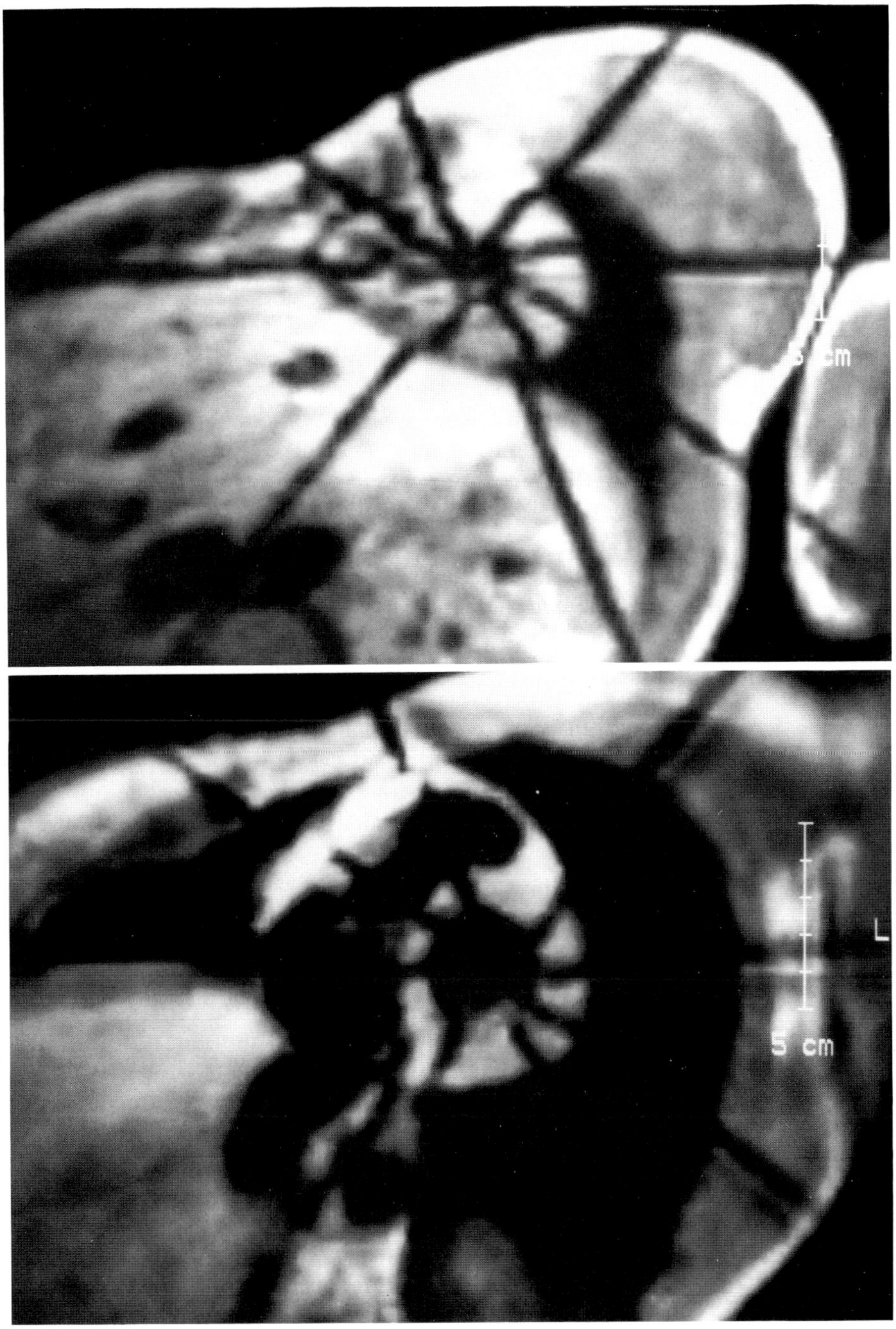

a

b

Fig. 11 a, b. A set of four radially oriented tags placed orthogonally to the short axis plane of the left ventricle were generated near end-diastole in a normal human volunteer. These two images represent **a** the midapical ventricular region and **b** the basal region of the left ventricle at 130 ms after tagging. Global rotation of the heart is demonstrated by the step-off noted between the original position of tag lines as visible in the chest wall or liver. In addition, deformation of the tags themselves reflects in-plane fiber rearrangement. Note the direction of the fiber rearrangement and the fact that the deformation of the tags from image A to image B is not symmetrical implying a degree of twist. This example demonstrates the potential of the technique in mapping fiber rearrangement throughout the left ventricle during the entire contractile phase of the cardiac cycle. (ZERHOUNI et al. 1988)

Obviously, the excited nuclei in the tagged regions will eventually return to their resting state. The time for the excited spins to return is in the order of the intrinsic myocardial longitudinal relaxation time T_1, which is about 500 ms. Therefore, if an image is acquired at any time before the excited spins have returned to equilibrium, a difference in signal intensity will be perceived between the tagged and non-tagged regions of the heart. Any movement of the heart between the time of tagging and that of imaging will be reflected by a displacement as well as deformation of the tag. [For a more formal description of the differences in signal intensity behavior the reader is referred to the original reference (ZERHOUNI et al. 1988).] Once the basic concept of the technique is matered, it is easy to recognize its versatility. Any number of tag lines can be generated in any number of patterns. Generally, images are best acquired in a plane orthogonal to the plane of tagging. As the technique is totally noninvasive, multiple experiments spanning multiple phases of the cardiac cycle and multiple regions of the heart examined in several planes can be performed leading to a full three-dimensional mapping of ventricular contraction. By studying the deformation of tag lines in multiple planes, it is possible to generate a global view of the fiber rearrangement in normal and abnormal contraction. Motions such as twist or shear can be quantified. As the method is still in its infancy, its full impact on the study of myocardial strain is not yet determined. Development of effective computer techniques to fully represent and analyze the data generated by such studies is still evolving. However, it is clear that the method has the advantage of generating an arbitrary number of markers that can be localized and tracked even in regions inaccessible to conventional markers. Computerized matching of slice to slice changes during normal and pathological contraction may lead to a better understanding of region to region interactions during such contraction. The totally noninvasive nature of the method also makes it immediately applicable to humans.

10.6.3 Range-Gated Doppler Ultrasound to Determine Strain

By sensing the Doppler shift of ultrasound reflected from moving biological structures, one can sense their velocity of motion. This technique has been used for quite a while to measure the velocity of flowing blood (BAKER 1970). By pulsing the bursts of ultrasound and receiving the reflected signal only at a specific time after sending a burst, one can also effectively set the distance (i.e., the range gate) from the transducer to the site at which one is measuring the velocity. Thus, it is in principle possible to map the velocity field of moving structures or fluids. By integrating velocity one obtains the changes in positions and thus the pattern of deformation in a tissue.

The advantage of integrating velocities is that one does not have to identify a specific ultrasonic echo arising from a particular interface; material interfaces are not required at all. Moreover, compared to tracking the echo from an interface, the method of integrating velocity is less sensitive to changes in echo amplitude, changes which often hamper tracking as an interface moves and changes orientation. On the other hand, one gives up the ability to measure absolute positions. Only changes in position can be obtained from integrating velocity (i.e., no constant of integration is available). For strain measurements, however, relative changes in length are the primary concern, so this limitation may not be a major handicap.

An initial application of this concept to study local cardiac wall motion has been to study local thickening of the myocardial wall under an epicardially placed transducer in dogs (HARTLEY et al. 1983). Again, only relative changes in thickness were measured, i.e., the thickening fraction. In this initial application, a velocity field was not measured; only the velocity at a single range-gated depth was determined. Since this range gate had to be set to a depth that always fell within the myocardium, the full thickness of the ventricular wall could not be measured.

For application to clinical measurements, initially even just to study myocardial thickening, for example, the requirement that the transducer be affixed to the epicardium would have to be overcome. This would necessitate having at least two range gates so that the relative velocity of the heart wall towards or away from the transducer could be separated from the thickening of the wall. A further advance would be to obtain data along multiple beams of ultrasound oriented in different directions through the same tissue space. In this way the two-dimensional or even three-dimensional measurements of strain that are possible with markers could in principle also be obtained via range-gated Doppler ultrasound. There is thus major developmental work required here before this technique could provide the detailed picture of deformations and strains that X-ray imaging of implanted markers now provides. The advantages of such development are numerous, however. Like MRI, the technique is noninvasive; moreover, measurements could be obtained rapidly, which would offer a distinct advantage over MRI.

10.7 Applications of Marker Motion Analysis to Other Organs

Studying the motion of embedded tissue markers is not only important in the heart, but also for any organ in which relative motion of tissues is a critical part of its function. The lung is another such organ, and several groups have utilized implanted markers to evaluate aspects of regional motion there. In one study (SIMON and MITZNER 1987; SIMON 1987), many local tetrahedra (see Sect. 10.5.4) were defined by an array of implanted spherical beads. For each tetrahedron, the observed motion of the four markers was translated into changes in local volume contained within the tetrahedron. By relating these volume changes to the location of the tetrahedron, the regional distribution of physical volume changes (i.e., ventilation) within the lung was obtained. In another study (CHEVALIER et al. 1978), the distances between pairs of embedded markers were compared – both when the lungs were in the thorax and when they were freshly excised (but in both cases expanded to total lung capacity) – to ascertain whether the presence of the thorax distorted the expansion of the lungs. A more recent study from the same laboratory (WEI et al. 1985) measured the magnitude of motion of embedded markers in lung parenchyma and tested how much of that motion was correlated with the heart beat. This study thus attempted to quantify a potential cardiogenic increase in the mixing of gases in the lung, a mechanism that had been suggested as an aid to pulmonary ventilation. All of these pulmonary studies employed biplane recording of X-ray images of embedded markers and used analysis methods identical or similar to that described in Sect. 10.5.5.

Studies of the dynamic mechanisms involved in swallowing have also been greatly aided by cine or videoradiography of implanted markers (KRAMER et al. 1987; HIIEMAE and CROMPTON 1985). Similar to studies in the heart, these studies also illustrated the advantages of imaging fixed anatomical points within an organ as opposed to previous techniques where only a radiopaque silhouette could be seen. For example, visualization of the changing silhouette of a radiopaque bolus passing through the pharynx has often been used in the past to study pharyngeal kinesiology. However, these silhouettes cannot reveal the motion of specific points on the wall of the pharynx (similar to the situation in the heart). Particularly, motions of a point in the pharyngeal wall that are directed longitudinally along the wall could be significant for deciding which of two competing mechanisms play a major role in swallowing, but such longitudinal motions would be most difficult to detect reliably from the silhouette of the bolus. To answer this question (PALMER et al. 1988), radiopaque markers were affixed by suction to the wall of the pharynx in volunteers, and single-plane (not biplane) videoradiograms were obtained. Motions of the markers projected into the plane of the image were analyzed frame by frame and showed large (and in some cases, predominantly) longitudinal components.

Motility at points lower in the digestive tract has also been observed using implanted radiopaque markers. In a classic study, GIANTURCO (1934) embedded lead shot in the gastric wall of a cat to outline the antrum of the stomach. He then observed the motion of these markers relative to ingested radiopaque boluses of fluid and solid masses of meat.

10.8 Future Directions of Motion Analysis Systems in Research and Clinic

Imaging of the motion of distinct, specific points in the walls of the heart (or other organs) has been required with increasing frequency as more sophisticated basic research questions have been asked. For animal studies, in which small spherical beads can easily be embedded, the development of computer automated systems for image analysis (Sect. 10.5.5) has already greatly expanded the feasibility of such studies by reducing the burden of data analysis by several orders of magnitude and improving the positional resolution of the data that can be obtained. For basic research questions, then, such existing systems appear to be sufficient.

For clinical studies of the motion of specific points, however, it is seldom feasible to implant the required markers. Thus, means for identifying points without implanting a bead must be sought and developed. Three techniques for accomplishing this in cardiac patients were presented in Sect. 10.6. The most promising two of these, involving magnetic resonance "tagging" or ultrasonic range-gated velocity measures, are only in the very initial stages of development. Much effort needs to be devoted to them before their full potential as clinical tools for dynamic analysis can be realized, but the reward will be greatly enhanced ability to "see" normal or pathological motions within the walls of the heart (or other organs).

Clinical analysis of local motion in the heart wall is primarily intended to estimate the functional consequences of regional ischemia. Correlating local functional deficits with the degree of reduction in myocardial perfusion and the resulting local changes in cellular metabolic and ionic state is therefore of key clinical importance. Imaging techniques exist to observe the distribution of all of these factors: perfusion, metabolism, and contractile motion. Thus, another avenue to advance the imaging of local myocardial motion will be development of radiological techniques that combine regional measurements of motion, metabolism, and perfusion. Simultaneous correlations among these variables should play a key role in future research and eventually in therapy.

References

Arts T, Meerbaum S, Reneman RS, Corday E (1984) Torsion of the left ventricle during the ejection phase in the intact dog. Cardiovasc Res 18: 183-193

Axel L (1984) Blood flow effects in magnetic resonance imaging. AJR 143: 1157

Baker DW (1970) Pulsed ultrasonic Doppler blood flow sensing. IEEE Trans Sonics Ultrasonics SU-17: 170-185

Brower RW, Ten Katen HJ, Meester GT (1978) Direct method for determining regional myocardial shortening after bypass surgery from radiopaque markers in man. Am J Cardiol 41: 1222-1229

Brower RW, Serruys PW, Bos E, Nauta J (1979) Regional myocardial shortening in relation to graft-reactive hyperemia and flow after coronary bypass surgery. J Thorac Cardiovasc Surg 77: 92-100

Brundage BH (1987) Ultrafast cardiac computed tomography: Where does it fit? Am J Cardiac Imag 1: 201-203

Buda AJ, Zotz RJ, Gallagher KP (1986) Characterization of the functional border zone around regionally ischemic myocardium using circumferential flow-function maps. J Am Coll Cardiol 9: 150

Canby RC, Evanochko WT, Pohost GM (1986) NMR imaging of the cardiovascular system. In: Fozzard HA, Haber E, Jennings RB, Katz AM, Morgan HE (eds) The heart and cardiovascular system, vol I. Raven, New York, pp 331-349

Chaitman BR, DeMots H, Bristow JD, Rosch J, Rahimtoola SH (1975) Objective and subjective analysis of left ventricular angiograms. Circulation 52: 420-425

Chevalier PA, Rodarte JR, Harris LD (1978) Regional lung expansion at total lung capacity in intact vs. excised canine lungs. J Appl Physiol 45: 363-369

Clayton PD, Jeppson GM, Klausner SC (1982) Should a fixed external reference system be used to analyze left ventricular wall motion? Circulation 65: 1518-1521

Dodge HT, Sheehan FH (1986) Quantitative angiographic techniques. In: Fozzard HA, Haber E, Jennings RB, Katz AM, Morgan HE (eds) The heart and cardiovascular system, vol I. Raven, New York, pp 351-368

Falsetti HL, Marcus ML, Kerber RE, Skorton DJ (1981) Editorial: Quantification of myocardial ischemia and infarction by left ventricular imaging. Circulation 63: 747-751

Fenton TR, Cherry JM, Klassen GA (1978) Transmural myocardial deformation in the canine left ventricular wall. Am J Physiol 235: H523-H530

Force T, Bloomfield P, O'Boyle JE, Khuri SF, Josa M, Parisi AF (1984) Quantitative two-dimensional echocardiographic analysis of regional wall motion in patients with perioperative myocardial infarction. Circulation 70: 233-241

Force T, Kemper A, Perkins L, Gilfoil M, Cohen C, Parisi AF (1986) Overestimation of infarct size by quantitative two-dimensional echocardiography: The role of tethering and of analytic procedures. Circulation 73: 1360-1368

Gallagher KP, Osakada G, Matsuzaki M, Miller M, Kemper WS, Ross J Jr (1985) Nonuniformity of inner and outer systolic wall thickening in conscious dogs. Am J Physiol 249: H241-H248

Garrison JB, Ebert WL, Jenkins RE et al. (1982) Measurement of three-dimensional positions and motions of large numbers of spherical radiopaque markers from biplane cineradiograms. Comput Biomed Res 15: 76-96

Gelberg HJ, Brundage BH, Glantz S, Parmley WW (1979) Quantitative left ventricular wall motion analysis: A comparison of area, chord and radial methods. Circulation 59: 991-1000

Gianturco C (1934) Some mechanical factors of gastric physiology. AJR 31: 735-744

Goodyer AVN, Langou RA (1982) The multicentric character of normal left ventricular wall motion. Implications for the evaluation of regional wall motion abnormalities by contrast angiography. Cathet Cardiovasc Diagn 8: 225-232

Halperin HR, Chew PC, Weisfeldt ML, Sagawa K, Humphrey JD, Yin FCP (1987) Transverse stiffness: A method for estimation of myocardial wall stress. Circ Res 61: 695-703

Hansen DE, Daughters GT, Alderman EL, Stinson EB, Baldwin JC, Miller DC (1987) Effect of acute human cardiac allograft rejection on left ventricular systolic torsion and diastolic recoil measured by intramyocardial markers. Circulation 76: 998-1008

Harrison DC, Goldblatt A, Braunwald E (1963) Studies on cardiac dimensions in intact, unanesthetized man. I: Description of techniques and their verification. Circ Res 13: 448-455

Hartley CJ, Latson LA, Michael LH, Seidel CL, Lewis RM, Entman ML (1983) Doppler measurement of myocardial thickening with a single epicardial transducer. Am J Physiol 245: H1066-H1072

Heikkila J, Tabakin BS, Hugenholtz PG (1972) Quantification of function in normal and infarcted regions of the left ventricle. Cardiovasc Res 6: 516-531

Hiiemae K, Crompton A (1985) Mastication, food transport, and swallowing. In: Hildebrand M, Bramble DM, Liem KF, Wake DB (eds) Functional vertebrate morphology. Harvard Univ. Press, Cambridge MA, pp 262-290

Holman BL (1980) Radioisotopic examination of the cardiovascular system. In: Braunwald E (ed) Heart disease. A textbook of cardiovascular medicine, vol I. Saunders, Philadelphia, pp 363-409

Hunter WC, Sugiura S, Douglas AS (1986) Systolic changes in local "shape" of the left ventricular wall. Proc Ann Conf Eng Med Biol 28: 124

Ingels NB Jr, Daughters GT, Stinson EB, Alderman EL (1975) Measurement of midwall myocardial dynamics in intact man by radiography of surgically implanted markers. Circulation 52: 859–867

Ingels NB Jr, Daughters GT, Stinson EB, Alderman EL (1980) Evaluation of methods for quantitating left ventricular segmental wall motion in man using myocardial markers as a standard. Circulation 61: 966–972

Ingels NB Jr, Hansen DE, Daughters GT, Stinson EB, Alderman EL, Miller DC (1987) Maximum midwall shortening is not oriented circumferentially in the left ventricular free wall of the transplanted human heart (abstract). Circulation 76: IV-540

Kisslo JA, Robertson D, Gilbert BW, von Ramm O, Behar VS (1977) A comparison of real-time, two-dimensional echocardiography and cineangiography in detecting left ventricular asynergy. Circulation 55: 134–141

Kong Y, Morris JJ Jr, McIntosh HD (1971) Assessment of regional myocardial performance from biplane coronary cineangiograms. Am J Cardiol 27: 529–537

Kramer SS, Anderson JH, Strandberg JD, Donner MW (1987) A permanent radiopaque marker technique for the study of pharyngeal swallowing in dogs. Dysphagia 1: 163–167

Levine RA, Gillam LD, Weyman AE (1986) Echocardiography in cardiac research. In: Fozzard HA, Haber E, Jennings RB, Katz AM, Morgan HE (eds) The heart and cardiovascular system, vol I. Raven, New York, pp 369–452

Lieberman AN, Weiss JL, Jugdutt BI et al. (1981) Two-dimensional echocardiography and infarct size: relationship of regional wall motion and thickening to the extent of myocardial infarction in the dog. Circulation 63: 739–746

Lima JAC, Becker LC, Melin JA, Lima S, Kallman CA, Weisfeldt ML, Weiss JL (1985) Impaired thickening of nonischemic myocardium during acute regional ischemia in the dog. Circulation 71: 1048–1059

MacKay SA, Potel MJ, Rubin JM (1982) Graphics methods for tracking three-dimensional heart wall motion. Comp Biomed Res 15: 455–473

Maughan WL, Jenkins RE, Ebert WL, Ciuffo A, Shoukas AA, Sagawa K (1984) Multiple marker cineventriculogrammetry: A new technique for simultaneous measurement of regional wall motion and overall geometry in animals. In: Sigwart U, Heintzen PH (eds) Ventricular wall motion. Thieme, Stuttgart, pp 14–23

McDonald IG (1972) Contraction of the hypertrophied left ventricle in man studied by cineradiography of epicardial markers. Am J Cardiol 30: 587–594

McDonald IG (1970) The shape and movements of the human left ventricle during systole. Am J Cardiol 26: 221–230

Meier GD, Ziskin MC, Santamore WP, Bove AA (1980 a) Kinematics of the beating heart. IEEE Trans Biomed Eng 27: 319–329

Meier GD, Bove AA, Santamore WP (1980 b) Contractile function in canine right ventricle. Am J Physiol 239: H794–H804

Palmer JB, Tanaka E, Siebens AA (1988) Motions of the posterior pharyngeal wall in swallowing. Laryngoscope 98: 414–417

Pandian NG, Skorton DJ, Collins SM, Falsetti HL, Burke ER, Kerber RE (1983) Heterogeneity of left ventricular segmental wall thickening and excursion in 2-dimensional echocardiograms of normal human subjects. Am J Cardiol 51: 1667–1673

Pohost GM, Canby RC (1987) Nuclear magnetic resonance imaging: Current applications and future prospects. Circulation 75: 88–95

Pohost GM, Okada R, Boucher CA, Bourge RC (1986) Radionuclide methods to assess cardiac function, perfusion, viability, and necrosis. In: Fozzard HA, Haber E, Jennings RB, Katz AM, Morgan HE (eds) The heart and cardiovascular system, vol I. Raven, New York, pp 309–329

Potel MJ, Rubin JM, MacKay SA, Aisen AM, Al-Sadir J, Sayre RE (1983) Methods for evaluating cardiac wall motion in three dimensions using bifurcation points of the coronary arterial tree. Invest Radiol 18: 47–57

Reiter SJ, Rumberger JA, Feiring AJ, Stanford W, Marcus ML (1986) Precision of measurements of right and left ventricular volume by cine computed tomography. Circulation 74: 890–900

Reiter SJ, Rumberger JA, Stanford W, Marcus ML (1987) Quantitative determination of aortic regurgitant volumes in dogs by ultrafast computed tomography. Circulation 76: 728–735

Rickards A, Seabra-Gomes R, Thurston P (1977) The assessment of regional abnormalities of the left ventricle by angiography. Eur J Cardiol 5: 167–182

Rittman EL, Kinsey JH, Robb RA, Gilbert BK, Harris LD, Wood EH (1980) Three-dimensional images of heart, lungs, and circulation. Science 210: 273–280

Robb RA, Lent AH, Gilbert BK, Chu A (1980) The dynamic spatial reconstructor: a computed tomography system for high-speed simultaneous scanning of multiple cross sections of the heart. J Med Syst 4: 253–288

Schwiep F, Cassidy SS, Ramanathan M (1986) In vivo canine right ventricular time-varying elastance. Proc Ann Conf Eng Med Biol 28: 127

Sechten U, Pflugfelder PW, White RD, Gould RG, Holt W, Lipton MJ, Higgins CB (1987) Cine MR imaging. Potential for evaluation of cardiovascular function. AJR 148: 239–46

Sheehan FH, Bolson EL, Dodge HT, Mathey DG, Schofer J, Woo H-W (1986) Advantages and applications of the centerline method for characterizing regional ventricular function. Circulation 74: 293–305

Sheehan FH, Stewart DK, Dodge HT, Mitten S, Bolson EL, Brown BG (1983) Variability in the measurement of regional left ventricular wall motion from contrast angiograms. Circulation 68: 550–559

Simon BA (1987) Dynamic distribution of pulmonary ventilation during high-frequency ventilation. PhD Dissertation, Johns Hopkins University, Baltimore

Simon BA, Mitzner W (1987) Redistribution of pulmonary ventilation during high-frequency (abstract). Fed Proc 46: 1424

Singer JR (1959) Blood flow rates by nuclear magnetic resonance measurements. Science 130: 1652

Smith WM, Starmer CF (1978) Error propagation in quantitative biplane cineroentgenography. Phys Med Biol 23: 677

Waldman LK, Fung YC, Covell JW (1985) Transmural myocardial deformation in the canine left ventricle. Normal in vivo three-dimensional finite strains. Circ Res 57: 152–163

Walley KR, Grover M, Raff GL, Benge W, Hannaford B, Glantz SA (1982) Left ventricular dynamic geometry in the intact and open chest dog. Circ Res 50: 573–589

Wei JH, Hoffman EA, Rittman EL, Wood EH (1985) Cardiogenic motion of right lung parenchyma in anesthetized intact dogs. J Appl Physiol 58: 384–391

Weiss JL, Bulkley BH, Hutchins GM, Mason SJ (1981) Two-dimensional echocardiographic recognition of myocardial

injury in man: comparison with postmortem studies. Circulation 63: 401–408
Wiseman MD, Hunter WC, Douglas AS (1987) Errors in calculation of local myocardial strain derived from positions of four implanted markers (abstract). Fed Proc 46: 836
Yin FCP (1981) Ventricular wall stress. Circ Res 49: 829–842
Young AA, Hunter PJ, Smaill BH (1989) Epicardial surface estimation from coronary angiograms. Computer Vision, Graphics and Image Processing (in press)
Zerhouni EA, Parish DM, Rogers WJ, Yang A, Shapiro EP (1988) Tagging of the human heart by magnetic resonance imaging: a non-invasive method of assessment of myocardial motion. Radiology 169: 59–63

11 Toward Computed Image-Controlled Electromechanical Stereotactic Brain Surgery

SUMIO UEMATSU, ARTHUR E. ROSENBAUM, and ASHOK J. KUMAR

CONTENTS

11.1 Introduction 191
11.2 Development of CT-Guided Stereotactic Surgery 192
11.3 The Stereotactic Frame 192
11.4 Surgical Planning and Applications 194
11.4.1 Biopsy of Brain Lesions 194
11.4.2 Drainage of Abscesses 194
11.4.3 Implantation of Radioactive Seeds 194
11.4.4 Thalamotomy for Movement Disorders 195
11.5 Stereotactic Brain Surgery Within the CT Scanner 195
11.5.1 Procedure 196
11.6 Thalamotomy with Combined Use of MRI, CT, and Cell-Unit Recordings at the CT Scanner Site 199
11.6.1 Current Technique 199
11.6.2 Future Integration of CT and MRI Images 202
11.7 Computerized Image Controlled Servomotor-Driven Stereotactic System 203
11.8 Technical Problems and Research Needs 203
11.8.1 Robotics in Stereotactic Brain Surgery 203
11.8.2 Problems with the Metallic Robot Arm 204
11.8.3 Analytic and Therapeutic Stereotactic Probe . . . 204
11.8.4 Elimination of the Stereotactic Frame 205
11.9 Focused Light Beam-Guided Brain Surgery . . . 205
11.10 Radiosurgery 205
11.11 Therapeutic Compounds Guided with Stereotactically Focused Magnetic Force 206
11.12 Conclusion 206
References 206

11.1 Introduction

The stereotactic technique developed by HORSLEY and CLARKE in 1908 was designed to explore deep-seated structures in the animal brain (HORSLEY and CLARKE 1908). Later, the technique was used in man in the treatment of Parkinson's disease. Selective destruction of subcortical structures was found to eliminate tremor and/or relieve rigidity (NARABAYASHI and OKUMA 1953). However, the target sites for this procedure were not only deep in the brain, but also adjacent to vital structures, such as the internal capsule and hypothalamus, and occupied very small areas. The probe needed to be placed with a precision measured in millimeters. Reaching the target's location was ensured by measuring the distance between two highly consistent structures, e.g., the anterior and posterior commissures, or from the foramen of Monro, visualized by the trapping of air within the ventricular system. The location of the target structure was estimated by using a brain atlas compiled from formalin-fixed autopsy brain specimens (SCHALTENBRAND and BAILEY 1959).

Advanced imaging techniques now allow direct visualization of the desired subcortical structures. Computed tomography (CT), magnetic resonance imaging (MRI), and to some extent positron emission tomography (PET) acquire signals that on Fourier transformation, result in a composite formed by elements called pixels. Each of the 65536 (256^2) to 1048576 (1024^2) pixels in an image is represented by a specific shade of gray (of computer-calculated intensity) in a specific location on the image. Additional processing software and/or hardware systems have been developed for further processing of the data forming the pixels, so that three-dimensional reconstructions can be generated for greater visual understanding of the target. In the future, holography should afford an even better three-dimensional perspective.

Present stereotactic procedures involve directing a probe along a single trajectory. The trajectory is made along the coordinates needed to reach the target, which are determined using a minimal portion of the vast pixel area. Yet, if all the pixel information were useable in probe guidance, electromechanical, robotic stereotactic brain surgery would be facilitated. Such a procedure might be called computed image-controlled electromechanical surgery (CICESS). This chapter reviews the develop-

SUMIO UEMATSU, M.D., F.A.C.S., Dept. of Neurosurgery, The Johns Hopkins University, School of Medicine, 600 North Wolfe Street, Baltimore, MD 21205, USA
ARTHUR E. ROSENBAUM, M.D., F.A.C.R., Dept. of Radiology and Radiological Science, The Johns Hopkins University, School of Medicine, 600 North Wolfe Street, Baltimore, MD 21205, USA
ASHOK J. KUMAR, M.D., Dept. of Radiology and Radiological Science, The Johns Hopkins University, School of Medicine, 600 North Wolfe Street, Baltimore, MD 21205, USA

ment of stereotactic brain surgery, its current status, and immediate problems to be resolved for future applications, such as CICESS.

11.2 Development of CT-Guided Stereotactic Surgery

Since the initial experiments with stereotactic neurosurgery by HORSLEY and CLARKE and clinical application by SPIEGEL et al. (1947), the principles of the technique have changed drastically. Originally, surgery targets within the brain were derived from brain atlases, which in turn were derived from data pooled from numerous autopsy specimens (SCHALTENBRAND and BAILEY 1959). Today, cross-sectional imaging, CT and MRI provide direct visualization of the previously radiologically invisible internal structures of the brain. Thus, the approximations inherent in extrapolating from the brains of cadavers have been obviated. The computed image displays a "slice" of the brain of the particular individual; the slice may be considered to be a grid of x and y coordinates. Moreover, as the body (brain) is moved further into or out of the scanner's gantry, the z ("depth") coordinate is derived. Thus, the image inherently contains the coordinates used for the stereotactic procedure (Fig. 1). As this imaging ability has progressed, a flurry of research and development has followed. Initially, portions of an existing stereotactic frame were adapted to the CT scanner (BERGSTROM and GREITZ 1976). Since the metal of the frame was not compatible with generating an image, PERRY et al. (1980), in a threefold development, advanced a CT-compatible frame, used the scanner's computer to calculate the coordinates of the trajectory, and provided active intraoperative verification of surgical progress. At the meeting of the American Society of Neuroradiology, in Toronto, Canada in 1979, BROWN et al. (1980) presented their concept of a stereotactic frame in which one portion was used for CT *coordinate determination*, and then was exchanged for another portion for *surgical use* in the operating room. The second portion contained the arc system and probe carrier, but was not CT compatible, and a hand-held calculator was used to complete the coordinates. These two camps, which espouse intraradiology vs. intrasurgery stereotactic procedures, have drawn much closer as the Brown-Robert-Wells frame has been redesigned for both localization and surgical CT compatibility and as Leksell and co-workers (Elekta AB, Stockholm) (LUNSFORD 1982) have redesigned their frame for CT compatibility (BOETHIUS et al. 1980), eliminating the need for the original Perry-Rosenbaum-Lunsford "CT" frame (PERRY et al. 1980). Other stereotactic frames have also evolved (HUK and BAUER 1980; LEKSELL and JERNBERG 1980; SHELDON et al. 1980; KOSLOW et al. 1981; BIRG and MUNDINGER 1982; GOERSS et al. 1982). An MRI-compatible frame was also developed by Leksell (Elekta AB) at the suggestion of PERRY et al. (1980).

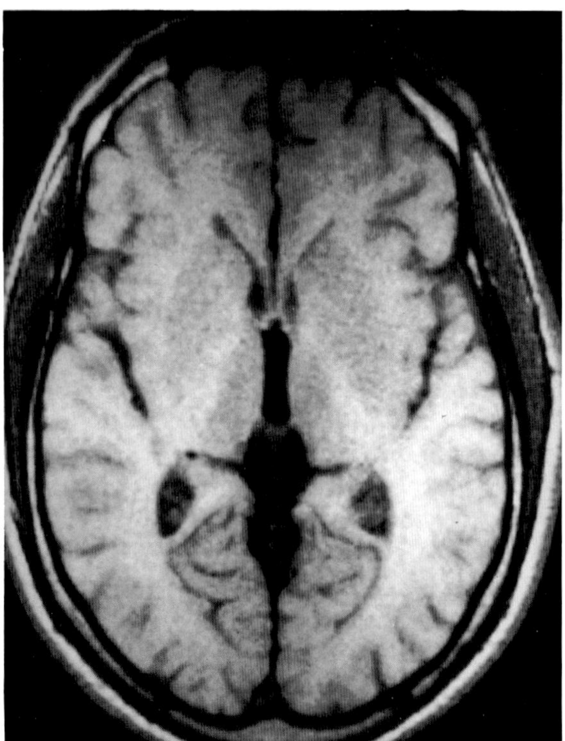

Fig. 1. Magnetic resonance image of the brain of a healthy individual. Note the defined gray and white matter and fissures with vessels. The anterior and posterior commissures, thalamus, basal ganglia, and internal capsule, important landmarks for stereotactic procedures, are clearly seen

11.3 The Stereotactic Frame

Current computed imaging technology requires that: (a) the stereotactic frame fit within the aperture of the CT gantry or within the bore of the MR scanner, (b) the frame provide the fiducial (reference) points necessary for computation of the coordinates, and (c) the frame produce no (or few) artifacts. To achieve these goals, three distinctly different frames have been developed; their distinctions are briefly described here. Originally, these appara-

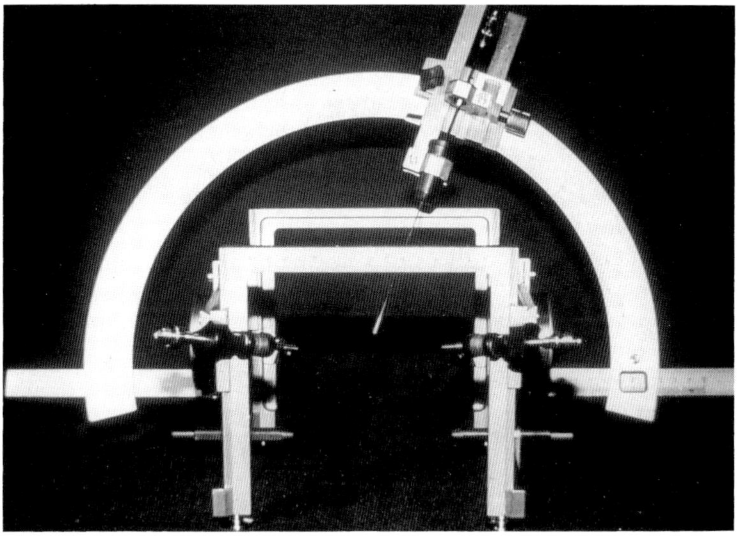

Fig. 2. A typical CT-MRI compatible stereotactic frame (Leksell) is shown. Note the arc containing arms superimposed on the head-holding frame. The probe carrier attached to the arc bar to direct the probe to the target point located in the center of the arc is demonstrated. The materials for the frame are aluminum alloy, carbon fiber, plastic, or fiberglass, which markedly reduce the artifacts formerly found when stainless steel was used in the construction

tuses were distinguishable by how the probe carrier was mounted. The most popular frames have been based on the arc or polar system (GILDENBERG 1987).

For example, the Leksell system employs a probe carrier fitted to an arc that is adjusted so that the target is always central (Fig. 2) (LEKSELL 1949); thus, the target is aligned with the center of the arc by adjustment of the supporting arms of the arc. No matter what angle is selected, insertion of the probe results in its arriving at the central target. In this system, spheroidal geometry is combined with rectilinear cartesian (x, y, z rectilinear) geometry.

The Todd-Wells apparatus also uses an arc system, but it is designed reciprocally, so that the arc system is fixed and the patient's head within the frame is moved to center the target zone of the frame in aligning the probe with the target (TODD 1967).

The later Wells design, the Brown-Roberts-Wells apparatus, consists of interlocking arcs. A calculator is used to define the spheroidal coordinates for determining the necessary adjustment of the frame to reach the target (BROWN et al. 1980). A pilot system also allows for checking the probe with the target before the surgical portion of the frame is applied to the retaining ring on the patient.

The Riechert and Mundinger system (RIECHERT and MUNDINGER 1955) is also an arc system, but instead of the target being at the center of the arc, the probe carrier is offset, and it is desirable to use a phantom or computer to adjust the apparatus. The phantom mechanically simulates the placement of the arc system on the head and the coordinates of the target.

Most of the frames currently available have been modified for use in both CT and MRI scanners. This was achieved by replacing the iron rods or feet with ones of aluminum alloy and the steel pins with fiberglass or carbon fiber pins, to eliminate artifacts. For example, if the copper strands of the coordinate indicator on the fiducial plate are replaced with a mixture of vegetable oil and copper sulfate powder, localization fiducials for either CT or MRI of the brain can be obtained. An excellent stereotactic map of the brain is thus obtained that is free of the distortion caused by removal and formalin fixation in the atlas-prepared brains. Target coordinates can also be derived from either axial or coronal scans. For localization in the sagittal plane, an indicator plate is attached to the vertex indicator of the frame. If desired, the scan can be made at a particular angle, such as the angle of the intended surgical approach to the brain, to visualize the brain structures that lie along the probe's trajectory (LEKSELL et al. 1985). We have prepared a simulation program for the target on each slice to preview the target's potential course (Siemens/Perry-Rosenbaum stereotactic software).

11.4 Surgical Planning and Applications

Computed tomography has already proved to be of great value as a guidance methodology in clinical stereotactic microtechniques that deal with localized or well-defined targets. CT has afforded precise planning of the trajectory followed by intraoperative monitoring of the probe's passage as it traverses each slice in the CT frame's "cubic" volume. This causes minimal trauma to intracranial vessels and functionally important brain structures. Although restrictions and interdictions are still inherent in the MRI environment, since MRI's hourly cost is currently approximately twice that of CT, MRI is particularly useful when very detailed anatomic planning is necessary and the particular structures are not optimally visualized on intravenously enhanced CT. Therefore, after the patient has been scanned by MRI, the image data are transferred to the CT environment for the actual operative procedure.

Standard applications for CT-guided stereotaxis include:

11.4.1 Biopsy of Brain Lesions

Stereotactic brain biopsy is indicated:

1. To differentiate malignant tumor from inflammatory masses.
2. To separate a primary brain tumor from a secondary (metastatic) tumor.
3. To determine the extent of microscopically discernible tumor infiltration, which may not be recognizable through imaging.
4. To aspirate cystic lesions, both to reduce their volume and to determine their cellular or tissue characteristics.

While CT and/or MRI are sufficiently accurate for localizing and determining the nature of mass lesions, they are not equivalent to formal pathologic diagnosis, which is the standard for most treatment. Thus cytologic and/or histologic verification is usually mandatory before therapy can commence. CT-guided stereotactic surgery can *safely* and reliably facilitate pathologic diagnosis (Apuzzo and Sabshin 1983).

11.4.2 Drainage of Abscesses

Computed tomography-guided aspiration provides a method for draining abscesses as small as 1 cm in diameter and for evacuating deep abscesses not amenable to standard surgical resection. When abscesses are multiloculated, each chamber may be viewed, aspirated, and reviewed the turn. One portion of the aspirated material can then be examined microscopically and another dispatched for culture and sensitivity studies to determine the appropriate antibiotic regimen.

11.4.3 Implantation of Radioactive Seeds

Precise placement of radioactive seeds within tumor tissue using the CT-guided stereotactic system continues to add an important dimension to the therapy of malignant tumors. The first implantation of a radioactive isotope in the brain was carried out by Frazier in 1914. He reported using 50–100 mg of radium seeds, implanted free-hand and removed the next day. By 1920, Frazier had treated 32 patients (Frazier 1920; Dyck 1984). In the ensuing years, however, the hazard of using these very energetic isotopes discouraged additional use. The combination of CT-guided stereotactic surgery and computerized three-dimensional dosimetry planning has revived interest in implanting radioactive seeds of lower energy (Gutin et al. 1981; Hosobushi et al. 1980; Mundinger 1958).

Depending on the nature of the tumor, the various isotopes used have included phosphorus 32 (^{32}P), cobalt 60 (^{60}Co), yttrium 90 (^{90}Y), iodine 125 (^{125}I), tantalum 182 (^{182}Ta), iridium 192 (^{192}Ir), gold 198 (^{198}Au), and radium 226 (^{226}Ra). Currently, for interstitial brachytherapy of solid tumors, most workers implant either ^{125}I or ^{192}Ir. These isotopes are available with gamma energies and tissue penetration characteristics that allow for selective tumor destruction, but they are still relatively safe for handling by health-care personnel. ^{192}Ir sources have a half-life of 74.2 days, a gamma energy of 300–610 keV, and a half-value for tissue penetration of 5 cm; ^{125}I has a half-life of 60.2 days, a gamma energy of 28–35 keV, and a 2-cm half-value for tissue penetration. The half-life of each of these isotopes is long enough that only a minor degree of decay occurs during the treatment period. The lower energy radiation of ^{125}I makes protection of visitors and hospital staff less problematic than when ^{192}Ir is used. Since the inverse square law indicates that the radiation dose to surrounding tissue dimin-

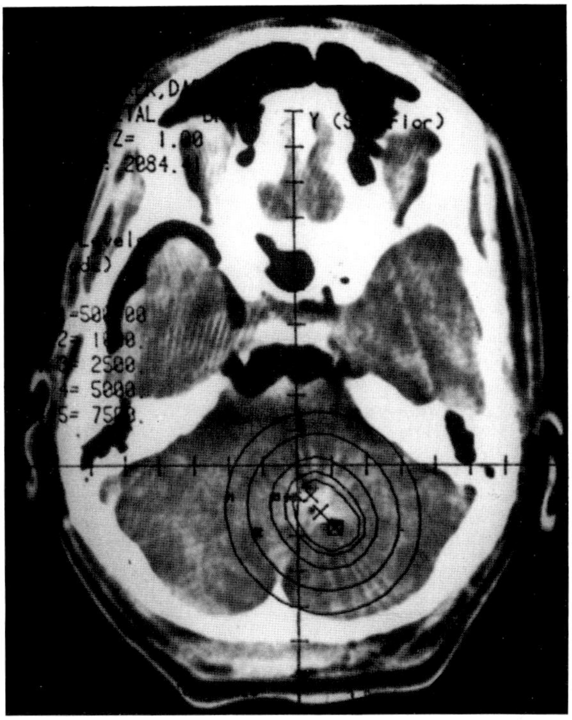

Fig. 3. Isodose curves of ^{125}I radioactive seeds implanted in a cerebellar tumor

ishes rapidly as the distance from the implanted source increases, the actual dose rate delivered to the target tissue will depend upon the number and activity of the sources implanted and on the geometric distribution of the implanted radiation sources. Detailed, physicist-derived computer-assisted dosimetry planning must be employed to avoid undertreatment of regions within a tumor or overtreatment and excessive necrosis of the surrounding normal brain (Fig. 3). Most workers currently use dose rates of 40–60 rad/h (1000–1500 rads/day). At these levels, interstitial brachytherapy can be shown to achieve a therapeutic ratio superior to conventional teletherapy. Moreover, destruction of recurrent tumor can be accomplished with relative safety, even in cases where the surrounding brain tissue has already received the maximum tolerated dose of external beam radiation therapy (Coffey and Friedman 1988).

Although none of the current therapeutic modalities can cure a highly malignant brain tumor (e.g., the life expectancy of patients with glioblastoma is 44 weeks on average), in such limited circumstances, seed implantation may offer the patient a better quality of life and the opportunity for further therapy (Greitz et al. 1986).

11.4.4 Thalamotomy for Movement Disorders

The pharmacologic treatment of Parkinson's disease seemed very promising after the introduction of l-dopa, but the therapeutic dilemma was not fully solved. Drugs are unable to delay progression of the disease, and the efficacy of the drug subsides over time. Matsumoto and his co-workers have shown that stereotactic thalamotomy can provide long-lasting relief from rigidity and/or tremor in approximately 80% of patients (Matsumoto et al. 1984).

For this procedure to be successful, precise target selection is essential. The most effective target is thought to be a specific area of the thalamus, the nucleus ventralis intermedius (Vim) (Ohye et al. 1982). Initial mapping of the thalamic nuclei, including Vim, was determined by ventriculography, which defined the classic landmarks, the anterior and posterior commissures, in the wall of the third ventricle. Vim is situated 12 mm lateral to the commissure line and 7 mm in front of the posterior commissure. (Ventriculography, once a powerful diagnostic technique before the introduction of CT, has been supplanted at most medical institutions in the United States by CT and MRI.)

Another important consideration for the treatment of movement disorders by thalamotomy is that since these are physiologic disorders, physiologic information should be used for the final target determination. Currently, this is achieved by neuronal cell-unit recordings (developed by Albe-Fessard et al. in 1961), made with a surgically introduced microprobe. The technique is complex and its use is currently limited to highly sophisticated stereotactic surgeons. In the future, physiologic targets are likely to be identified by their metabolic activity on PET or MRI of specific neurotransmitters in the basal ganglia.

11.5 Stereotactic Brain Surgery Within the CT Scanner

At the Johns Hopkins Hospital, stereotactic surgery has been performed with the patient within the CT gantry in neuroradiology since 1984 (Fig. 4). The neuroradiologic CT environment has been designed to satisfy the standard operating room requirements for air handling, anesthetic gas delivery and scavenging systems, cardiovascular monitoring, surgical lighting, suction and electrocautery, and surgical scrub facilities. Conventional sterile technique is

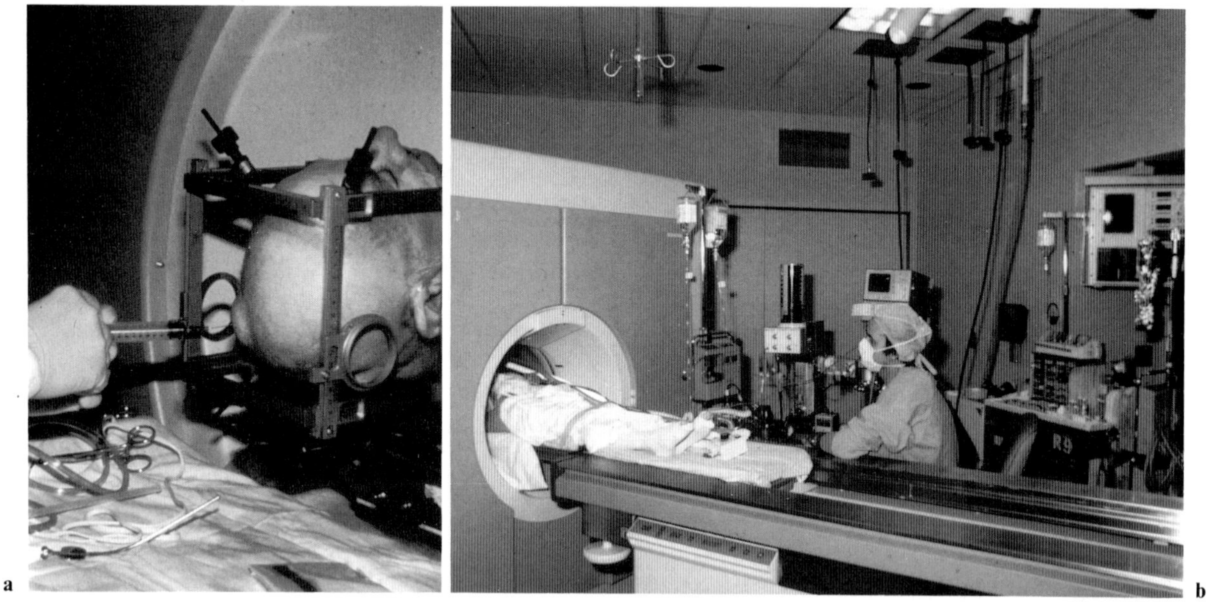

Fig. 4. **a** View of a patient and the stereotactic frame in the CT gantry opening. **b** The anesthesiology group closely monitors the patient and controls general anesthesia during CT-guided stereotactic brain surgery. Note the ceiling-mounted laser and physiologic monitors

followed. The team includes neuroradiologic technologists, neuroanesthetists, neurosurgeons, neuroradiologists, and neurocytologists (Uematsu et al. 1987b). Lunsford, Stuhldreher, and Rosenbaum designed a neurosurgical operating room that contains a CT stereotactic scanner (General Electric 8800); its overall utilization is lower than that of a radiology-based scanner that does conventional CT when stereotactic procedures are not being performed.

11.5.1 Procedure

It is our preference to perform stereotactic surgery under general anesthesia; the alternative is to perform it under local anesthesia with sedation. An artifact-free Leksell MRI stereotactic frame was adapted to the CT scanner, and the Siemens/Perry-Rosenbaum stereotactic software program is used. After placement of the stereotactic frame and fiducial reference plates, iodinated contrast material is injected intravenously, and the patient is scanned to localize the lesion, to select the target, and to compute the stereotactic coordinates. Based on these coordinates, the probe entry site is marked on the scalp. The probe is advanced through a burr hole toward the target. Some surgeons prefer the smaller twist drill hole. The somewhat larger burr hole allows us to visualize the superficial brain arteries and veins and to coagulate any calvarial or scalp bleeding better. When the probe has advanced to a point 8 cm short of the planned target, a confirmatory CT slice and biopsy are made. Probe advancement and corresponding CT scanning are then made 4 mm above the target, at the target ("0" mm), and 4 and 8 mm beyond the target, so that typically five biopsies are obtained.

The specimens are examined by a cytopathologist at the scanner area, providing the surgeon with immediate information about the nature and sufficiency of each specimen. Portions of the specimens are also transferred to the pathology laboratory for further processing (e.g., histopathologic sectioning, biomarkers, etc.). Surgical closure and a final CT scan follow.

The advantages of carrying out the procedure at the scanner site become obvious when problems are encountered during surgery. For example, when an unexpected sample of crystal-clear fluid instead of tumor tissue was extracted through the biopsy needle, immediate explanation was needed. The probe had been anticipated to be already in the midbrain, a surgically dangerous region (Fig. 5a). On injecting a small quantity of air it was learned that the cavity from which the crystal-clear fluid returned communicated with the cerebrospinal fluid pathway around the brain stem, the ambient cistern of the subarachnoid space. The side-opening of the probe was then directed toward the wall of the fluid-filled

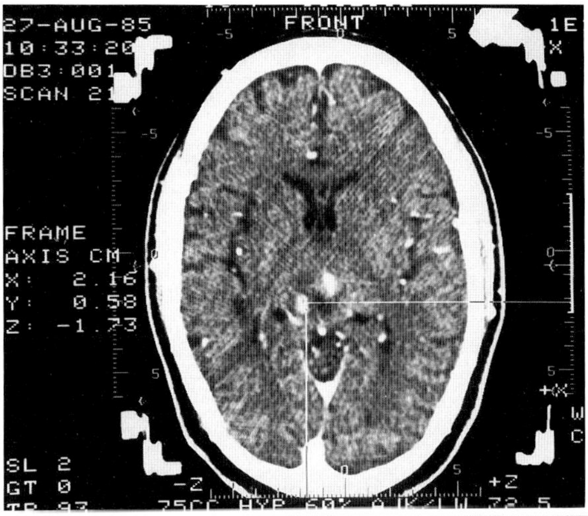

a

Fig. 5. **a** CT of a 16-year-old girl with a 2-week history of diplopia. In the neonatal period, she developed transient left hemiplegia immediately after ventriculoperitoneal shunt placement for hydrocephalus. CT scan revealed areas of increased density in the midbrain. A target was selected on the medial edge of one of the lesions. Note the area of decreased density medial to the lesion. Two lines, meeting at the target, were drawn from the x and z coordinate scale on the monitor screen. The coordinates of the target were x, 2.16; y, 0.58; z, – 1.73 mm. **b** Because unexpected crystal clear fluid flowed out from the probe as the probe entered the target site, 0.5 cc air was injected. A scan immediately after the air was injected uncovered a cystic cavity filled with air. A magnified schematic drawing overlaid on the photograph depicts our biopsy probe suctioning the tissue and cutting out minute amounts of the wall tissue of the cystic lesion. Simulations of the scales of the frame and the positive and negative directions of the x, y, and z axes are generated on the image by the Siemens/Perry-Rosenbaum software

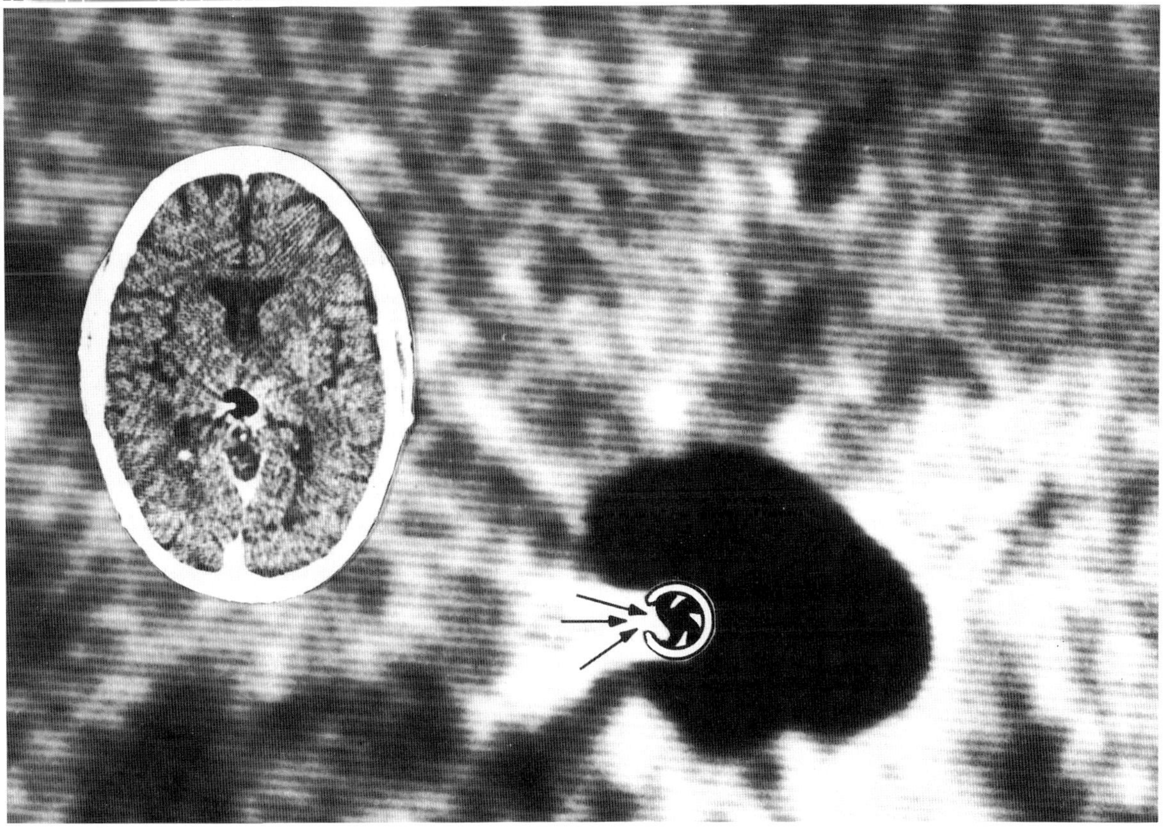

b

cyst to enable biopsy of that tissue (Fig. 5b). Subsequent histologic study of that tissue led to the pathologist's diagnosis of cystic transformation of an iatrogenic hematoma resulting from the insertion of a ventricular catheter 15 years earlier (UEMATSU et al. 1987a).

Another advantage of intraoperative scanning is monitoring of the progress and completeness of aspiration of a brain abscess (Fig. 6). As the abscess is emptied, the cavity begins to collapse, and the wall may obstruct the aspiration probe's opening. In such cases, a scan with the probe in place will show how the side-opening of the probe should be redirected to evacuate the remaining abscess fluid. Intraoperative scanning is especially valuable when the brain abscess lies next to the ventricular system, since inadvertently advancing the probe into the ventricle would seed the inflammatory pus into the cerebrospinal fluid, inducing ventriculitis!

Intraoperative scanning may also allow stereotac-

6

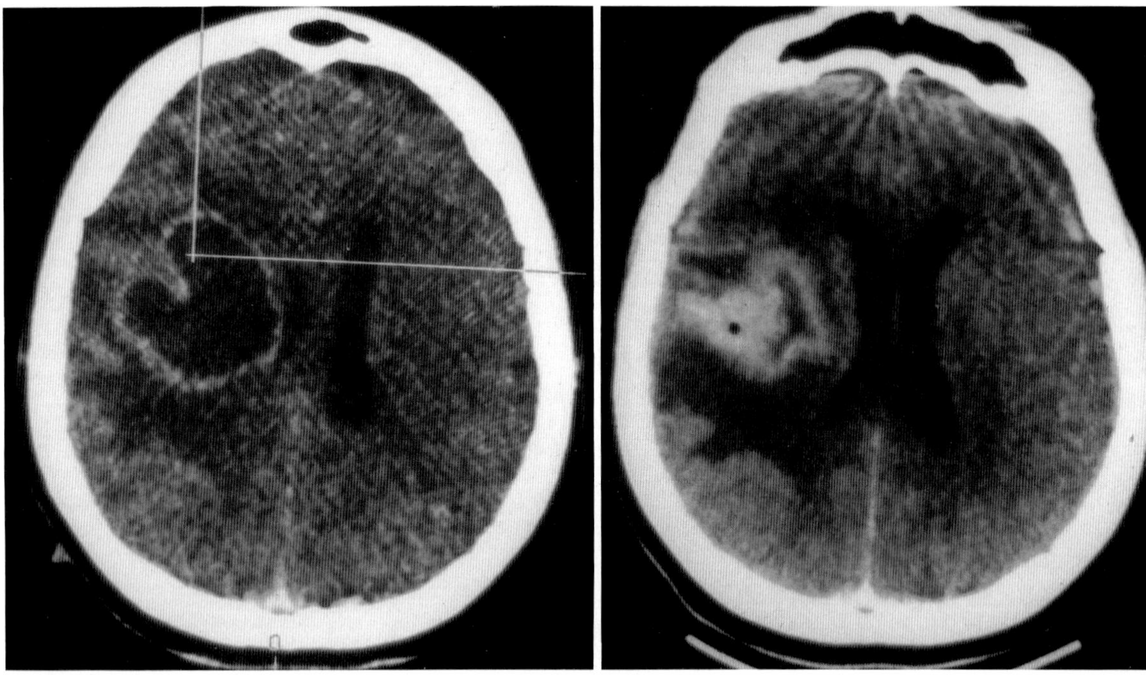

a b

7

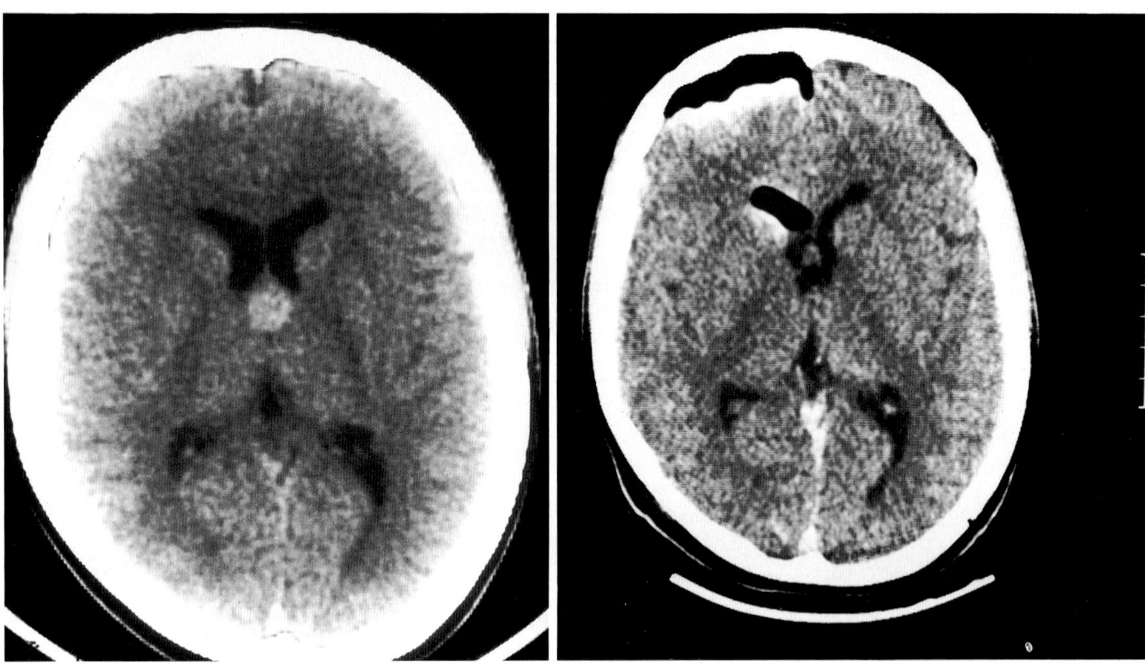

a b

Fig. 6. **a** CT scan of a brain abscess before aspiration. A target site is indicated at the crossing point of the *horizontal* (x) and *vertical* (z) *lines*. **b** Collapsed abscess cavity with a hole created by small amount of air trapped in the probe trace. **a, b** Note proximity of the ventricular wall to the abscess wall

Fig. 7. **a** CT of a colloid cyst of the third ventricle in a 24-year-old white female who complained of severe nocturnal headache. Note complete obstruction of the foramen Monro. **b** CT scan taken immediately after aspiration of the cyst, with the patient's head still in the gantry opening. Note opening of the ventricular fluid passage. The cyst is gone, yet the important structure for memory function has been left intact in the third ventricle

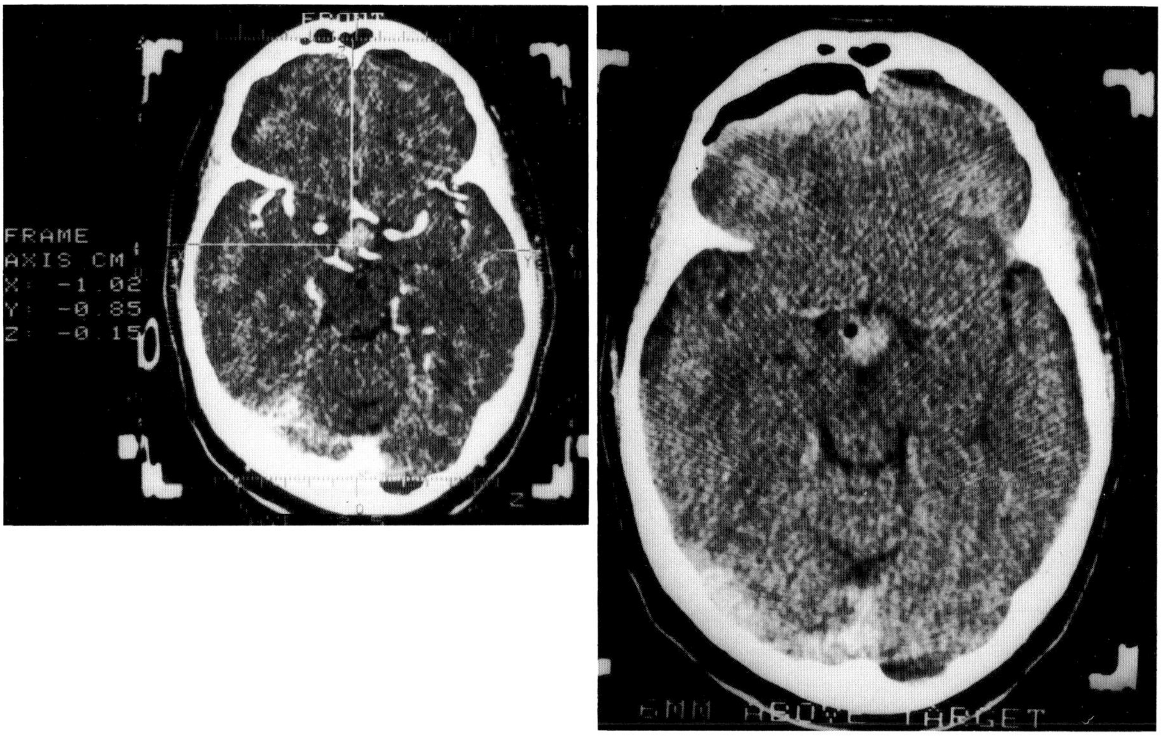

Fig. 8. **a** CT scan of the brain of a 30-year-old engineer with a brain lesion in the area of the hypothalamus. The lesion is surrounded by the cerebral arteries composing the circle of Willis. The target for biopsy was chosen in the central area of the lesion, away from the arteries. **b** Intraoperative CT scan before application of the aspiration force ensured the appropriate location of the probe to avoid accidental trauma to the vessels. A small amount of air injection upon removal of the probe confirmed successful biopsy, with the air-filled hole created by tissue removal. No demonstrable hemorrhage was seen. The patient was subsequently treated with radiation and is free of symptoms and doing well 1 year later

tic aspiration of a colloid cyst of the third ventricle (Fig. 7) or of lesions surrounded by multiple vessels (Fig. 8) (UEMATSU et al. 1989).

11.6 Thalamotomy with Combined Use of MRI, CT, and Cell-Unit Recordings at the CT Scanner Site

In 1987, UEMATSU et al. reported on thalamotomy in the treatment of a movement disorder that used MRI for target determination and intraoperative CT for coordinate calculation and probe placement (Fig. 9). A microelectrode was used for physiological assessment of the brain structures along the course of the thalamotomy probe. Final target determination was confirmed by cell-unit recording (Fig. 10). MRI provided excellent delineation of the gray and white matter, internal capsule, basal ganglia, and thalamus. Moreover, high-contrast midsagittal sections showed the commissures and the adjacent regional structures for calculating the target coordinates. Since ferromagnetic instruments were used during stereotactic surgery, which would have endangered both the patient and personnel during MRI scanning, the surgical portion of the procedure was performed using the CT scanner table.

11.6.1 Current Technique

The first step is to precisely delineate the anterior-posterior commissure line (AC-PC line), as observed on a midsagittal MRI scan (Fig. 11), and, using a cursor, to define and measure that line at the MRI console. The AC-PC line is then extended anteriorly to the frontal skin surface and posteriorly to the occipital skin surface. The distance from the intersection on the frontal skin surface to the upper edge of the frontal sinus is then measured. The distance from the occipital intersection skin surface to the inion is also measured (Fig. 11). These measurements are then related to the patient's scalp. Using an image-intensified fluoroscope, the patient's inion and the superior margin of the frontal sinus are

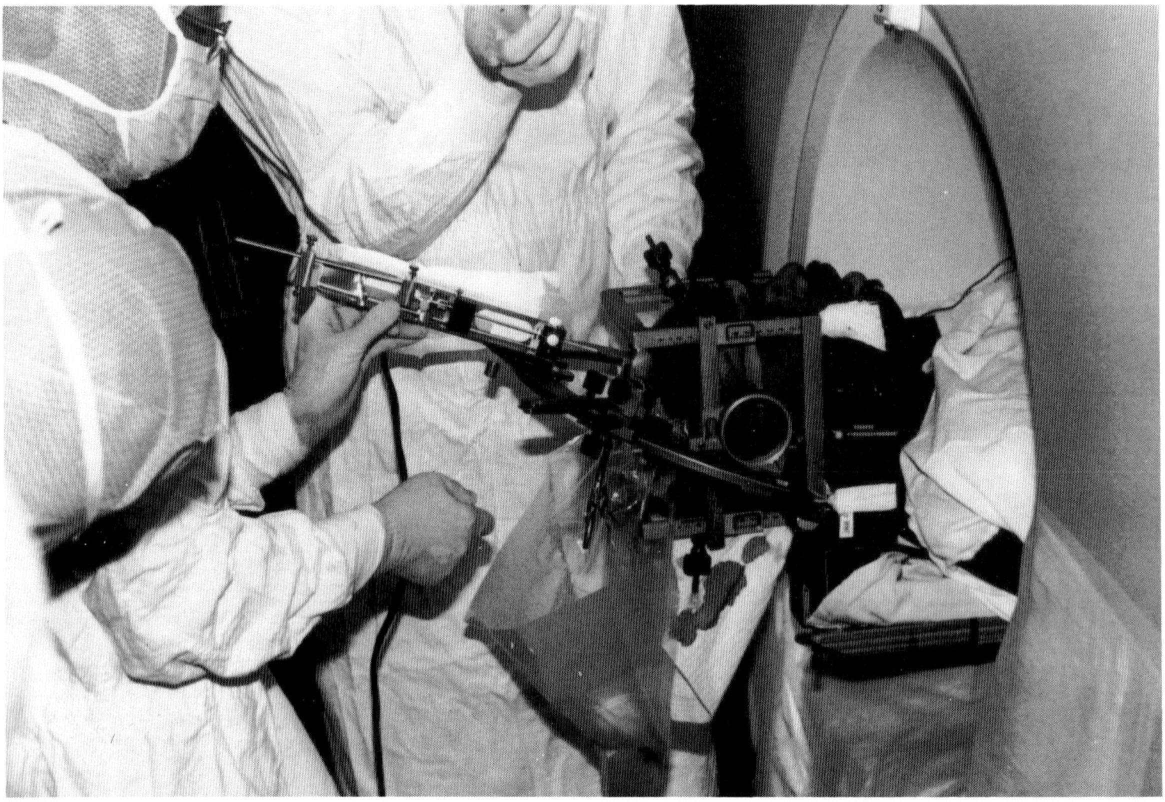

9

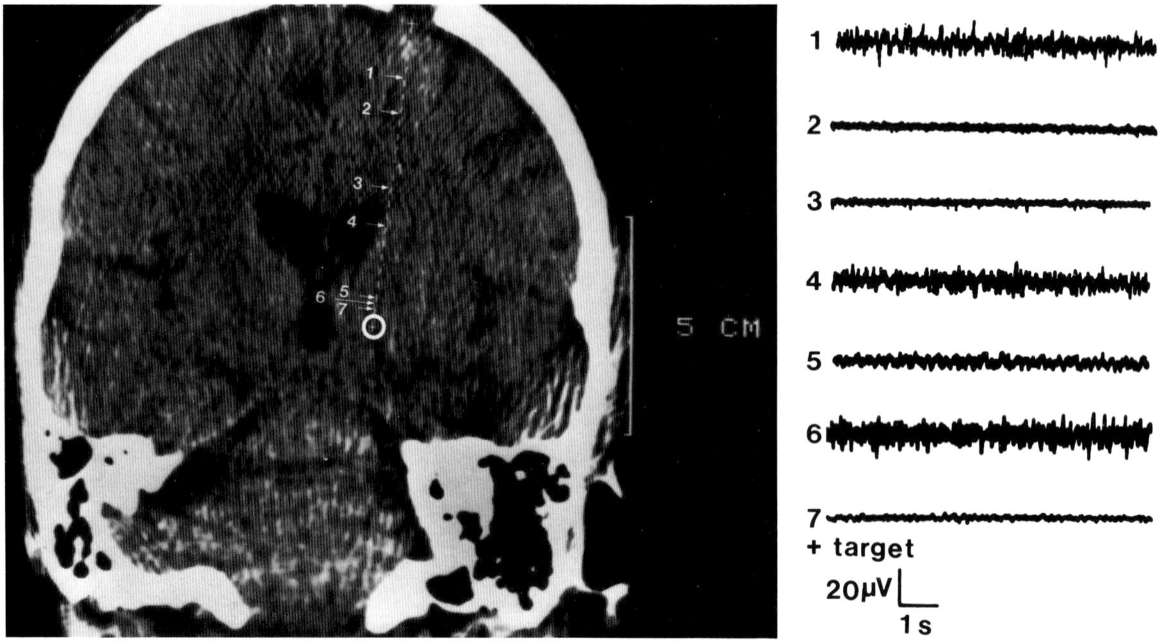

10

Fig. 9. Stereotactic thalamotomy at the CT gantry site. Note how the head-holding frame holding the microelectrode and the head of the patient extend out of the CT gantry opening

Fig. 10. CT scan along the planned probe trajectory. The numbers correspond to electrophysiologic recordings displayed on the right and recorded at distances of 67.2, 57.6, 37.2, 27.6, 7.6, 6.9, and 5.2 mm, respectively, from the target

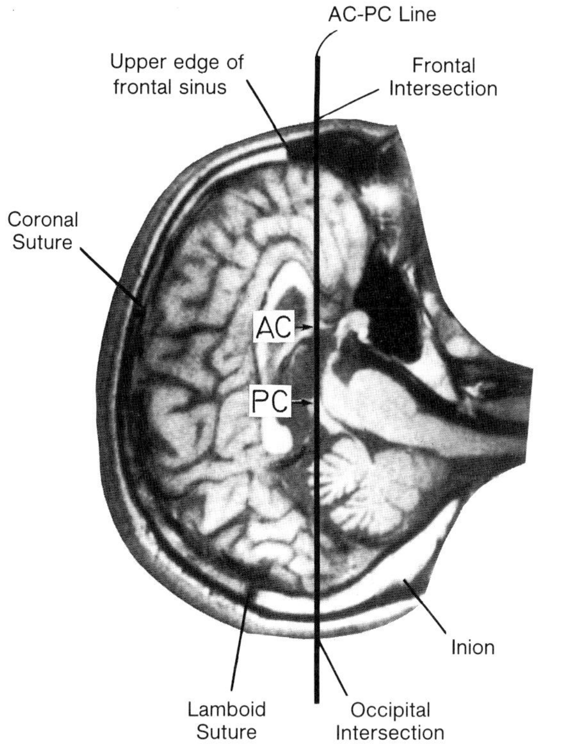

Fig. 11. Sagittal plane MRI scan used to transfer the AC-PC line to the scalp with its anterior and posterior elongations

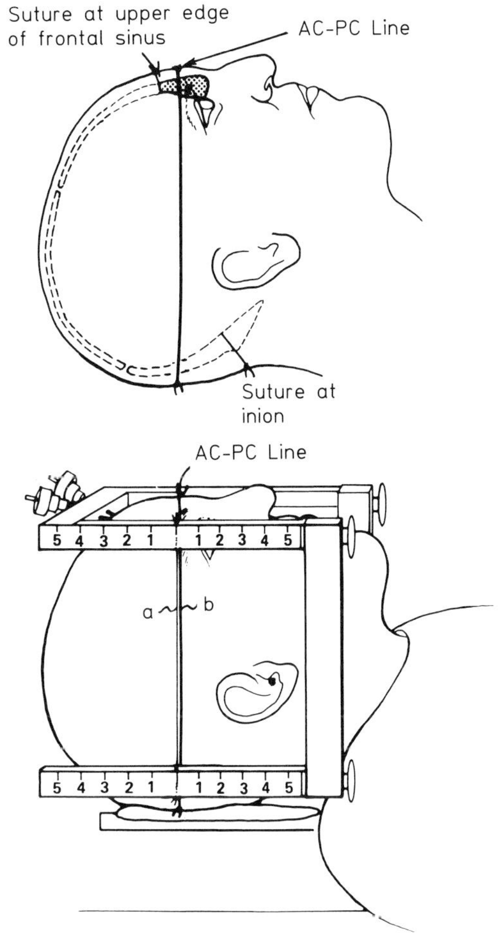

Fig. 12. The *upper portion* of the figure shows the wire wrapped around the scalp along the AC-PC line. The *lower portion* demonstrates how the vertical wire **(a)** attached to the frame at 0 of the x axis and the AC-PC line wire **(b)** on the scalp are matched and superimposed. Alignment was confirmed by fluoroscopy and the frame was affixed to the patient's head in that position

identified. The scalp overlying them is then infiltrated with a local anesthetic. A superficial-to-deep wire suture is placed over each of these bony landmarks. The points where the projected AC-PC line intersects the frontal and occipital scalp are marked after comparison with the MR image. The frontal scalp, AC-PC, and occipital scalp markings are connected by a long wire suture placed in the patient's scalp and wrapped around the head. The Leksell stereotactic frame is then placed over the patient's head. Again under fluoroscopic guidance, the wire superimposed over the AC-PC line on the scalp is adjusted by moving the patient's head until the wires on the right and left sides are perfectly aligned in the frame. The head is then affixed to the frame in this position by four pins, two frontally and two occipitally (Fig. 12). The CT gantry is positioned at 0°. Precise orientation of the scanning plane is achieved by superimposition of a light/laser beam on the CT gantry along the MRI-derived AC-PC line. Serial, nonoverlapping axial scans 2 mm thick are made above and below that line using the built-in software program (Fig. 13). The CT

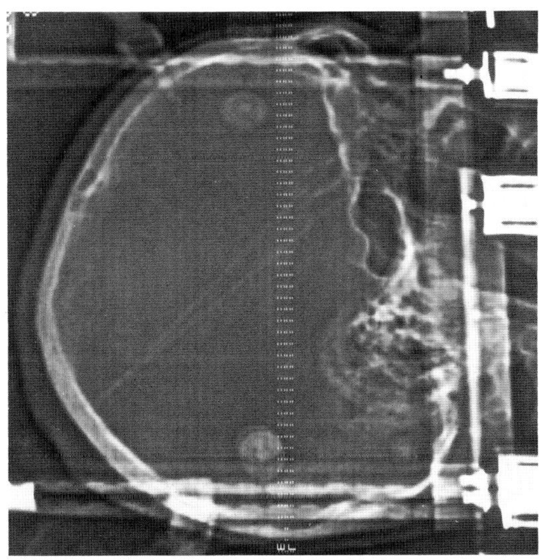

Fig. 13. CT with each scan level 2 mm apart as the target was ▷ neared with the AC-PC line in the center, as planned

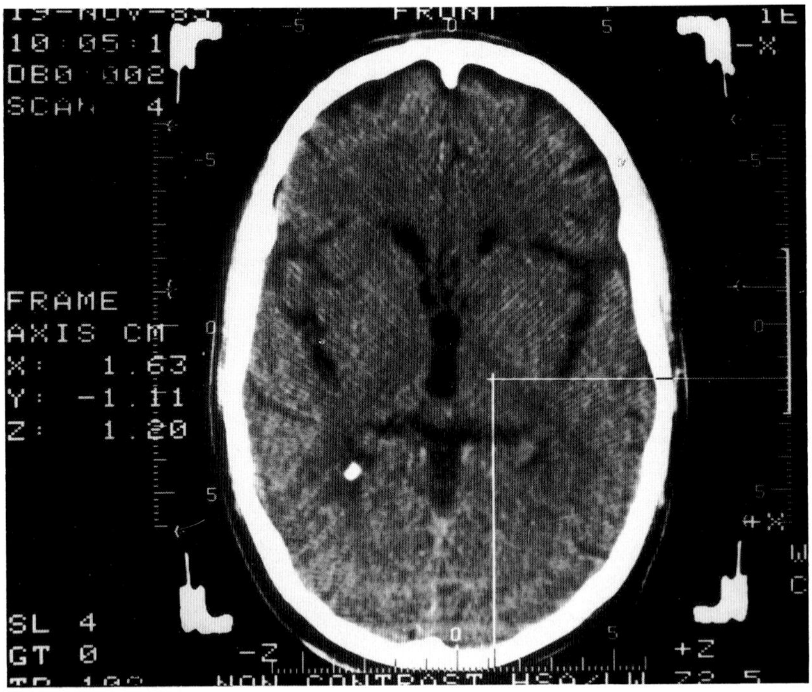

Fig. 14. A CT scan 2 mm below the AC-PC line was chosen to define the target. The precise target (Vim) was located by superimposing the CT film over the MR image to identify the relative location of the internal capsule and the thalamus. The coordinates of the Vim are determined from this

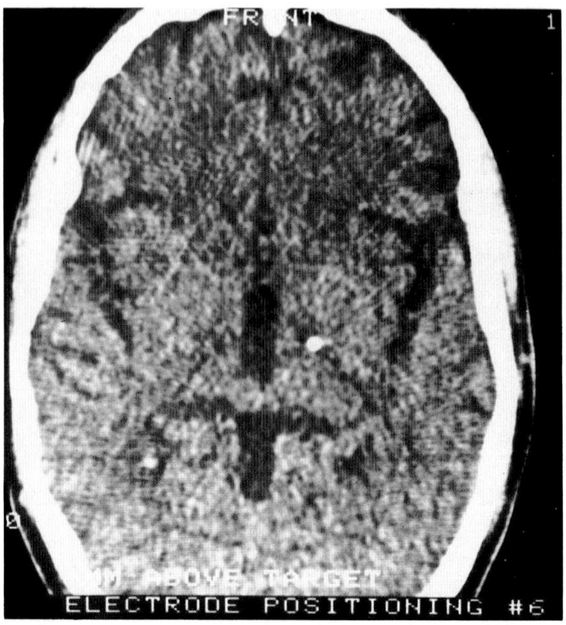

Fig. 15. Before the radiofrequency lesion was made, a confirmatory CT scan was made with the probe in place. Note that the probe tip is precisely at the planned target site

images are reviewed on the screen and an optimal slice is selected. Figure 14 shows a film of an image made 2 mm below the AC-PC line, in which a theoretical target was selected. The CT film and the previously obtained MRI film are compared, including superimposing them, for better identification of the internal capsule, particularly its medial rim, on CT. Superimposition of a magnification-corrected transparent stereotactic brain atlas over the CT film further assists in defining the position of the Vim. After the target site is selected by the cursor on the CT screen, the fiducial sites are integrated so that the scanner, frame, and plane of the CT sections are in synchrony. The CT coordinates (x, y, z) are then determined by the computer and displayed. The CT-derived x, y, and z coordinates are then transferred by the surgeon onto the stereotactic frame (Figs. 15, 16).

11.6.2 Future Integration of CT and MRI Images

Magnetic resonance imaging is currently the optimal neuroradiologic technique for safely and accurately defining the anterior and posterior commissures to derive the AC-PC line. CT is currently the optimal technique for probe and electrode guidance during stereotactic thalamotomy.

Two or more defined methods of CT-MRI guidance for stereotactic surgery are likely to become

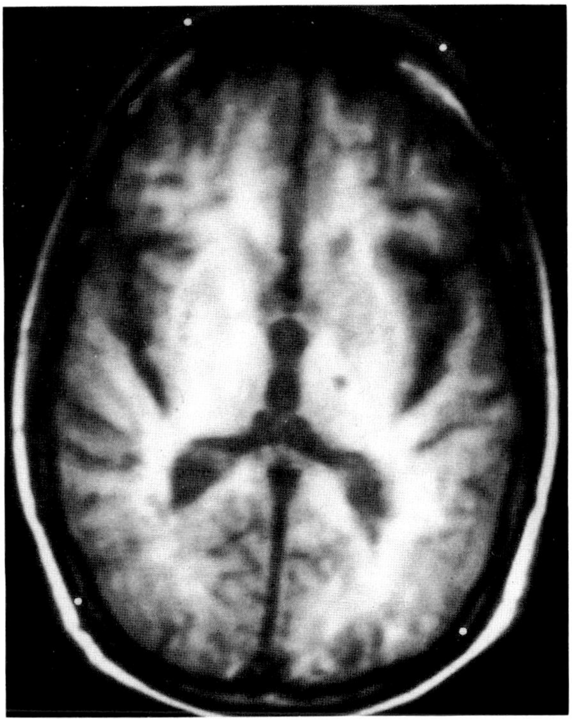

Fig. 16. MRI of the same patient 6 months after Vim thalamotomy. The radiofrequency lesion is seen as a hypointense dot that is well matched with the planned and actual target site

available. The first, an indirect method, would require the MRI-defined AC-PC plane to be externalized, so that the skin could be accurately marked, as in CT. Then the various MRI slices would be matched with CT slices to confirm the target location. A CT stereotactic software program would again define the stereotactic coordinates.

The second, a direct method, would require the AC-PC plane and level to be defined on MRI (with or without the MRI-CT stereotactic frame in situ), after which the MRI image data would be integrated with the CT image data (i.e., via a PACS work station). With the capacity to provide precise superimpositions, the stereotactic coordinates could be readily mapped by high-resolution MRI, and intraoperative CT scans could be generated to determine the probe/electrode position and intraoperative therapeutic results, while MRI's superior anatomic information could be accurately applied as necessary. PET and analog images that have been digitized can also be integrated with CT. The hazards of ferromagnetic instrumentation, including anesthesia equipment and support usage peculiar to MRI, would be avoided, while CT's currently lower cost (as compared to MRI) would apply (UEMATSU et al. 1987b).

11.7 Computerized Image-Controlled Servomotor-Driven Stereotactic System

KELLY developed a novel CT-controlled stereotactic system capable not only of biopsy but also of resection of deep-seated brain lesions (KELLY and ALKER 1980). The core part of the system consists of external and internal arcs driven by the servomotor on the modified Todd-Wells stereotactic head-holder stationed on the operating table. The external arc holds a laser scope and the internal arc holds a scope-shaped brain retractor. Movement of the laser beam within the target field of the brain is electronically controlled by the cursor on the CT or MR images on the cathode ray tube (CRT) in the operating room. Since the position of the laser beam in relation to the outline of the lesion is simulated by a cursor on the CRT, the surgical procedure can be directed precisely to the area demonstrated by the computed images. This minimizes the amount of retraction or resection of normal brain tissue while maximizing resection of the pathologic tissue seen on the CT or MR images.

This technique not only allows resection of a deep-seated brain tumor, but also enables selective resection of the amygdalum and hippocampus in the treatment of intractable seizures. Although surgery may not be the ideal treatment for a malignant brain tumor or seizure disorder, the approach described here has undoubtedly encouraged further research and development of the computer-controlled surgical approach. Even at the present state of development, this approach has decreased surgical morbidity by minimizing trauma to the brain.

11.8 Technical Problems and Research Needs

11.8.1 Robotics in Stereotactic Brain Surgery

It is clear that current stereotactic procedures depend heavily on "nuts and bolts" manual operation by a highly skilled neurosurgeon. However, to reduce the technical difficulties, attempts have been made to use a robotic system. For example, KWOH et al. (1985, 1988) reported clinical use of a robotic system for stereotactic biopsy of brain tumors. From 1984 to 1986, one of us (SU), in collaboration with Aloka, Tokyo, and Japan Radio Company, Ueda City, Japan, explored the utility of robotics using a series of model experiments (Fig. 17).

For stereotactic procedures, the electromechanical arm of a robot should have at least six joints, to

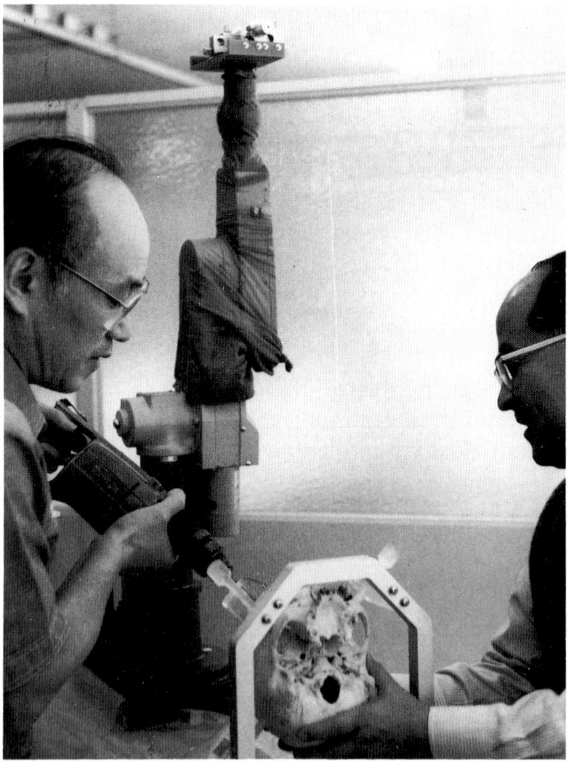

Fig. 17. View of the model experiment using a dry skull. A burr hole is being made 25 mm lateral to the midline and just anterior to the coronal suture. The robot arm is in an upright position. The hand part of the robot is on the top, attached to a probe holder, and the forearm and arm parts are covered with sterile stocking to avoid contamination. (Robot used in this experiment was Puma 260, Kawasaki-Juko, Kawasaki, Japan.)

Fig. 18. Diagram of the robotic control system. *A*, Target in the brain. *B*, Integration site of robotic and CT tables. *C*, Table holding the robot. *D*, CT table

allow a range of motion that includes rotation, flexion, and extension, similar to that of the human arm (Fig. 18). The advantage of robotics is to eliminate the relatively bulky frame currently used. The patient's head requires restraint from motion as before, but a less elaborate technique can be used.

The robot may be stationed on a detachable table docked at the head of the CT table. The robot and the table need to be very firmly integrated so that there is not the slightest displacement during surgery and the geometric relationships between the CT scanning system, the robot arm, and the target in the brain are preserved.

The model experiments confirmed that the robot's accuracy in reaching targets was very satisfactory for clinical application. For example, the model experiment for thalamotomy had an overall error defined by the probe tip from the target of 0.3 ± 0.2 mm on the x coordinate and 0.3 ± 0.4 mm on the y coordinate.

11.8.2 Problems with the Metallic Robot Arm

The major concern about a robotic system is its safety. If accidental failure of the electrical system occurs, the system must stop instantly, without jerking, as the robot arm stops moving. Also, disconnection of the robot arm from the probe or surgical instrument in the brain must be accomplished readily and easily whenever necessary.

11.8.3 Analytic and Therapeutic Stereotactic Probe

The stereotactic approach could be further expanded by adapting a probe equipped with trans-

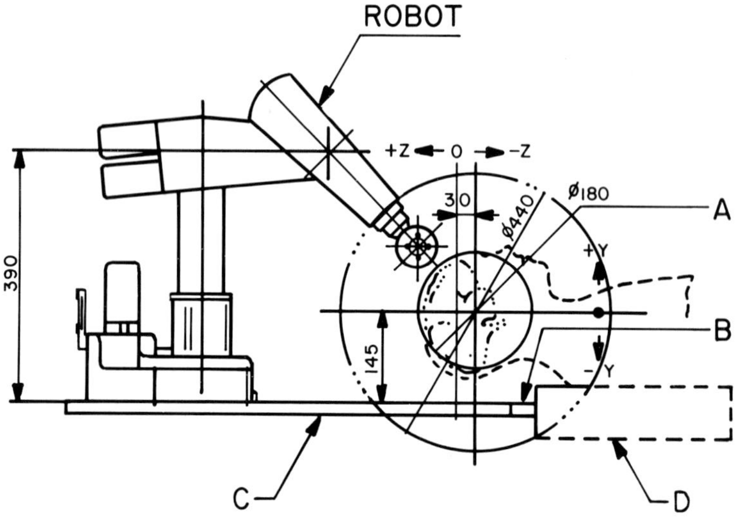

ducers or sensors (pressure, thermocouple, ultrasound, and Doppler) for tissue analysis, or by using a fiberoptic or infrared scope to inspect intraventricular or cystic cavities. A therapeutic probe with a radiofrequency-heat system, mechanical suction system, or ultrasound-homogenizer system could be used to remove tumors or destroy cerebral arterial plaque. A probe capable of injecting biologic "glue" could be used to repair a ruptured aneurysm or to construct collateral blood flow by adding synthetic vessels. These procedures would require miniature stereotactic instruments (two or three) that could be introduced to target areas. Such instruments could also be used to place clips on vessels and/or to construct anastomoses (RAND and MOSS 1973).

The CT-guided stereotactic procedure is currently limited to a single trajectory or target, for several reasons:

1. It is very time consuming to set up the manually operated stereotactic frame in more than a few trajectories, and more than one burr hole would probably be needed.
2. Repetitive, multiple probe insertions may result in brain trauma or hemorrhage.
3. Current stereotactic frames restrict mobilization of the probe and contain a single probe carrier.

11.8.4 Elimination of the Stereotactic Frame

For stereotactic procedures, the geometric relationship between the target point in the brain and the pixel points on tomography must be maintained. This is currently accomplished by fixing the patient's head in the stereotactic frame, which is fastened to the CT table. This firm fixation is needed to ensure constancy of the target locus. However, stereotactic procedures without a frame are facilitated as intercerebral reference points are used for target coordinate control.

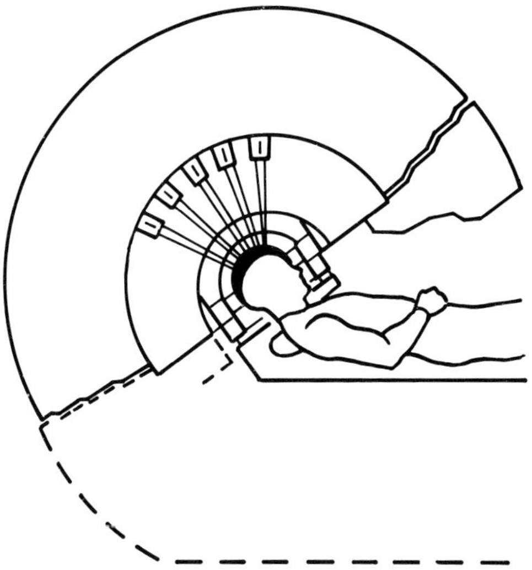

Fig. 19. Schematic drawing of "gamma-knife" (after LEKSELL 1983).

11.9 Focused Light Beam-Guided Brain Surgery

To decrease the potential risks of the mechanical arm, a computer-directed light beam can be used. The beam projects onto the exposed brain, aiming at the lesion underneath. The beam is projected from a built-in light source in the operating microscope. Microscope movement is controlled by the computed image-controlled electromechanical system (CICES). The surgeon's hand is guided to the brain lesion by the stereotactic light beam. This allows the surgeon to approach the lesion with minimal retraction of the brain and to circumvent major blood vessels or vital structures underneath the exposed brain.

Composite CT, MRI, PET, and digitized conventional images can be viewed by the team as the procedure progresses, and the surgeon can ask the CICES to project the light beam on the surgical field as indicated by cursor movement on the CRT. For stereotactic CT, a larger gantry opening (i.e., 70 cm diameter) and a high speed high resolution CT scanner (e.g., Somatom Plus) can be used, so that the entire surgical procedure may be conducted within the scanner without the need to remove the probe during scanning. Three-dimensional display of both CT and MR images is already available and very likely to be added to the existing stereotactic program.

11.10 Radiosurgery

Radiosurgery is based on stereotactic radiation of target structures in the brain. The technique does not require an incision or opening of the skull. Accelerated monoenergetic heavy particles, accelerated electrons, supervoltage roentgen radiation, neutrons, and various gamma-emitting nuclides are directed at the target tissue. The technique, which was introduced by Leksell in 1951, is now commonly called the "gamma-knife".

Incorporation of the CICES into radiosurgery promises a closed stereotactic approach to the brain (Fig. 19).

11.11 Therapeutic Compounds Guided with Stereotactically Focused Magnetic Force

Focused electromagnetic force, stereotactically directed to target tissue, could be used to attract ferromagnetic therapeutic compounds into a target. For example, chemotherapeutic agents compounded with magnetic substances could be used as anticonvulsants, or even as neurotransmitters. Such agents could make it possible for antibiotics to penetrate the blood-brain barrier or an abscess wall. Anticonvulsants could be concentrated in higher doses in the seizure focus. Delivery of a particular neurotransmitter to a specific cerebral nucleus for treatment of a movement disorder would be possible. Similarly, analgesics could be brought into the involved organ to alleviate pain.

11.12 Conclusion

Physicists, computer scientists, neuroradiologists, and neurosurgeons are indeed fortunate to be practicing in this era of rapidly evolving computerized imaging. The challenge will be to ignite our collective imaginations to advance new possibilities and opportunities for "electro"-microbrain surgery.

Acknowledgments. The authors, and especially Sumio Uematsu, express appreciation to Mr. Rokuro Uchida, President of Aloka Ltd., for encouragement and support throughout the robotic model experiments conducted from 1984 to 1986. The authors are also grateful to Mr. Torii and his associates at Japan Radio Co. for assisting in and preparing the model experiments at their factory. The final model experiment, in November 1986, was partially sponsored by Codman & Shurtleff, Birmingham, MA. We also express our grateful appreciation to Mrs. Jo Ann Barsda, Ms. Maria Caughlin and Ms. Marge Eddy for their assistance in preparation of the manuscript.

References

Albe-Fessard D, Arfel G, Guist G, Hardy J, Voureh G, Hertzog E, Aleonard P (1961) Identification et delimixation precise de certaines structures sous-corticales de l'homme par l'electrophysiologie: Son interet dans la chirurgie stereotaxique des dyskinesies. CR Acad Sci (Paris) 253: 2412-2414

Apuzzo MLJ, Sabshin JK (1983) Computed tomographic guidance stereotaxis in the management of intracranial mass lesions. Neurosurgery 12: 277-285

Bergstrom M, Greitz T (1976) Stereotaxic computed tomography. AJR 127: 167-170

Birg W, Mundinger F (1982) Direct target point determination for stereotactic brain operations from CT data and the setting parameters for polar-coordinate stereotactic devices. Appl Neurophysiol 45: 387-395

Boethius J, Bergstrom M, Greitz T (1980) Stereotaxic computerized tomography with a GE 8800 scanner. J Neurosurg 52: 794-800

Brown RA (1979) A computerized tomography-computer graphics approach to stereotaxic localization. J Neurosurg 50: 715-720

Brown RA, Roberts SR, Osborn AG (1980) Stereotaxic frame and computer software for CT directed neurosurgical localization. Invest Radiol 15: 308-312

Coffey RJ, Friedman WA (1988) Stereotactic applications: general overview. In: Heilbrun MP (ed) Stereotactic neurosurgery. Williams & Wilkins, Baltimore, p 17

Dyck P (1984) Historical review. In: Dyck P (ed) Stereotactic biopsy and brachytherapy of brain tumors. University Park Press, Baltimore, p 3

Frazier CH (1920) The effects of radium emanations upon brain tumors. Surg Gynecol Obstet 31: 236-239

Gildenberg PL (1987) Whatever happened to stereotactic surgery? Neurosurgery 20: 543-553

Goerss SJ, Kelly PJ, Kall BA, Alker GH Jr (1982) A computed tomographic stereotactic adaption system. Neurosurgery 10: 375-379

Greitz T, Lax I, Bergstrom M, Arndt J et al. (1986) Stereotactic radiation therapy of intracranial lesions. Methodologic aspects. Acta Radiol 25: 81-89

Gutin PH, Phillips TL. Hosobuchi Y et al. (1981) Permanent and removable implants for the brachytherapy of brain tumors. Int J Radiat Oncol Biol Phys 7: 1371-1391

Horsley V, Clarke RH (1908) The structure and functions of the cerebellum examined by a new method. Brain 31: 45-124

Hosobushi Y, Phillips TL, Stupar TA et al. (1980) Interstitial brachytherapy of primary brain tumors; preliminary report. J Neurosurg 54: 416-418

Huk W, Bauer U (1980) A new target device for stereotaxic procedures within the CT scanner. Neuroradiology 19: 13-17

Kelly PJ, Alker GJ Jr (1980) A method for stereotactic laser microsurgery in the treatment of deep-seated CNS neoplasms. Appl Neurophysiol 14: 172-177

Koslow M, Abele MG, Griffith RC, Mair GA, Chase NF (1981) Stereotactic surgical system controlled by computed tomography. Neurosurgery 8: 72

Kwoh YS, Reed IS, Chen JY, Shao HM, Truong TK, Jonckheere E (1985) A new computerized tomographic-aided robotic stereotaxis system. Robotic Age

Kwoh YS, Edmond JH, Jonckheeri A, Hayati S (1988) A robot with improved absolute positioning accuracy for CT guided stereotactic brain surery. IEEE Trans Biomed Eng No 2. 33: 153-160

Leksell LA (1949) Stereotaxic apparatus for intracerebral surgery. Acta Chir Scand 99: 229-233

Leksell L (1983) Stereotactic radiosurgery. J Neurol Neurosurg Psychiatry 46: 797-803

Leksell L, Jernberg B (1980) Stereotaxis and tomography. A technical note. Acta Neurochir 52: 1-7

Leksell L, Leksell D, Schwebel J (1985) Stereotaxis and nuclear magnetic resonance. J Neurol Neurosurg Psychiatry 48: 14-18

Lunsford LD (1982) Innovations in stereotactic technique coupled with computerized tomography. Contemp Neurosurg 4 (15): 1-6

Matsumoto K, Shichiijo F, Fukami T (1984) Long-term follow-up review of cases of Parkinsons's disease after unilateral thalamotomy. J Neurosurg 60: 1033-1044

Mundinger F (1958) Contributo alle indicazione, alle dosimetra ed alla tecnica di applicazione di radioisotopi per l'irradiazone interstiziale dei tumorii cerebrali. Anat e Chir 3: 21-38

Narabayashi H, Okuma T (1953) Procaine oil blocking of the globus pallidus for the treatment of rigidity and tremor of parkinsonism. Proc Jpn Acad 29: 310-318

Ohye C, Hirai T, Miyazaki M, Shibazaki T, Nakajima H, (1982) Vim thalamotomy for the treatment of various kinds of tremor. Appl Neurophysiol 45: 275-280

Perry JH, Rosenbaum AE, Lunsford LD, Swink CA, Zorub DS (1980) Computed tomography-guided stereotactic surgery: conception and development of a new stereotactic methodology. Neurosurgery 7: 376-381

Rand RW, Moss JA (1973) Treatment of cerebral aneurysms by stereotaxic ferromagnetic silicone thrombosis. Bull Los Angeles Neurol Soc 38: 21-23

Riechert T, Mundinger F (1955) Beschreibung und Anwendung eines Zielgerätes für stereotaktische Hirnoperationen (II. Modell). Acta Neurochir [Suppl] (Wien) 3: 208-337

Schaltenbrand G, Bailey P (1959) Introduction to stereotaxis with an atlas of the human brain, vol II. Year Book Medical, Chicago; Thieme, Stuttgart

Sheldon CH, McCann G, Jacques S, Lutes HR, Frazier RE, Katz R, Kuki R (1980) Development of a computerized microstereotaxic method for localization and removal of minute CNS lesions under direct 3-D vision. J Neurosurg 52: 21-27

Spiegel EA, Wycis HT, Marks M, Lee A et al. (1947) Stereotaxic apparatus for operations on the human brain. Science 106: 349-350

Todd EM (1967) Stereotaxic surgery of the basal ganglia. In: Todd-Wells manual of stereotaxic procedures. Codman and Shurtleff, Randolph, MA

Uematsu S, Rosenbaum AE, Erozan YS et al. (1987a) Intraoperative CT monitoring during stereotactic brain surgery. Acta Neurochir (Wien) 39: 18-20

Uematsu S, Rosenbaum AE, Delong MR et al. (1987b) Magnetic resonance planned thalamotomy followed by X-ray/CT-guided thalamotomy. Acta Neurochir (Wien) 39: 21-24

Uematsu S, DeLong M, Nauta H, Jankel W, McArthur J, Rosenbaum A, Narabayashi H (1989) Microphysiological recordings at CT gantry site during stereotactic thalamotomy. Stereotact Funct Neurosurg 52: 183-190

Subject Index

Abscess, drainage with CT stereotaxis 194, 198
Academics
  career development 12, 13
  commitment 9
  environment 4, 5, 9, 10, 14
  growth and development 1, 4
  image 4
  incentives 15
  migration to private practice 14
  opportunities 1, 5
  responsibilities 18
  role models 4, 5
Administrators (university)
  and radiology contributions 15, 16
  being informed 3, 10
  research expectations 3
Advanced Technology Laboratories Inc. 159, 161, 166
Aloka Tokyo LTD 203
Alzheimer's disease
  cortical atrophy 26, 28
  pattern recognition 39
  PET studies 127
American Medical Association 4
American Society of Neuroradiology 192
Angiography
  flow imaging with MRI 78
  for cardiac wall motion 181–183
Animal care and use committee 22
Animal research
  facilities 21, 22
  issues regarding 22
  models 22, 122
Apple/Macintosh 47
Artificial intelligence 2, 23, 67
Atherectomy catheters
  Kensey 149
  prototype devices 149
  Simpson 147–149
Autoradiography
  for chemotherapy 133
  with image registration 34

Basic scientists
  alienation of 4
  appointments in clinical departments 4
  funding of research 4
  integrating with clinicians 4, 10
  multidisciplinary contributions 4, 12
  responsibilities in clinical departments 4, 13, 15
BCNU
  intraarterial vs intravenous delivery 133, 134
  NMR spectroscopy for tumors 105
  PET studies of 133
  pharmacokinetics of 133, 134
  toxicity/complications 133–135
Bile acids, oral use for gallstones 142
Biliary drainage 141
Biopsy, CT guided 194, 197
Blood brain barrier
  breakdown in tumors 133
  PET determination of 121
Blood flow
  determination with NMR 96, 102, 106
  determination with PET 121
  determination with ultrasound Doppler 160–164
Brain
  cortical atrophy 26, 28
  ventricular shape analysis 28, 29
  surgery (see stereotactic brain surgery)
Brain tumors
  chemotherapy of 133, 134
  CT volumetric analysis 65
  MRI and PET overlays of 34
  NMR spectroscopy of 109
Brown-Roberts-Wells stereotactic head frame 192, 193

Calibration cube for image distortion analysis 178
Cancer (see tumors)
Cardiac imaging (also see cardiac wall motion, cardiac wall thickness, myocardial deformation, myocardial markers)
  chamber outlines 170, 171
  overview 169
  with angiography 181
  with MRI 183–186
Cardiac ventricular torsion 174
Cardiac ventricular volume 174
Cardiac wall motion (also see myocardial markers)
  contrast ventriculography and its limitations 170–172
  rationale for studying 170
  torsion 174
  transit time sonomicrometry 174
  using angiographs 181
  using Doppler ultrasound 186
  using MRI 183–186
Cardiac wall thickness (also see myocardial deformation, myocardial markers)
  echocardiographic determination 172, 173
  using angiography 181
  using surface markers 173
Career development
  monitoring progress 13
  role of research 4
Cemax Medical Systems 48
Center for devices and radiological health 166
Chairman
  creating academic environment 10
  participating management role 10
  responsibilities and role in academics 10
Chemical shift imaging (CSI) 80, 81, 98
Chemoembolotherapy 132
Chemotherapy, intraarterial 132–135
  applications 132
  clinical acceptance 132
  considerations for protocol design 132
  CT guided stereotaxis 206
  drug streaming problems 132, 134, 135
  factors to consider 132
  for fibrinolysis 143
  liver 132, 134
  pharmacokinetics in brain tumors 133, 134
  rationale for 132
Chemotherapy, response measured by NMR 102, 107, 109, 110
Cholecystectomy 141
Cholecystitis 141
Cholecystolithiasis, recurrent 142
Coarctation, balloon dilatation 137
Compartmental modeling 119
Computers
  expanding role 47
  impact on diagnostic radiology 47
  robotic brain surgery applications 191
  work stations 26, 43, 47
Corometrics/Aloka ultrasound 155, 160
Cray supercomputer 43

CT stereotaxis
  applications 194
  intraoperative scanning 197
  radioactive seed implants 194
Cyberware laboratories 51, 58
Cyclophosphamide 103
Cystic duct
  patency and gallbladder
    ablation 141, 142
  occlusion 142

Dementia
  cortical atrophy 26
  volumetric changes 30
Departmental
  economics 1, 2
  major decisions 1, 2
  structure 2
Dimensional Medical System 48
Dopamine receptors 119
Doppler
  blood flow determinations 160–163
  tissue deformation detection 186
  with stereotactic probes 204
Dotter, Charles
  role in stents 144
  role in thrombolysis 143

Economics 1, 2
  health care costs 2
  deterrent to academics 14
  research equipment costs 16
Edge detection threshold 48, 60
  image frequency component 38
Eigenimaging 39
Electron spin resonance imaging 88
Extracorporal shockwave lithotripsy
  (ESWL) 141

Faculty
  composition 4, 14
  research time 9, 14
Faraday shielding 97
Fellowship programs,
  neuroradiology 2
  research component 19, 20
Femur, 3-D imaging 61
Fiducials for image registration 30,
  31, 201
Flow imaging
  MRI 78
  ultrasound 160–164
Fluorouracil 96, 105
Food and Drug Administration
  (FDA) 73
Fourier shape decomposition,
  harmonic amplitudes in image
  analysis 27
Fourier transformation 94
Fourier transform NMR
  spectroscopy 94
Free induction decay (FID) 70, 71, 94

Gallbladder, ablation 141–143
Gallstones
  dissolution 141, 142
  fragmentation with ESWL 141
Gamma knife 205
General Electric Co. 2, 48, 73
Glucose metabolism
  coupling with oxygen
    metabolism 122
  PET determination of 119,
    121–123, 127
Gradient coils 74, 75
Gradient screening 78

Haloperidol 124
Health Maintenance Organizations
  (HMO) 1
Huntington's disease, PET
  measurements in 125, 127
Hybrid color display
  color composition techniques
    41
  hue, saturation, intensity (HSI)
    scales 41
  pseudocolor to separate image
    features 41
Hyperthermia
  monitoring response with NMR
    spectroscopy 107, 108, 110
  therapy using ultrasound 167

Imaging-3D
  brain 42
  combining images 66
  educational applications 64
  for brain surgery 191
  fractures 50–55
  grants to support research 21
  hip and acetabulum 50–54,
    59
  history 48, 49
  liver 66
  muscle and soft tissue 56, 57
  oncology 58, 63
  orthopedics 57–62
  prosthetic design 57–62
  radiation therapy planning 62
  sacrum 55
  shoulder 54, 55
  spine 55
  surgical planning 56
  techniques 41, 42, 49, 50
  tumor volumetrics 65
  volume visualization 49
Image analysis
  diagnostic error rates 24
  edge detection 38, 43
  error analysis 24
  functional nature 2, 25
  harmonic amplitudes 26–28
  image segmentation 38–40
  importance of 2
  investments in 2, 8, 9
  linear filtering 39
  morphology transformation 26
  opportunities 2
  pattern recognition 38–40, 67
  quantitative shape analysis 26–28
  ROI analysis 25
  signatures and signature data
    banks 25
  spatial statistical pattern recognition
    techniques 38
  texture analysis 23, 25, 26, 29
  thresholding 42
  visual inspection scanning 24
Image registration 25, 29, 65
  conformal mapping 30
  external fiducials 25, 30, 31, 201
  for stereotactic brain surgery 202, 203
  from multiple imaging
    modalities 29, 32, 37
  image overlay 29, 36, 67
  redirected sampling 25
  rescaling and resampling 36
  techniques of 30–36
  use of 3-D coordinates 31
Image (tissue) segmentation 38
Industry, funding support 17
Inter and multidisciplinary approach
  to rationale for 15–19
  research 4, 10, 15, 16
Interventional radiology (also see
  atherectomy catheters,
  chemotherapy, gallbladder,
  gallstones, lasers, thrombolysis,
  stents, valvuloplasty)
  efficacy-functional evaluation
    of 150
  role in radiology 131
Irradiation (see radiotherapy)

Japan Radio Company 203

Kawasaki-Juko 204

Lamor frequency 94
Lasers
  argon 138
  CO_2 139–140
  combined with angioplasty 139
  combined with thrombolysis 139
  Excimer 140
  hot tip 139
  Nd:YAG lasers 138
  perforations with 140
  problems associated with research
    into 138
  sapphire tip 139
  with photoreactive dyes 140
Left ventricular hypertension
  during aortic valvuloplasty 137
Leksell stereotactic head frame 192,
  193
Linear-filtering 39
Lithotripsy (also see extracorporal
  shockwave lithotripsy)
  ultrasound use 167
Liver tumors 65, 132, 134, 135
Lung tumors 24

Magnets
  high field 74, 90
  shielding 74
  types 73, 74

Magnetic resonance imaging
  3-D imaging 65, 66, 67
  biological effects 85, 86
  brain tissue-CNS differentiation 26
  cardiac 169, 183–186
  developmental history 69, 70
  hardware 72–76
  holography 89
  image analysis for tissue differentiation 39, 40
  image overlays with PET 37
  information provided 76
  microscopy (high resolution) 74, 83, 84
  non medical applications 86–88
  principles and theory 70, 71
  rapid (fast) imaging 77
  sodium imaging 79, 96
  solids 85
  techniques
    chemical shift 74, 80, 81
    echo planar 75, 77, 81
    gradient echo 72
    projection reconstruction 72
    real time imaging 78
    spin echo 72
  timing diagrams 72, 73
Medical students, attraction to radiology 3
Mental retardation, PET studies in 121
Methylspiperone 119
Methyl-tert-butyl-ether (MTBE) 142
Monooctanoin 142
Morphometry analysis
  definition 26
  erosion applications 26
Multinuclear imaging 79
Myocardial deformation (also see myocardial markers)
  techniques for measuring 173
Myocardial infarction, PET determinations 122
Myocardial markers
  cineradiographic system calibration 176
  computer x-ray tracking of 181
  dewarp distortions 180
  marker motion 176, 181
  six marker approach 176
  tetrahedron approach 176
  triplet approach 175
  using MRI tagging 183–186

NASA (National Aeronautic and Space Administration) 24
National Cancer Institute (NCI) 21
National Institutes of Health (NIH) 3
  medical imaging research funding levels 3, 5
National Oceanic and Atmospheric Administration (NOAA) 24
Neuroreceptors
  blockade 124, 127
  imaging with PET 123–125
Nitinol 144, 146
NMR sequences
  chemical shift imaging (CSI) 80–82
  DEPTH 97
  DRESS 82
  ISIS 98
Nuclear magnetic resonance imaging (see magnetic resonance imaging)
Nuclear magnetic resonance microscopy 74, 83, 84
Nuclear magnetic resonance spectroscopy,
  basic principles 70, 71, 93, 94
  biological significance of ^{31}P spectra in tumors 95
  ^{13}C spectra 95, 97, 112
  ^{19}F spectra 96
  ^{1}H spectra 95
  ^{39}K spectra 96
  ^{23}Na spectra 96
  continuous wave NMR (CW-NMR) 94
  detectable nuclei in living systems 95
  deuterium spectra 96
  DRESS technique 82
  future role 111–113
  monitoring cancer therapy 93, 102–108
  pH determinations 95
  phosphorous spectral components 94, 95
  reaction rates of metabolites 96
  role in interventional radiology 150
  spatial localization 82, 98
  spectral characterization 94
  techniques of 17
  tumors
    bioenergetic characterization from ^{31}P spectra 95
    cellular subpopulations 101
    criteria for model for study 99
    future applications 111–112
    human tumors 108–109
    hypoxia 101
    indicator of recurrence 110
    oxygenation 110
    perfusion 101, 102
    presence/absence of PCr
    response to therapy 102–108, 110–112
    to mesure blood flow and perfusion 96, 101, 102
    to monitor drug pharmacology/metabolism 96, 106, 109
    untreated growth 100, 101
    variability in spectra 99
Oral bile acids 141
Orthopedic prosthetic devices, design using 3-D imaging 57–62
Oxygen metabolism, PET measurements of 121

PAC's (picture archiving and communication systems) 23, 24
Parkinson's disease
  cortical atrophy 26
  CT stereotaxis and treatment 195
  PET measurements in 124
  statistical pattern recognition and 39
Patent ductus arteriosus, transcatheter treatment 135
Pattern recognition 67
Pendergrass Radiology Laboratory 24
Perry stereotactic head frame 192
Pharmacokinetics, intraarterial chemotherapy 133, 134
Phoenix Medical Systems 48
Phosphate metabolites in NMR spectra 95
Phospholipid metabolism and NMR 95, 101
Pixar imaging 47, 49, 50, 53, 65
Positron emission tomography (PET),
  basic principles 117, 118
  ^{11}C-BCNU chemotherapy 133
  blockade studies 123, 124
  blood flow measurements 121
  commercial package centers 127
  for interventional radiology 150
  future applications 125–127
  kinetic modeling 119–121
  monitoring therapy 127
  neuroreceptor studies 123–125
  radiopharmaceuticals available (list) 119
  role and utilization in health care systems 126
  tumor imaging 32, 34, 37
Prewhitening 38
Prolactinoma NMR image/spectra of 98
Prostate, ultrasound examination 166
Psychosis, PET studies in 125

Quantum Medical Systems 162–164

Radiotherapy
  planning using 3-D imaging 62
  response monitored with NMR spectroscopy 106, 107
  with CT guidance and stereotaxis 205
Radioactive seeds
  CT stereotaxis and 194
  interventional radiology and 132
  planning using 3-D imaging 62
Radiofrequency coagulation 142
Radiofrequency coils 74–76, 97, 98
Radiofrequency heating, therapeutic application 204
Radiologist
  changing role 1, 2, 7
  loss to private practice 3, 14
  providing functional data 2
  role models 4
Radiopaque markers (to study movements)
  heart 174–183
  intestine and stomach 187

lung 187
pharynx 187
use of computers to follow movement 181
Region of interest (ROI)
manual identifications 25
templating 34
Relaxation times, definition T_1, T_2 70, 94
Research,
animal considerations 21–22
flexibility 8
funding
balance 18
departmental 17, 18
extramural peer reviewed 5, 17
industrial 17
private sources 17, 18
importance 4
incentives for clinicians 15
monitoring 14
multidisciplinary interaction 2, 4, 10, 15, 16
obstacles to 14
planning 10, 11
program development 7–9
rationale 15, 16
role in clinical department 3–5, 7
space needs 8
time allocation 14
training (see training programs)
setting goals 10–13
Research grant support,
competition 3, 18
funding levels 3, 5
opportunities 3
Research program development,
commitment 9
concerns regarding 9
cost considerations 8, 16
defining goals 10
directions 9
factors to consider 8
flexibility 8
importance for radiology 8
integrating clinical and basic research 15
investments in 8
planning 10
rationale for 10
role of department chairman 10
trends 8
Research training programs
basic scientists 20
examples of 21
faculty 19
fellows 19
grants for 20
importance 18
need for 3, 13, 14, 15
postdoctoral 18–21
predoctoral 20
residents 18, 19
Residents
"burn-out" 3
nonacademic interest 3
research in residency 18, 19
two tract training system 19
Resolution
MRI 69
PET 24, 30
Spectroscopy 24
Resonance 94
Riechert-Mundinger stereotactic head frame 193
Robotics for stereotactic brain surgery 203, 204
Role models 3

Sacrum, 3-D evaluation 55
Schizophrenia
cortical atrophy 26
PET measurements in 124
Sclerosants 142, 143
Septostomy (atrial)
Rashkind approach 135
stationary balloon technique (Mitchell) 137
Serotonin, PET applications 123
Siemens Medical Systems 48, 49
Single photo emission tomography (SPECT) 117–119, 126
SKE postulate (signal and parameters known exactly) 38
Spatial localized spectroscopy 98, 99
Spatially localized spectroscopy 82, 83, 98
Spine, 3-D evaluation 55
Statistical pattern recognition, and multidimensional discrimination 38
Stents (intravascular)
applications 144, 146
coronary artery stents 147
flexible stents 147
for aneurysms 146
for portocaval shunts 146
Gianturco stent 145, 146
Palmaz stent 145
properties of ideal stent 144
thermal memory alloy stent 146
Wallstent 146
Stereotactic brain surgery
CT guided 195
frames 192, 193
historical perspective 191, 192
light beam guided 205
procedures 196–199
robotics 203, 204
servomotor driven central systems 203
Stereotactic probes, therapeutic applications 204, 205
Stereotactic head frames 192, 193
Stereotaxis applications (also see CT stereotaxis)
transforming and scaling images 28–30
use with analytical and therapeutic probes 204–206
Streptokinase 143
Stroke
PET measurements 122
volumetric brain changes in 30
Sun Microsystems 47, 49, 65, 75
Superconductors 89, 90

Teaching 14
Technology
impact on radiology 1
transfer 2, 24, 140
Tenure tract systems 14
Thalamotomy 195, 199, 202
Thrombolysis
potential future agents 144
with streptokinase 143
with T-PA 143
with urokinase 143
Tissue plasminogen activator (T-PA) 143, 144
Todd-Wells stereotactic head frame 193
Toshiba America Inc. 161, 165
Tourette's syndrome, PET imaging of 124
Tracker catheter 135
Training programs 2, 3, 14, 18–20
Trancept Systems 47
Transducers, ultrasound 157–159, 164
Tumors (also see specific organs i. e., brain, liver, lung)
bioenergetic status by NMR 95
blood flow 96, 102, 106
cell population types 101
CT stereotaxis 194
experimental
RIF-1 99, 102–107
9L-glioblastoma 100
104E myeloma 100
16/c adenocarcinoma 100
MDA-MB231 101
Nunn osteogenic sarcoma 110
R3-230AC 108
VX-2 133
heterogeneity and NMR spectroscopy 101
monitoring regression 39, 126
oxygenation 110
volumetric analysis with 3-D imaging 65
NMR spectroscopy of 94–113
pH 102
radioactive seed implants 132, 194
treatment
intraarterial chemotherapy 132–134
ultrasound therapy 167
using stereotaxis 194, 195, 205, 206

Ultrasound
analog scan converters 156
bistable systems 156
cardiac imaging 170–174
digital scan converters 156
Doppler applications
blood flow 160–164
color flow images 162, 163
flow direction 162

dynamic focusing 158
early generation
equipment 156–158
intracavity transducers 164, 165
linear array scanners 157, 158
m-mode operation 160
modern transducers 158
phased array sector scanning 158
signal conditioning 157
spectral analysis 163, 164
static (digital) scanners 157

Urokinase 143

Valvuloplasty
aortic valve 137
balloon design 137
complications 137
mitral valve 137
pulmonary valve 135, 136
Vasodilatation,
pharmacoangiography 132
with BCNU 134

Volume graphics (visualization) 48, 49
Volume rendering technique 56
Volumetric analysis
cardiac ventricles 174
normal brain structures 26
tumors 65

Water suppression for ^{1}H-NMR
spectra 95
Work stations 44, 47, 49